COVID-19 Syndemics and the Global South

This book focuses on syndemics in the Global South and uses COVID-19 as a window to understand clusters of disparities and disease comorbidities. The pandemic has exposed and multiplied structural inequalities and certain subpopulations were more exposed to COVID-19 as well as experienced greater morbidity and mortality. The effects of the pandemic differ between countries but have had an especially major impact, although in varying ways, in the Global South. The contributions in this volume explore the differential impacts of COVID-19 at individual, community, national, or regional levels, considering how structural violence is institutionalized in a way that creates vulnerable situations and disproportionate suffering. The book will be of interest to anthropologists and sociologists as well as to those working in global and public health.

Inayat Ali leads the Department of Public Health and Allied Sciences at Fatima Jinnah Women University, and is Assistant Professor in the Department of Anthropology at FJWU, Pakistan. He is also Research Fellow in the Department of Social and Cultural Anthropology at the University of Vienna, Austria.

Merrill Singer is Emeritus Professor of Anthropology at the University of Connecticut, USA.

Nicola Bulled is Assistant Research Professor at the Institute for Collaboration on Health, Intervention, and Policy (InCHIP), University of Connecticut, USA.

Routledge Studies in Health and Medical Anthropology

https://www.routledge.com/Routledge-Studies-in-Health-and-Medical-Anthropology/
book-series/RSHMA

COVID-19 Syndemics and the Global South
A World Divided

Edited by Inayat Ali, Merrill Singer, and Nicola Bulled

Routledge
Taylor & Francis Group

LONDON AND NEW YORK

First published 2024
by Routledge
4 Park Square, Milton Park, Abingdon, Oxon OX14 4RN

and by Routledge
605 Third Avenue, New York, NY 10158

Routledge is an imprint of the Taylor & Francis Group, an informa business

British Library Cataloguing-in-Publication Data
A catalogue record for this book is available from the British Library

ISBN: 9781032430164 (hbk)
ISBN: 9781032430171 (pbk)
ISBN: 9781003365358 (ebk)

DOI: 10.4324/9781003365358

Typeset in Sabon
by codeMantra

To global frontline healthcare providers and caregivers
in the fight against COVID-19

Contents

Figures

Contributors

Inayat Ali is Incharge of the Department of Public Health and Allied Sciences at Fatima Jinnah Women University and Assistant Professor in the Department of Anthropology at FJWU, Pakistan. Also, he is Research Fellow in the Department of Social and Cultural Anthropology at the University of Vienna, Austria.

Chiemezie S. Atama is Senior Lecturer in the Department of Sociology and Anthropology University of Nigeria, Nsukka. She is also the Founding/Executive Director of Equity Watch Initiative [E-WIN], a non-governmental organization that is committed to promoting gender equality and empowering women and girls.

Laurel Baldwin-Ragaven is Professor of Family Medicine at the University of the Witwatersrand and the Clinical Head of Family Medicine at the Gauteng Provincial Department of Health, South Africa.

Nicola Bulled is Assistant Research Professor at the Institute for Collaboration on Health, Intervention, and Policy (InCHIP), University of Connecticut, USA.

Lorena Nunez Carrasco, PhD, is Associate Professor in Sociology at the University of the Witwatersrand, Johannesburg. Her current research explores the linkages between migration and health, focusing on illness experiences, including HIV/AIDS. She has researched African Initiated Churches and published on faith, illness, subjectivity, and the urban space. She is interested in the topic of death in the context of migration and displacement, and at present, she is researching experiences of mourning in the context of the COVID-19 pandemic.

Richard Chenhall is Professor of Medical Anthropology in the Melbourne School of Population and Global Health at the University of Melbourne, Australia.

Jennifer A. Cook is Research Associate at the Tower Center for International Affairs and Public Policy, Southern Methodist University, Dallas, Texas, USA.

Obinna J. Eze is a doctoral student in the Department of Sociology and Anthropology, University of Nigeria, Nsukka.

Peter van Heusden is a senior bioinformatician working at the South African National Bioinformatics Institute (SANBI), Cape Town, South Africa.

Kezia Lewins is Lecturer, specializing in Medical Sociology, at the University of the Witwatersrand, Johannesburg, South Africa.

Gracsious Maviza is MA candidate in the School of Public Health, University of the Witwatersrand, Johannesburg, South Africa. She is currently researching the experiences and narratives of loss and grief during COVID-19.

Vuyokazi Myoli is MA candidate in the School of Public Health, University of the Witwatersrand, Johannesburg, South Africa. She is currently researching the experiences and narratives of loss and grief during COVID-19.

Mary Grace A. Pelayo is a health social scientist, researcher, and community trainer in the Philippines.

Kimberly G. Ramos is a healthcare professional in the Philippines.

Louis Reynolds is a retired pediatric intensive care and lung specialist, and Associate Professor and member of the Advocacy Committee of the Department of Pediatrics and Child Health, University of Cape Town. He is a member of the People's Health Movement.

Ian Christopher N. Rocha is a health social scientist, global health researcher, and healthcare professional in the Philippines.

Kate Senior is a medical anthropologist based in Australia. She has extensive experience working with remote Aboriginal communities, with an emphasis on understanding the way that people live and conceptualize health and well-being and the barriers they face when accessing health services.

Merrill Singer is Emeritus Professor of Anthropology at the University of Connecticut, USA.

Storm Theunissen is MA candidate in the School of Public Health, University of the Witwatersrand, Johannesburg, South Africa. She is currently researching the experiences and narratives of loss and grief within Afrikaans families during COVID-19, and how the pandemic has affected the grieving rituals of these families.

Preface

This volume begs a brief note. It was back in 2021, when the lead editor Inayat Ali conceptualized this idea and extended the proposal to Merrill Singer to co-author a volume on COVID-19 in the Global South from the syndemic perspective. Singer readily embraced the proposition, setting the wheels in motion for what would become an illuminating journey of knowledge creation. Given her expertise on syndemics and work in various countries, Nicola Bulled was invited to join this endeavor. We then began inviting our authors to write chapters for the book. It has taken us around two years to complete the volume. In between many things changed, including the title of this book and the status of the pandemic. Originally, the book contained 14 chapters from different countries of the Global South, but due to various reasons, a few of our authors could not contribute. Yet, the resulting compilation remains a testament to its original intent. Bursting with diverse viewpoints, the volume serves as a catalyst for stimulating discussions surrounding COVID-19 while providing a profound analytical framework applicable not only to this pandemic but also to other outbreaks, epidemics, or silent pandemics. Through the synergy of these scholars' contributions, the volume encapsulates the essence of the syndemic perspective and its application to the intricacies of global health challenges.

This edited volume is a result of provocations and interests caused by a continuously changing and evolving pandemic. The provocation is significantly due to the diverse effects of the pandemic, especially in the Global South. In an age defined by global connectivity and communication, the pandemic has starkly highlighted the persistent divisions within our world or worlds. The book in your hands or on your electronic devise, titled *COVID-19 Syndemics and the Global South: A World Divided*, delves into the intricate interplay of socio-cultural, economic, (geo-)political, and ecological factors that have given rise to the differing effects of COVID-19.

Critical medical anthropology has already examined the complex structural influences that shape health outcomes and disease trajectories. This volume follows the same line. Using syndemics perspective, this work sheds light on the "biosocial" occurrences, where biological and social worlds intersect to underscore the susceptibility of certain people, communities, and countries to diseases and their disproportionate consequences. Through this lens, the book unveils the evident and preventable health inequities that endure across populations and within societal subsets. This framework, combined with the understanding of "structural violence," provides a basis for comprehending the diverse expressions of COVID-19 and its extensive implications.

As the pandemic traverses nations, the Global South emerged as a center of attention. The book challenges established perceptions of the Global South as merely an underdeveloped concept, choosing instead a more nuanced interpretation rooted in historical legacies of colonialism and neo-imperialism. The Global South is not uniform; its nations differ in politics, economics, and demographics. Despite this diversity, the Global South framework serves as a valuable tool to address deep-seated inequities and historical imbalances among nations. While globalization may appear to blur North-South divisions, the book argues that these divisions persist and continue to shape the lives of individuals globally. Recognizing the limitations and analytical usefulness of the Global South concept, the authors carefully navigate these intricacies.

This volume acknowledges the dynamic nature of COVID-19, an ever-evolving phenomenon that progressed through various strains, immune responses, and societal reactions. This "evolving syndemic process" drives the authors' exploration and analyses of interconnected disease and societal processes, capturing the present and recent past to inform future considerations.

Although in May 2023, the WHO chief declared an end to COVID-19 as a global health emergency, but the emergencies will still continue, especially in the Global South. This unfortunate fact is highlighted by the appearance of a new variant of the COVID-19 virus called EG.5 or, informally, as Eris (nicknamed after the Greek goddess of strife and discord). A descendant of Omicron, Eris is already the dominant coronavirus subvariant in several countries, currently infecting more people than any other single strain. Although apparently the pandemic is said to be "over" (for the moment), the disease has made the lives of many people more challenging and may continue to do so in the future.

In the end, we would like to thank to our authors who have contributed to this volume, and who have been always there to respond to our emails to deal with their chapters. Their responsiveness in addressing emails and their commitment to refining their chapters have been invaluable. We also extend our sincere thanks to the anonymous reviewers whose insightful comments played a pivotal role in enhancing the quality of this work. Their feedback has been instrumental in refining our ideas and perspectives. Our appreciation extends to our publisher for accepting our volume proposal and demonstrating patience throughout the process, as we meticulously crafted the final manuscript. Last but certainly not least, we wish to acknowledge and express our deep gratitude for the unwavering patience and support of our family members. Their understanding and encouragement have been integral in propelling us forward on this rewarding journey of completion.

Introduction

*Nicola Bulled, Merrill Singer,
and Inayat Ali*

Critical medical anthropology has paid significant attention to the structures of social relationships that shape, reshape, produce, reproduce, and influence the course of a disease. Traditionally, medical anthropology regarded health conditions as consequences of local ecologies, cultural configurations, or psychological factors. Such explanations became regarded as inadequate as scholars, inspired by critical theories of postmodernism, Marxism, and deconstructionism of the latter part of the 20th century, argued that they failed to consider the structures of social relationships that unite and influence individuals and communities. Rather than focusing only on local cultural systems, critical medical anthropology considers how large-scale political, economic, and cognitive structures constrain individuals' decisions, shape their social behavior, and affect their risk for disease. As noted by Singer and Baer (2012, pp. 39–40), "CMA [critical medical anthropology] focuses on the social origins of illness, such as the ways in which poverty discrimination, stigmatization, violence, and fear of violence contribute to poor health." In doing so, the critical medical anthropology perspective regards regional variation of disease distribution as a product of complex interactions involving global political-economic inequality, culture, society, and nature.

These perspectives of the entanglements of biosocial and structural events have become mainstream medical anthropology drawing attention to social justice and disparities in health across populations. For example, Alex Nading's (2014) nuanced work examining dengue in Nicaragua shows us how vulnerabilities are intimately tied to global economies, local politics, shared constructs of disease and disease risk, and perceptions of responsibilities of neighbors, citizens, and governments. Paying attention to such interactions reveals significant unjust and preventable health inequities across populations and between population subgroups.

Such inequities are repeated in the case of coronavirus diseases 2019 (COVID-19) despite the increasing (inter)connectedness in what remains a divided world. Certain subpopulations were more exposed to COVID-19 and experienced more infection-related morbidity and mortality. Structural factors such as poverty, population density, unequal access to treatments

DOI: 10.4324/9781003365358-1

and vaccine distribution, economic disparities, and social marginalization significantly enhanced the effects of the pandemic. In addition, various and varying comorbidities have played a significant role in intensifying the effects of infection. In this regard, COVID-19 is not just one pandemic but "many pandemics" (Ali, 2021; Mendenhall, 2020) substantially influenced by time and place. The effects of the pandemic differ between countries of the world but have had an especially major impact, although in varying ways, in the Global South.

COVID-19 in the Global South

The Global South is not just a metaphor for low economic and industrial development. It refers to the entire history of colonialism, neo-imperialism, and distinguishable socio-cultural and economic changes that shape and perpetuate major differences in living standards, life expectancy, and access to resources (Dados & Connell, 2012). The conception of the Global South has its roots in the work of analysts like Walter Rodney, who examined the processes of underdevelopment in Africa. Rodney (1972) asserts that the creation of the Global South was not simply a consequence of colonial conquest or internal factors. Rather, it entailed the active underdevelopment of subordinate areas through the extraction of raw natural resources and labor for the benefit of the core or dominant nations of the world system (Frank, 1969). It was the direct product of unfolding processes of capitalist expansion and the integration of dominated (e.g., colonial) societies into the capitalist world system (Wallerstein, 1989).

The emergence of the idea of the Global South marks a critical historical juncture dating to the mid-1970s with the re-invigoration of neoliberalism and the global restructuring of the geography of inequality and oppression. Some have asserted that the processes of globalism have broken down many of the barriers separating the Global North and South (Pouliot & Thérien, 2018). This assertion, however, has been refuted by marshaling compelling examples of the historical force and continuing impact of North–South fault lines on the lives and well-being of people around the world (Amzat & Razum, 2022).

We recognize that Global South is a construct consisting of many different nations with differing politics, economics, histories, demographics, and environments that are relevant to local expressions of a disease. Inequalities are not limited to the North/South divide and there are power asymmetries within Global South nations. We adopt a definition of the Global South that calls attention to historic patterns of inequity in the distribution of power, resource control, and health and as such includes spaces and communities in developed nations shaped by exploitation, oppression, and neocolonial relations, such as Indigenous Australians, African Americans, Latinx, and immigrant communities. In this volume, contributors pay attention to local and regional differences as these are critical to varied disease expressions. We adopt the Global South conceptual framework with keen sensitivity to its limits as well as its analytic utility.

In this volume, we present original contributions by anthropologists, epidemiologists, and other health researchers, offering cases of COVID-19 syndemics in the Global South. These critical inquiries pose unsettling questions and explorations that reveal various visible and invisible syndemic entanglements.

The Syndemic Framework

A syndemics approach recognizes that disease clusters are significantly related to socio-cultural, economic, political, and ecological factors. As a concept developed by critical medical anthropologists, the syndemics approach takes into account shared characteristics within a community including health-related perceptions, beliefs, and practices and their interface with "local biologies" (Lock, 1993), "societal memories" (Ali, 2020), local ecologies, and socio-cultural configurations. In addition to recognizing the influences of social and structural factors, syndemics theory uniquely centralizes biology and specifically disease interactions as contributing to disease clusters, in so doing combining established theories of social determinants of disease and comorbidities. Syndemic epidemics, involving the synergistic adverse interaction of two or more diseases or health conditions, are not random, rather they tend to develop under conditions of health inequality caused by poverty, stigma, stress, or structural violence. They can involve physical and behavioral health, as well as communicable and non-communicable diseases.

An argument for syndemic arrangements first investigates why certain diseases cluster together; second, it examines the pathways through which two or more diseases interact biologically in individuals and within populations, and, as a consequence, increases their overall disease burden; and third, it assesses the ways in which social environments, especially conditions of social inequality and injustice, contribute to disease clustering and interaction as well as to the vulnerability of populations. As such, applying the syndemic framework involves showing how diseases or other health conditions interact adversely to increase the burden of disease in a population, interactions that are promoted by socio-cultural, political, and economic conditions.

COVID-19 has been regarded as a syndemic (Horton, 2020) as it complies with this definition, albeit with distinct biological and social arrangements in different contexts (Mendenhall, 2020; Singer et al., 2022). For example, research has shown that diabetes increases the likelihood of an adverse COVID-19 outcome, and conversely that COVID-19 infection can contribute to the development of diabetes and all of the health complications it introduces (Xie & Al-Aly, 2022). In communities already burdened with diabetes epidemics, an epidemic that most heavily affects poorer sectors of the population who are reliant on calorie-dense diets and have limited access to routine healthcare management, COVID-19 has proven fatal (see Singer and Cook, Ali, and Bulled in this volume). Given that social conditions and sharply unequal social relations can contribute to the clustering, formation, and progression of diseases like COVID-19 and diabetes, a biosocial concept like syndemics offers a holistic approach to address these often-entwined conditions (Mendenhall & Gravlee, 2021).

Organization of the Book

The book is divided into four sections to address the evolving and syndemogenic nature of COVID-19. The first section addresses known social and institutional structures that supported the emergence of COVID-19 syndemics in the Global South. In Chapter 1, Singer and Bulled use the three case studies of Lagos, Nigeria, the Haredi of urban Israel, and Manila, Philippines, to explore why cities in the Global South became epicenters for COVID-19-associated syndemics. The chapter presents more than just a comparative overview of present disease burdens and COVID-19 control responses and looks beyond urban characteristics that support high levels of communicable and non-communicable diseases. The authors introduce the historic role of the Global North in establishing the current conditions of global inequity which contributes to urban-associated diseases, initially during the eras of colonialism and post-colonial neoliberal restructuring, then during the corporate shift in the North to relocate production and hazardous materials recycling processes to the South, and finally during the consolidation of the global food system that has resulted in a reliance on calorie-dense foods. In Chapter 2, Ali examines the syndemic of COVID-19, diabetes, and chronic kidney disease in Pakistan. Ali argues that historical legacies of exploitation and disparity under British colonialism including economic corruption and healthcare system restructuring created a class system in which individuals are made more vulnerable in the face of poverty, malnutrition, and disease. COVID-19 could infect anyone, but its effects are critical for those who are already facing various vulnerabilities. Closing out this section, Singer and Cook, in Chapter 3, assess the adverse bidirectional syndemic interactions between diabetes and COVID-19 in Mexico and in US/Mexico border areas. COVID-19/diabetes syndemics have emerged in communities throughout the Global South (see Chapters 2, 6, and 9) for many of the same reasons discussed by Singer and Cook. Extensive changes in diets in recent decades in these communities are driven by several interlinked political and economic factors, including rapid urbanization (driven by climate change, neoliberal governance, and economic restructuring), foreign direct capital investment, and the global food marketing system.

The second section explores how COVID-19 amplified existing syndemics in communities in the Global South. In Chapter 4, Rocha, Pelayo, and Ramos present the effects of COVID-19 and COVID-19 control policies on tuberculosis (TB) management in the Philippines, the most affected country in the Western Pacific Region. Strict lockdown measures disrupted TB case finding, reduced TB treatment plans, and curtailed TB contact tracing. COVID-19 management efforts also diverted healthcare services and healthcare funding, already overstretched and inadequate, away from TB. Given the physiological interactions between COVID-19 and TB, the syndemic amplified existing health inequities. In Chapter 5, Senior and Chenhall shift our perspective to consider how the media and public health rhetoric convey and construct the political and structural contexts of the lived experiences of disease. In Australia, as elsewhere, COVID-19 exposed gaps in health between high and low socio-economic groups, yet rhetoric remained focused on individual responsibility and blame, consistent with the new public health neoliberal agenda. Consequently, Aboriginal Australians and other at-risk populations, already politically and economic marginalized, became further socially marginalized.

Chapters 6 and 7 present the complex social, political, economic, and health challenges of South Africa. In Chapter 6, van Heusden, Lewin, Reynolds, and Baldwin-Ragaven delve into South Africa's 25-year-old democracy and the challenges it faces, encompassing issues like HIV/AIDS, unemployment, food insecurity, and climate change. Amid crumbling infrastructure, corruption, and strained healthcare, the emergence of SARS-CoV-2 compounded the difficulties. They show how the South African state in a pattern of "organized abandonment" failed in its constitutional mandate to provide quality healthcare and address legacies of inequity that resulted in pre-COVID-19 syndemics and set the stage for devastating COVID-19 outcomes. In Chapter 7, Nunez Carrasco, Maviza, Myoli, and Theunissen explore the impact of COVID-19 syndemics on three diverse South African communities: amaXhosa in the Eastern Cape, white Afrikaans-speakers, and Zimbabwean migrants. The amaXhosa community faced elevated risks due to high rates of HIV, TB, and chronic conditions like diabetes, leading to increased COVID-19 susceptibility and mortality. Overwhelmed public healthcare facilities worsened chronic disease treatment disruptions and limited food access for the impoverished amaXhosa. Afrikaner groups experienced unemployment and financial strain, resorting to borrowing and community aid. Apartheid legacies hindered middle-class Afrikaners from using public healthcare, exacerbating COVID-19 and mental health challenges. Zimbabwean migrants, unable to return home, faced heightened exposure due to work requirements. Syndemics highlight diverse biosocial factors and interactions while unveiling long-term social impacts of concurrent epidemics.

In the third section, the chapters present new syndemics that have emerged because of the COVID-19 pandemic, both as biological interactions with COVID-19 and as a result of changed social contexts in relation to COVID-19 control policies. In Chapter 8, Bulled describes the iatrogenic syndemic of COVID-19/diabetes/"black fungus" in India resulting from the indiscriminate use of steroids to treat COVID-19 patients in response to an overwhelmed health system. The social inequities in India created the ideal context for syndemic outbreaks, with marginalized groups at greatest risk given poor living conditions, increasing exposure to black fungus and COVID-19, existing health conditions including undiagnosed diabetes, and overreliance on poorly regulated pharmaceuticals given limited access to quality health care. Atama and Eze explore the unprecedented increase in gender-based violence in Nigeria due to COVID-19 pandemic-related stress and control measures in Chapter 9. In Nigeria, and in many communities globally, women were heavily impacted by lockdown efforts, which limited their ability to work and earn wages, increasing their financial dependence on others including men who may treat them violently, had reduced access to gender-based violence support programming or supportive social networks, and heightened levels of anxiety due to the health risks posed by COVID-19 infection.

The final section presents future considerations for COVID-19 syndemic management. In Chapter 10, Singer addresses the increased threat of adverse syndemic interactions between environmental diseases of the Anthropocene and COVID-19 faced by children in the Global South. Poor living conditions, including inadequate sanitation and running water and overcrowding facilitate the transmission of SARS-CoV-2 to children. In addition, children are especially vulnerable to various environmental risks, including climate change, air pollution, toxic chemicals exposures, and e-waste resulting in poor overall health that worsens COVID-19 morbidity and mortality. Furthermore, the diversion of resources from child health, such as routine vaccines, to address the pandemic among adults will make children more vulnerable to disease. This chapter calls attention to the value of assessing and responding to the ecosyndemics of childhood in overcoming barriers to improving child health in the Global South.

Notably, COVID-19 has been called an "ever changing pandemic" Yazel, Bishop, and Britt (2022). Over time, various strains and sub-strains of SARS-CoV-2 have appeared, diffused, become dominant, and faded, to be replaced by other strains. With each wave of infection, the pandemic has changed, depending on the infectious and pathogenic characteristics of the dominant strain, the immunological status of populations (levels of infection-blocking antibodies), and societal and medical responses to the pandemic (e.g., vaccination rates, maintenance of risk-reduction behaviors, treatment). As the face of the pandemic has changed, and changed again, so too have the local and regional syndemics that comprise it. Under such conditions, we recognize syndemics as dynamic phenomena that have different features over time. We refer to this newly described feature as the "evolving syndemic process." Changes at multiple levels from the microscopic to the societal have shaped and will continue to shape COVID-19-involved syndemics potentially creating variance in syndemic expression, disease composition, and impact across locations.

One key factor that may impact the evolving syndemic process is the emergence of new infectious diseases (EIDs), a disproportionately common event in the Global South (e.g., Zika, Ebola, SARS, Nipah, Marburg, multi-drug-resistant tuberculosis). Jones and colleagues (2008, p. 992) advocate for the

> re-allocation of resources for 'smart surveillance' of emerging disease hotspots in lower latitudes, such as tropical Africa, Latin America, and Asia, including targeted surveillance of at-risk people to identify early case clusters of potentially new EIDs before their large-scale emergence.

For these reasons, this book describes the present and recent past of ongoing intertwined disease and societal processes. Writing in a dynamic pandemic is fraught as the future is never quite what you thought it would be. Still, to have some basis for anticipating and preparing for the future, you must grasp the present. This is the goal of this volume which is informed by the realization that the next chapter of the COVID-19 pandemic and the role of syndemics therein has yet to be written.

References

Ali, I. (2020). *Constructing and Negotiating Measles: The Case of Sindh Province of Pakistan*. Vienna: University of Vienna.

Ali, I. (2021). Syndemics at play: chronic kidney disease, diabetes and COVID-19 in Pakistan. *Annals of Medicine, 53*(1), 581–586. https://doi.org/10.1080/07853890.2021.1910335.

Amzat, J., & Razum, O. (2022). The war in Europe viewed from the South: a global health concern. *International Journal of Public Health, 67*, 1605184.

Dados, N., & Connell, R. (2012). The global south. *Contexts, 11*(1), 12–13.

Frank, A.G. (1969). *Latin America: Underdevelopment or Revolution*. New York: Monthly Review Press.

Horton, R. (2020). Offline: COVID-19 is not a pandemic. *The Lancet, 396*(10255), 874. https://doi.org/10.1016/S0140-6736(20)32000-6.

Jones, K., Patel, N., Levy, M., Storeygard, A., Balk, D., Gittleman, J., & Daszak, P. (2008). Global trends in emerging infectious diseases. *Nature, 451*(7181), 990–993. https://doi.org/10.1038/nature06536.

Lock, M. (1993). Cultivating the body: anthropology and epistemologies of bodily practice and knowledge. *Annual Review of Anthropology, 22*(1), 133–155.

Mendenhall, E. (2020). The COVID-19 syndemic is not global: context matters. *Lancet, 396*(10264), 1731–1731. https://doi.org/10.1016/S0140-6736(20)32218-2.

Mendenhall, E., & Gravlee, C. (2021). How COVID, inequality and politics make a vicious syndemic. *Scientific American*. https://www.scientificamerican.com/author/clarence-c-gravlee/.

Nading, A.M. (2014). *Mosquito Trails: "Ecology, Health, and the Politics of Entanglement"*. University of California Press. Oakland, CA.

Pouliot, V., & Thérien, J.P. (2018). Global governance in practice. *Global Policy, 9*(2), 163–172.

Rodney, W. (1972). Problems of third world development. *Ufahamu: A Journal of African Studies*, 3(2). http://dx.doi.org/10.5070/F732016395.

Singer, M., & Baer, H. (2012). *Introducing Medical Anthropology: A Discipline in Action* (2nd ed.). AltmaMira Press. Lanham, MD.

Singer, M., Bulled, N., & Leatherman, T. (2022). Are there global syndemics? *Medical Anthropology*, 41(1), 4–18. https://doi.org/10.1080/01459740.2021.2007907.

Wallerstein, I. (1989). *The Modern World-System III. The Second Era of Great Expansion of the Capitalist World-Economy, 1730–1840s*. London: Academic Press.

Xie, Y., & Al-Aly, Z. (2022). Risks and burdens of incident diabetes in long COVID: a cohort study. *Lancet Diabetes and Endocrinology*, 10(5), 311–321. https://doi.org/10.1016/S2213-8587(22)00044-4.

Yazel L., Bishop C., & Britt H. (2022). Adapting during the ever-changing pandemic environment: A one year examination of how health education specialists remain adaptable. *American Journal of Health Education*, 53(3), 142–148. https://doi.org/10.1080/19325037.2022.2048746.

1 Sick in the City

COVID-19 and the Syndemics of Urban Life

Merrill Singer and Nicola Bulled

Most of the over 4 billion people living in cities around the world, especially those dwelling in informal settlements in the Global South, suffer from diseases linked to features of contemporary city life, including inadequate housing, poor sanitation, and waste management, unhealthy and insufficient diets, inadequate exercise, crowding, poor air quality, and urban heat island effects. In response to the awareness of these health-related challenges, the subfield of urban health emerged as a component of international public health in the mid-1980s. One product of this work is the term "urban penalty," which has been proposed to describe the particular health burdens of living in cities for many people (Gould, 1998). At an ever-increasing pace since the Industrial Revolution, cities have developed into the epicenters of a dual health burden comprising interacting communicable and non-communicable diseases, first in the Global North and then in the Global South.

The hallmarks of urbanization (e.g., constructed environments, high population size and density, impervious surface cover, urbanized lifestyle activity levels, and fossil fuel-based transportation and manufacture) have also been identified as drivers of urban-associated diseases (UADs) (Flies et al., 2019). UADs have been defined as "any disease that increases in prevalence or severity due to urban living or urban growth or is expected to increase due to future urbanization trends" (Flies et al., 2019). Understanding the urban features that are risk or protective factors for health offers direction for the development of appropriate interventions and preventive measures needed by an increasingly urbanized global world (Vlahov & Galea, 2003).

The most frequent and serious UADs tend to be discussed as individual and distinct conditions (e.g., Harpham & Molyneux, 2001; King et al., 2003; Miller, 2001). This orientation reflects the traditional biomedical view of diseases as discrete, disjunctive, and nameable entities in nature. But diseases do not exist in isolation. They are mixed with other diseases in populations, and this complexity is manifest in sufferer experience and management.

DOI: 10.4324/9781003365358-2

This mixing pattern involving three diseases is evident in the following statement by a woman patient interviewed in an urban Kenyan hospital:

> Because of my [HIV] disease, I was so sick and I thought I was dying. I tried many medicines but they did not work. I went to [the public hospital] and they did a scan to my stomach. I was diagnosed with stomach ulcers. I even called my daughter and told her that I was going to die. The pain I was going through was so much, I had never had such a pain before. This depressed me a lot.
>
> (Mendenhall et al., 2015, p. 17)

Syndemics research – which focuses on complex disease interactions and the social/ecological forces that shape them – emerged in the mid-1990s among urban-based anthropologists and colleagues as a critical biosocial corrective to the medical silo-ization of diseases. Based on studies of urban drug users, one of the leading voices Singer (1996, p. 99) argued that substance abuse, violence, and AIDS "are not merely concurrent, in that they are not wholly separable phenomena." Instead, they comprise a syndemic of closely linked and interdependent health threats in the context of urban poverty. This chapter explores the question: why have cities in the Global South become epicenters of syndemics? We draw on three case studies – Lagos, Nigeria, the Haredi of urban Israel, and Metro Manila, Philippines – involving but not limited to COVID-19, to show how and why syndemics significantly shape urban health and health inequalities in the Global South and beyond, and to suggest responses to urban syndemics and the role of anthropology in this effort.

Our Bodies, Our Cities

The urban environment is significantly different from the kinds of places in which humans evolved as a species, and this difference has consequences for health. At most, cities are about 4,000 years old, while the hominid line dates to over 4 million years ago. While urban life has changed us, our genetic history was largely shaped by selection for non-urban habitats and lifeways. This misfit with a novel ecosystem is a factor in the most prominent diseases of the city as reflected in the risks of urban life caused by pollution, emotional stress, epidemic and endemic infectious diseases, heat stress, sedentary lifestyles, and diet. These common features of urban life place heavy burdens on bodies that evolved in adaptation to mobile foraging lifeways in low-density, relatively egalitarian populations.

In cities, our bodies encounter multiple, historically new challenges. The array, configuration, and intensity of health threats vary within and across cities. While these differences reflect local/global histories, geographic, climate, and geopolitical location, demography, size, distribution of health and social inequalities, age structure, industrial development, transportation systems, and government policies among other factors, threats to health tend to intersect and complicate a city's health burden.

Because of physiological plasticity, the human body is highly adaptable to changing environmental stressors. In local settings with long exposure, for example, people living in the Argentinean Andes have genetically adapted to a level of arsenic exposure through their drinking water that would cause many populations to suffer high rates of disease (Schlebusch et al., 2015). But there are limits to human adaptability which if surpassed can result in body damage, disease, or death (Dow et al., 2013; Sherwood & Huber, 2010).

The Biosocial Nature of Syndemics

Historically, predominant biomedical and epidemiological perspectives have stressed an isolated focus on the identification and/or treatment of a singular presenting disease even though most patients are "individuals with multiple coexisting diseases" (Valderas et al., 2009). To address this issue, Feinstein (1970, p. 455) introduced the term "co-morbidity" to label the co-occurrence of diseases, while noting that "Co-morbidity can alter the clinical course of patients with the same diagnosis by affecting the time of detection, prognostic anticipations, therapeutic selection, and post-therapeutic outcome of the index disease." Syndemics research differs from merely documenting comorbidity by focusing attention on the synergistic effects of multiple health conditions and how these conditions are rooted in the features of specific social and environmental contexts. The concept of syndemics emerged among urban researchers because it was in the city that they readily encountered numerous cases of the negative effects of interconnected hierarchies of inequality and multiple diseases of diverse origin. Although several researchers have drawn attention to specific urban syndemics (Ellis et al., 2021; Heckert, 2019; Illangasekare et al., 2013; Singer et al., 2006), and Moen and colleagues (2020) observe that "Syndemics often disproportionately affect urban communities," no one has fully articulated why cities are frequent sites of syndemic production, a goal of this chapter.

Syndemics emerge in local or regional settings because they reflect specific intersections of population demographics, disease configurations, and social and environmental factors. Thus, the syndemics of residents of Soweto, a township of the City of Johannesburg, South Africa, with over 1 million residents (Mendenhall, 2014), are different from those of men who have sex within the border city of Tijuana, Mexico (Pitpitan et al., 2016), and both of these differ from the syndemics of patients in a Nairobi, Kenya, hospital (Mendenhall et al., 2015), or among male sex workers in Ho Chi Minh City, Vietnam (Biello et al., 2014). These examples exhibit distinct risk contexts, group behaviors, encompassing political and economic factors, and health complexes and, hence, different syndemics.

Syndemics of the City

Cities, especially poorer cities, and the poorest sectors of all cities, are epi-centers of syndemics because they foster synergies of intersection. On the one hand, they facilitate disease clustering and interaction, as well as physical vulnerability. City residents face a concentrated array of health stressors, including toxic exposures from manufacture, vehicular transportation, and other sources, the spread of infectious diseases in dense populations, chronic diseases linked to urban diets and diminished physical activity, emotional stress from violence, noise, economic vulnerability, political precarity, and other sources, and anthropocentric climate change impacts. These factors combine to weaken body systems increasing susceptible to synergistic dis-ease. On the other hand, cities magnify the intersection of multiple axis (e.g., ethnicity, gender, class, sexual orientation) of inequality and injustice. In cit-ies, the interconnected nature of hierarchical social categorizations gener-ates overlapping systems of health-damaging disadvantage. Of course, cities can provide access to healthcare and other vital resources including public health promotion, but these are not equitably accessible across or within cit-ies. Research on health in cities has adopted three approaches: rural/urban contrasts, intercity comparisons, and intracity comparisons. The latter two of these approaches call attention to the intersection of locality and hierar-chy, ideas that are critical to the syndemics understanding of varied disease interactions shaped by context. The role of cities as syndemogenic locations is illustrative in the following three case studies.

Syndemics of Poverty in Lagos, Nigeria

Lagos, Nigeria, a port city surrounded by water, is one of the fastest-growing and most populous cities in the world. Since 1960, the population of Lagos has grown 100-fold, and now exceeds 20 million residents. Sixty-five per-cent of Lagosians are urban poor who reside in informal settlements with no or limited access to essential services. The poorest sections of Lagos are characterized by harrowing population density and overcrowding, decay-ing housing, low wages and high unemployment, inadequate waste disposal, air pollution, poor healthcare access, and insecure residential status (Aliu et al., 2021). Homes are often densely populated, with estimates that in Lagos "more than 75% of urban slum dwellers live in one room households with a density of 4.6 persons per room" (Adelekan, 2009, p. 6).

There are over 100 slum areas and informal settlements scattered across Lagos. Typical is Makoko, a disorderly settlement of crowed tiny houses with little privacy. Some homes are on dry land, others are built in the water on stilts separated by countless narrow canals that people use to move about by canoe. It is unknown how many people live in Makoko as there has never been an official census. Estimates range widely from 100,000 to over a mil-lion (Adeshokan, 2020). Most people in Makoko survive as fishermen or fish sellers. Homes are constructed with whatever materials can be salvaged. Household waste and raw sewage are dumped into the fetid water beneath people's homes. The air is permeated by the smell of rotting fish, garbage, and feces. There is no hospital in Makoko. According to Baale Jeje Aide Albert, a local leader, "Many pregnant women have died in canoes on their way to Island Maternity [Hospital]" (Bakare, 2020). Living conditions endured by many Lagosians have been described as "breeding grounds for diseases such as tuberculosis, hepatitis, dengue, pneumonia, malaria, cholera, and diarrheal diseases" (Akinwale, 2018). Additionally, residents of Lagos' informal settlements are at high risk for asthma, heart disease, diabetes, depression, and substance abuse. The precarity of life for the poor is well-expressed by Lagos resident Joyce Ugbede to Oxfam (Mayah et al., 2017): "Nothing is permanent here, except suffering."

The creation of Lagos as a sprawling metropolitan area and its current precarity dates first to the area's use as a slave trading port and then subsequently as a colony of Britain, a subordinate status that continued until and after Nigeria's independence in 1960. During the latter decades of the 19th century, Nigeria was under the thumb of the Royal Niger Company. Local leaders were forced to sign agreements ceding control of land "to mine, farm, and build" with the Company. The treaties became the constructed legal fiction justifying Britain's "'right' to impose its will on Nigeria" in the interest of advancing imperial economic gain (Inyang & Bassey, 2014, p. 1946). The wealth extracted from its colonies in raw materials, minerals, and food items helped to fund the take-off of the Industrial Revolution in Britain while causing significant changes in the social, economic, and political structures of colonized territories. British colonial rule and expropriative economic activities exacerbated differences of class, region, language, gender, and community across Nigeria (Metz, 1991).

Nigeria has continued to suffer the burden of its colonial history. Within a context of frequent internal conflict, civil war, violent coups, and fragile governance, the country has been dominated by powerful domestic elites in alliance with multinational organizations. Notes Kwarteng (2012), "Ethnic and religious conflict has been a consistent feature of modern Nigerian politics. Another is the extent of corruption that has pervaded the country." This legacy of colonialism, and the shift from colonial to neocolonial fragility, is a product of strategizing "by the departing colonial power in order to perpetuate British traditional economic influence and control in the emergent independent Nigerian state" (Attah, 2013, p. 71). With its significant oil reserves, Nigeria suffers from what has been called a resource curse, "the adverse effects of a country's natural resource wealth on its economic, social, or political well-being" (Ross, 2015, p. 40). Despite the great need for vital life-fostering resources in the Nigerian population, most of the profits of oil sales go to multinationals and Nigeria's elites. This is a primary force behind the grinding poverty in the city. Moreover, already facing annual flooding, as a low-lying coastal city Lagos is threatened by significant sea level rise due to climate change. Not only has oil extraction despoiled parts of Nigeria's environment (e.g., the Niger delta) and fueled the ever-worsening air pollution in Lagos, it is driving the melting of glaciers and the potential submergence of the city (Princewill, 2021). These are some of the key social and ecological forces steering the emergence of syndemics in Lagos.

There are multiple disease components in the syndemics of Lagos. The water surrounding Lagos puts its residents at risk for water-borne diseases like malaria. In the build up to World Malaria Day in 2021, Lagos's state commissioner of health, Akin Abayomi announced that the city was suffering from approximately 700,000 diagnosed malaria cases annually, comprising 70% of all outpatients in the state public healthcare facilities, with many more undiagnosed cases that are never seen by healthcare providers. According to Abayomi, "Malaria is prevalent in [two] vulnerable groups – children under five years and pregnant women, where the infection can be profoundly more severe" (Nigeria Premium Times, 2021). A syndemic risk for people with malaria is co-infection with helminths. A review by Mwangi and colleagues (2006) suggests that helminth infection creates a cytokine milieu that makes sufferers more susceptible to clinical malaria. Yazdanbakhsh and colleagues (2001) add that the presence of T-regulatory cells increases during helminth infection, which, if present in sufficient numbers, facilitates malaria development upon exposure. A study of intestinal helminths and malaria parasites in over a 1,000 randomly selected children from Lagos found four helminth parasites: *Ascaris lumbricoides* (30%), *Trichuris trichiura* (18%), hookworm (0.7%), and *Strongyloides stercoralis* (0.3%), as well as the malaria parasite, *Plasmodium falciparum* (36%) (Adeoye et al., 2007). At the same time, infection with helminths, co-infection with other diseases (e.g., Lassa fever, HIV, COVID-19) (Soyemi, 2021) and insufficient and inappropriate diet put pregnant women in Lagos at risk for "complex syndemics involving more than two diseases in adverse interaction" (Singer, 2013).

While COVID-19-associated syndemics comprising various disease components (e.g., diabetes, heart disease, cancer) have occurred around the world, in Lagos hunger has become a key factor driving infection and outcome. After Lagos had its first confirmed cases of COVID-19, the federal government imposed a five-week lockdown that restricted movement and required all except essential services to close. For the resource poor and socially marginalized, the impact was devastating. Rising food prices left many parents struggling to feed their families. Adeleke Adekunle, a volunteer with the Nigerian Slum/Informal Settlements Federation, told Human Rights Watch (Ewang et al., 2021), "We have many people who work today to eat tomorrow... The lockdown came quickly, and everyone said, 'How are we going to survive?' In two or three days, people were out of cash and food items." When the lockdown ended, people found they were even poorer than before the outbreak began and the daily struggle to survive had intensified (Ewang et al., 2021). Lagos confronted a second and third wave of COVID-19 infections, the last involving the more contagious Delta variant.

On August 11, 2021, Lagos set a record for new COVID-19. By August, the city was recording six COVID-19 deaths a day and the positivity rate of those tested for the SARS-CoV-2 virus had risen eightfold to about 9% (Osae-Brown & Sguazzin, 2021).

The virus is a special risk for those suffering from undernutrition. Kurtz and colleagues (2021) examined the interaction between malnutrition and COVID-19 in hospitalized patients and found a higher odds for severe COVID-19 for children between six and 17 years with history of malnutrition and even higher odds of severe COVID-19 for adults between 18 and 79 years with history of malnutrition. In a study of patients with COVID-19, Bedock and colleagues (2020) found that the prevalence of malnutrition was significantly higher in patients with more severe infections who were admitted to the intensive care unit than in the other patients (66.7% vs. 37.5%, respectively). Undernutrition impairs the immune system, potentially making people more vulnerable to infections like COVID-19 (Holdoway, 2020). Significant protein malnutrition in small children causes atrophy of the thymus and long-lasting immune defects including diminished functional T-cell counts. Malnourished children suffer disproportionately from various infectious diseases and from exacerbated disease (Schaible & Kaufmann, 2007).

The spread of COVID-19 in Lagos has raised concerns about the impact on tuberculosis (TB) patients in a country that is fourth among the high-burdened countries for TB and one of just six countries that accounts for 60% of new TB cases globally. As the U.S. Centers for Disease Control and Prevention (CDC) (2021) reports, there is growing evidence that patients with chronic respiratory diseases like TB are at heightened risk for severe illness or dying from COVID-19 (Adejumo et al., 2020). It is already known from research on Lagosians with TB that they suffer with a substantial burden of diabetes comorbidity. A study in Lagos of 480 TB patients found that 12.3% also had diabetes (Ogbera et al., 2015). Diabetes is syndemically linked with TB as dual diagnosis is associated with an increased risk of TB drug resistance, treatment failure, and recurrence of TB (van Crevel et al., 2018).

As indicated here, the syndemics of Lagos are multiple, complex, and entwined. They form a supersyndemic (a set of interacting syndemics), which collectively increases the burden of disease and critical health outcomes within particularly vulnerable sectors of the city's population.

The COVID-19 Syndemic among the Haredi of Urban Israel

The Haredi (those who are "fearful"), the strictly orthodox Jews of Israel, are overwhelmingly urban dwellers who live primary in the capital city of Jerusalem (27%), Bnei Brak (16.4%), a city located east of Tel Aviv on the central Mediterranean coastal plain of Israel, and Modi'in Illit, Beitar Illit, Elad, and Beit Shemesh (22% combined). In 1948, the Haredi accounted for about 1% of the Israeli population. By 2020, the Haredi population numbered approximately 1,175,000, which constitutes 12.6% of the total population of the country. Because of their large families and a 4% per year growth rate, they are projected to reach 16% of Israel's population by 2030 (Malach & Cahaner, 2021). Comparatively, as a result, the Haredi population is very young with almost 60% under 20 years of age, compared with 30% for the general population.

While sharing many social and behavioral attributes, the Haredi do not constitute a homogenous group as they are divided into subgroups with their own histories, leaders, and social rules and practices. Generally, however, they tend to isolate from the broader population of Jerusalem culturally and socially and there is a history of tensions with the wider society, which have been magnified by the arrival of COVID-19. In Jerusalem, Haredi neighborhoods comprise most of the northwest sector of the city, while the large Ramot neighborhood in the northwest of Jerusalem has a mixed Haredi/non-Haredi population. Bnei Brak, one of the poorest and most densely populated cities in Israel, is among the top ten densely populated urban areas in the world. Over half (53%) of the Haredi population of Israel lives below the poverty line according to the Israeli Central Bureau of Statistics, far higher than the 9% poverty rate among non-Haredi Jews. The average monthly per capita income among Haredi society is about half of the average for non-Haredi Jews and only a little higher than the Arab population of the country (Zaken, 2018).

Because of their young population, the Haredi have a lower death rate than the general Israeli population. However, when the COVID-19 pandemic hit, the Haredi suffered particularly high infection rates comprising 26% of cases, more than double their proportion of the Israel's population (Malach & Cahaner, 2021). Additionally, they had higher hospitalization and mortality rates (0.07 per 10,000 persons) compared to Israelis generally (0.01), even higher than Israel's subordinated Arab population (0.02) (Khitam et al., 2021; Waitzberg et al., 2020). Haredis over the age of 65 have died of COVID-19 at over four times the number in the same age group in the general population. Shomrim, an Israeli investigative journalism nonprofit organization, reported that 1.3% of Haredi over age 65 has died of COVID-19 at this point in the pandemic, compared to 0.27% (1 in 373) of those over 65 in the general population (JTA & Staff, 2021). The vulnerability of Haredi seniors is reflected in the fact that while Haredi over the age of 65 account for only 3% of the Israeli population, by the end of 2020 they comprised 52% of COVID-19 patients in this age group (Sharon, 2020). These patterns are especially pronounced in Bnei Brak, which has an older Haredi population than other Haredi communities. The COVID-19-associated mortality rate among those 70–74 years of age in Bnei Brak is 4.9 deaths per 1,000 population (Sharon, 2020).

These high rates of infection and mortality have been explained in terms of vaccine hesitancy based on distrust of the government and medical institutions, having large multigenerational families living together in small, crowded apartments, and regularly attending unmasked indoor communal activities (e.g., prayer, Torah study, weddings, bar mitzvahs, and holiday and circumcision celebrations). Even Haredi who are sick with COVID-19 prefer to remain at home with their families and volunteer home-care providers. Notably, COVID-19 is not the first infectious disease outbreak among the Haredi in recent years. For example, there have been several eruptions of measles and mumps in Israel that disproportionately struck Haredi families (Stein-Zamir et al., 2008). Israel's 2018 measles outbreak, for example, began in a Haredi community in Safed in northern Israel.

Overall, health is an understudied issue in the Haredi community. Several studies, however, do provide suggestive information on chronic diseases likely involved in COVID-19 syndemics among the Haredi. The prevalence of diabetes among the Haredi is 15–18%, which is twice that of Israel's total population (Israel Center for Disease Control, 2017). Mixed method research with Haredi women found they report higher rates of diabetes and overweight, and lower physical activity rates compared with the general population (Leiter et al., 2019). Despite these disease rates, Haredi who have diabetes have been found to go years after diagnosis without talking about their illness with relatives, friends, or members of their religious community except their spouses and physicians. They explain the topic of sickness is very personal and they fear the spread of rumors about their health, rumor being a common feature of close-knit communities. The consequence, however, is a constraint on social support which is helpful in managing diabetes (Levkovich et al., 2021). Additionally, research on cardiovascular disease risk factors and health behaviors of Haredi women in Israel found that 30% were over-weight and 24% were obese (Body Mass Index [BMI] of 30.0 or higher). Haredi women reported higher rates of combined overweight and obesity as well as obesity alone compared with the general Israeli female population. Having increased number of children was associated with higher BMI (Leiter et al., 2020).

Of note, in December 2020, the Israeli Health Ministry reported that over 90% of those who had died of COVID-19 (a highly disproportionate number of which were Haredi) were suffering from chronic UADs like heart disease, high blood pressure, and diabetes (The Times of Israel, 2020). Specifically, the Ministry data showed that 34% had high blood pressure, 25% had diabetes, and 21% had heart conditions. These data support the assertion of a COVID-19-associated syndemic among the Haredi. There has been a nearly universal finding that chronic cardiometabolic diseases, including diabetes, cardiovascular conditions, and obesity produce a more severe infection course in COVID-19 patients, including pneumonia, respiratory failure, septic shock, multiorgan failure, and death (Cai et al., 2020; Du et al., 2020; Grasselli et al., 2020; Hill et al., 2020; Onder et al., 2020; Zhou et al., 2020). People with diabetes, for example, tend to have impaired immune function (Casqueiro et al., 2012). While there are several pathways of diabetes/immune system interaction, including the role excess of body fat in immune misfunction, available evidence shows that in diabetes, patients' critical neutrophil actions are compromised while antioxidant systems and humoral immunity may be depressed, diminishing the ability to fight infection (Delamaire et al., 1997). Hill and colleagues (2021) note, "It has become clear that the coexisting COVID-19 pandemic and the growing obesity epidemic combine to fit the definition of a syndemic and represent a global challenge" of public health.

The COVID-19-associated syndemic among the Haredi involves an entwined set of historic political forces, social factors, and diseases. The deepest roots of the syndemic lie in the historic adoption by the Haredi of defensive structuring as a reaction to intense and enduring anti-Semitic attacks in their counties of origin, bolstered by perceived hostility from non-orthodox Jews following migration to Israel. Defensive structuring entails a sociocultural adaptation "that recurs with great regularity among groups that perceive themselves as exposed to stress of long duration" from the surrounding social environment with which they cannot cope directly or forcefully (Siegel, 1970, p. 11; Singer, 1982). Features of defensive structuring include central authority over group members by a specially knowledgeable and respected elite (i.e., each group's exalted rabbi), conformity and subordination of the individual to the group, a high rate of endogamy, strong embrace and defense of group cultural identity symbols (the Torah, group dress patterns, holiday traditions), strict performance of group rituals, use of an in-group language (Yiddish), and explicit rules of conduct. In Israel, defensive structuring is manifest as the maintenance of an insular, close-knit, and close-contact lifeway that includes considerable distrust of the government and the public health establishment. As a result, the Haredi are at heightened risk for exposure to the SARS CoV-2 virus and resulting higher infection rates. They are made further vulnerable through the development of comparatively elevated rates of chronic disease comorbidities among their elderly members, conditions—commonly linked to poverty—that weaken the body immune system among other damages. This interacting set of biosocial factors has led to comparatively higher syndemic-driven morbidity and mortality among elderly Haredi since the emergence of COVID-19.

The Syndemic of the *Pasaway* in Manila, Philippines

Manila is the commercial, industrial, financial, cultural, and administrative center of the Philippines. In 2018, Manila was listed by the Globalization and World Cities Research Network as an "alpha-" global city, ranking it seventh in economic performance globally and second regionally (Bouchet et al., 2018). It is the fastest-growing city and one of the most densely populated in the world, estimated at 42,857 people per square kilometer or 111,000 people per square mile, with an average population growth rate of 1.75%. The total population of Metro Manila in 2022 was 14.4 million people.

Its rapid growth has challenged the city's infrastructure. Water services and trash disposal are heavily burdened by the large population, with much

sewage being dumped directly into storm drains, septic tanks, or open canals and overfilled trash dumps spilling toxic leachates into ground water
and the bay (Asian Development Bank, 2004). Most services throughout the
city have been privatized (Baker, 2012; Mimmi & Ecer, 2010; Morin et al.,
2016). In addition, in recent decades a shelter crisis has erupted in Metro
Manila, widely recognized as a problem of the rapidly growing population.
The informal settlement of land has taken place in Metro Manila since the
late 16th century; however, it was not until the early 20th century that informal communities began to be associated with makeshift housing and unsanitary conditions (Alcazaren et al., 2011).

The roots of many of Manila's current urban problems can be traced back
to actions taken by the colonizers of the Philippines argues Von Einsiedel
(2020), former Commissioner for Planning for Metro Manila. The Spanish
implemented three major actions during their colonial rule that decimated
the economic potential of Filipino natives: (1) *Reduccion* or deliberate resettlement; (2) privatization of land ownership; and (3) the Manila-Acapulco
Galleon Trade. *Reduccion* involved the resettlement of the population from
small thriving communities, referred to locally as *barangay*, into larger but
more compact neighborhoods to reduce their number for easier government
control and to ease conversion from Islam to Catholicism. By privatizing
land that was previously considered communal property, the Filipino peas-
antry were forced to become tenants, sharecroppers, and paid or unpaid farm
laborers. Finally, as the native population was excluded from participation in
the Manila-Acapulco, Mexico Galleon Trade, the resulting economic prosperity was confined to Spaniards. While the Galleon trade brought prosperity
to Manila and opened it up to world trade, it came at a heavy price for the
majority of Filipinos (von Einsiedel, 2020). Under American rule, many modern amenities were brought to urban life in Manila; however, little was done
to alter the inequitable socio-economic structure established by the Spanish.
For example, church lands purchased by Governor William Howard Taft in
1903, to be subdivided and sold to tenants of the estates was not accompanied by a program of financial assistance to peasant farmers. As such, much
of the land was purchased by the Filipino elite, Americans, and US corporations. In addition, the Tydings-McDuffie Law or the Philippine Rehabilitation
Act and the Bell Trade Act, both enacted by the US Congress on April 30,
1946, two months before Philippine independence, ensured that the Philippines would continue to be under American control economically. Bell Trade
Act ensured the continuation of US control over the Philippines exchange
rate and included a "parity clause" which granted rites of Philippine public
resources to US citizens or corporations. Consequently, Philippines remained
economically exploited, with the country's natural resources used to develop
and support the commercial and industrial interests of the US.

The more recent expansion of Manila in global trade has increased demand for the commercial, industrial, and residential development of land, resulting in land value increases of 25% annually in the 1990s (Shatkin, 2004).

Much of this value increase has been attributed to the specific structural distortion of land prices, a consequence of the legacy of concentrated urban landownership by Filipino elites and speculative investment encouraged by the existing property tax system (Mendiola, 1983; Strassmann et al., 1994). In addition, the concentration of agricultural land ownership in the hands of wealthy elites and the growth of Metro Manila as a global export-oriented manufacturing hub has resulted in high rates of rural-urban migration (Kahl, 2006; Shatkin, 2004). As a result, from 2000 to 2006, the proportion of households living in informal settlements increased by more than 81%, with approximately one-third of city dwellers residing in slums (NEDA, 2011). Slums are characterized as crowded areas with inadequate housing, infrastructure and service provision, and insecure residential status.

Metro Manila's industrial growth has been insufficient to support the expanding labor force causing an increasing number of people to work informal temporary low-paying jobs (Alcazaren et al., 2011; Ofreneo, 2013). Consequently, low-income housing in the form of informal settlements occupies marginal areas of the city with high hazard exposure, such as low-lying coastal areas, along and within river channels and on steep hillsides (Baker, 2012; Few, 2003). These slum communities are subject to frequent low-intensity flooding and regularly suffer from flood-related economic losses and illness (Porio, 2011). Housing is often constructed from makeshift/temporary materials unable to withstand the forces from wave or flood inundation, typhoon winds, or settlement fires. It is estimated that one-fifth of informal settlers in Metro Manila live in hazard-prone areas along waterways and the coastline and suffer disproportionately from the impacts of flood hazards (Clapano, 2013; Porio, 2011; Zoleta-Nantes, 2002). Efforts to address the housing crisis in Metro Manila have been ongoing since the early 1900s. Strategies have ranged from the criminalization of squatting, forced evictions, relocation (typically to locations far from livelihood-earning opportunities), the provision of socialized housing and, in a few cases, granting of land rights (Alcazaren et al., 2011).

The poor living conditions of slum dwellers have been linked to high rates of disease. When access ways are flooded due to poor drainage, residents of slums often have to pass through polluted waters. This results in skin conditions, enteric disease, and diarrhea. Slum dwellers also have significantly higher rates of infant and under 5-mortality (29 and 40 per 1,000 live births, compared to 16 and 21 per 1,000 in non-slum populations) (piMetrics, 2017). Managing routine health conditions impacts already limited household financial resources. In a study of Metro Manila's slum dwellers, more than 20% of respondents indicated having to take loans on a regular basis for the purpose of buying medicine and seeking medical services (Morin et al., 2016). Although medicines are available for free from health centers, studies indicate that this resource is rarely accessed (Porio, 2011). In addition, only 49% of urban slum dwellers of PhilHealth insurance company members compared to 61% of non-slum residents (piMetrics, 2017).

The urban poor are also more at risk for TB mortality (Shimazaki et al., 2013). WHO estimated that the Philippines has the third highest prevalence of TB in the world in 2019, with up to 1 million active cases (Weiler, 2019). Around 70 people die from TB in the country every day. The overcrowded living conditions of the urban poor exacerbates the spread of TB (Reyes & Amores, 2014). Furthermore, the urban poor often avoid seeking healthcare given indirect expenses like the cost of transportation, or fear of income loss when forced to take leave (Zimmerman et al., 2022). Drug-resistant TB has further complicated the situation as treatment often requires travel to multiple health facilities and hospitals to collect the different prescriptions necessary for successful treatment, at significant personal cost (Bernardo et al., 2022). Despite government efforts to address the TB epidemic, including expanding digital solutions (National Tuberculosis Control Program, 2020), implementing specimen and medication transportation programs to alleviate the financial burdens related to TB treatment (WHO, 2021), 42% of households with TB were still suffering "catastrophic costs" associated with the disease (Florentino et al., 2022).

Philippines' urban TB crisis is supporting a growing HIV epidemic. Philippines had the fastest-growing HIV epidemic in the western Pacific region between 2010 and 2017, with a 174% increase in HIV incidence. Men who have sex with men in urban cities account for more than 80% of all new infections (Gangcuangco, 2019). While HIV treatment hubs are primarily located in major urban centers, access to medicines for prevention and treatment remains limited. The COVID-19 pandemic worsened the crisis, with a noted 60% decline in HIV testing in 2020, a 37% decline in average number of newly diagnosed HIV cases, a 28% decline in HIV treatment initiation, with only 61% of Filipinos living with HIV on antiretroviral therapy (Alibudbud, 2021). Stringent COVID-19 control policies in Manila and other urban spaces contributed to lower accessibility to testing and treatment centers, given travel restrictions and limited public transportation (Hapal, 2021). In addition, government budget measures were reappropriated and realigned to address COVID-19.

COVID-19 significantly compromised the delivery of many essential health services. Health practitioners in the Philippines consider people living with diabetes as particular collateral victims of the pandemic. Military imposed lockdowns and resulting loss of jobs, transportation shut downs, and the realignment of health services towards COVID-19 prevented people with diabetes from accessing treatments or routine monitoring, forcing them to resort to home remedies and rely on neighbors for medical advice (Quinto et al., 2021). Not all patients could access telemedicine services, loss in employment made drugs unaffordable, and access treatment programs were temporarily halted (Arcellana & Jimeno, 2020). Furthermore, non-operative outpatient management, including wound monitoring, was suspended. As such, orthopedic centers that treat people with diabetes were unable to prevent diabetic foot ulcers which progressed to severe soft tissue infections that required amputations. An estimated three-fold increase in emergency major amputations occurred from 2017 to 2020, and another two-fold increase from 2020 to 2021 (Robredo & Cembrano, 2022).

The inadequate urgency in diabetes care in the Philippines can be traced back to before the onset of the COVID-19 pandemic. The national insurance system does not cover comprehensive diabetes care in a preventive model and private insurance companies only offer limited diabetes coverage. Most patients rely on out-of-pocket expenses (Tan, 2015). In addition, subsidies for maintenance medication from the rollout of the primary benefit package for diabetes are considered deficient (Dayrit et al., 2018). Social and structural support for lifestyle modification is also scarce. Adequate nutrition is often unaffordable, particularly for low-income patients and public spaces especially in slum neighborhoods are not conducive for safe physical activity (Arcellana & Jimeno, 2020). Consequently, diabetes is the fourth leading cause of mortality in the Philippines and deaths due to diabetes increased by 7.8% from 2019 to 2020 (Philippine Statistics Authority, 2021), and by 17.5% from 2020 to 2021 (Philippine Statistics Authority, 2021). One out of every five Filipinos has abnormal glucose levels, with diabetes prevalence rising 3% since 2013 (Villegas-Florencio, 2021). The presence of diabetes among COVID-19 patients significantly increased the risk of mortality, respiratory failure, duration of ventilator dependence, severe/critical COVID-19, critical care hospital admission, and length of hospital stay (Espiritu et al., 2021).

The Philippine response to COVID-19 was one of the longest and strictest in the world, with some observers and scholars describing the government response as "draconian," "militarized," and "police-centric" (Maru, 2020). Quarantine rules specified that only one person per family was authorized with a "quarantine pass" to leave the household to purchase essential goods. The police and military were brought in to impose lockdown measures. Images of special action forces operating checkpoints reinforced by their armored personnel carriers or tanks were a common sight (Mayol et al., 2020). Lockdown measures were implemented notwithstanding issues or concerns relating to income, livelihood, food security, space, or population density. While lockdown measures were implemented indiscriminately, they were noticeably more intense in places where population density was high, namely urban poor areas (Hapal, 2021).

Violators of government policies were punished. Among those arrested were residents of Sitio San Roque, Quezon City (the largest city in Metro Manila), who on April 1, 2020, gathered to receive relief goods (Hapal, 2021). While queuing, the police came and arrested 21 residents who were charged with violating the *Bayanihan to Heal as One Act* and later released on bail amounting to 17,500.00 Philippine pesos (approximately USD 350.00) per person. Several days after, the police raided the soup kitchen feeding the residents of Sitio San Roque and tore down placards protesting or pleading for help from the government. On April 16, 2020, President Rodrigo Duterte threatened that if the lack of discipline among Filipinos persisted, "the military and the police will take over. I am ordering them now to be ready. The police and the military will enforce social distancing and curfew. They will. It is just like martial law too. You choose" (Presidential Communications Operations Office, 2020). Overall, from March 17 2020 to August 11 2020, the police apprehended 303,859 quarantine violators, of these 47% were warned, 25% fined, and 28% were charged (One News PH, 2020).

Hapal (2021) argues that the government's reliance on draconian measures corresponded with Duterte's war on drugs narrative, focused on discipline and order. This approach invariably produced contradicting binary archetypes. Healthcare professionals, frontline workers, police, military, and law-abiding citizens were positioned as virtuous contributors to the war on COVID-19. In contrast, the *pasaway*, an importune, stubborn, obstinate person, violated government-imposed health protocols. In popular discourse, *pasaway* often pertains to resource poor people, specifically young, out of school or unemployed men (Jensen et al., 2013). During the pandemic, it was used to describe people who violated stay-at-home orders, did not wear masks, did not practice social distancing, argued with authorities, or displayed any other errant behavior (Philippine Daily Inquirer, 2020). The *pasaway* has been repeatedly blamed by the government for the accelerated rate by which the virus spread all over the Philippines. Notes Hapal (2021, p. 234),

> Theoretically speaking, one could think of the *pasaway* as an empty signifier, able to unite a range of different negative traits with implicit class contempt. In this way, the *pasaway* helps to stabilize the middle class as well as legitimate violent actions dealt to the underclass.

For the Philippines government, disciplining the population became more important than any other disease control measure including testing, tracing, scaling up the healthcare system, vaccines and various other prevention or treatment technologies (Hapal, 2021). Emphasis was placed on disciplining and apprehending the *pasaway*, the poor, slum dwellers, the marginalized and vulnerable, above everything else to protect law-abiding citizens. In so doing, their disease containment measures create a syndemic founded on inequity whereby the *pasaway* was increasingly at risk for multiple interacting health morbidities and mortalities including TB, HIV, enteric disease, diabetes, and COVID-19.

Conclusion: Responding to Urban Syndemics Globally

Cities shape every aspect of the health and well-being of their residents including the experience of urban precarity and risk. As Susser (2021, p. 404) observes, "the anthropological analysis of the 'urban' is pivotal to the understanding of how contemporary precarity is made and experienced." But even as the world struggles with a common pandemic, precarity is not a uniformity, and cities, their residents, and their diseases are varied. So too their syndemics. Focusing on three case studies – Lagos, Nigeria, the Haredi of urban Israel, and Metro Manila, Philippines – in this chapter, we have called attention to the critical role of a diversity of syndemics to the precarity of urban life, particularly so for people in the Global South and the poor everywhere.

Syndemic research was initiated by anthropologists engaged in applied urban health research with the objective of not only understanding syndemics, but also playing a role in alleviating the suffering they cause. Initial efforts in this regard involved working in and with activist-oriented community-based organizations to both address the structural issues driving AIDS-associated syndemics and to implement prevention efforts. Subsequent work has shown that because of their holistic and up-close-and-personal engaged approach to research, anthropologists have been particularly effective in identifying and fully describing syndemics, their experience among sufferers, their pathways of biological and biosocial interaction, and their embeddedness in injustice and inequality.

Moving forward on these fronts in the urban contexts in which most people in the world now live entails addressing two concerns. First, to date, we have few adequate accounts of syndemics that include both the biological (and bio behavior) and biosocial components. Second, fewer still are the number of analyses of the ecosyndemogenic features of cities, that is, explanations of how urban conditions magnify the likelihood of syndemics emerging and the burden of disease and social suffering they create. While the last 25 years of syndemics work has been promising, there is much to be understood about disease interaction and the role of social conditions and relations in this process. There are as well three questions of importance to advancing social response to syndemics, namely: (1) Can policy changes like Universal Health Coverage (Sustainable Development Goal 3.8) effectively diminish the impact of syndemics among the urban poor in the Global South?; (2) In light of the devastating impacts of climate change and COVID-19, how can the syndemics emerging in the cities of the Global South be ameliorated?; and (3) Have grassroots social movements been a force in diminishing urban syndemics?

References

Adejumo, O., Daniel, O. J., Adepoju, V. A., Femi-Adebayo, T., Adebayo, B. I., & Airauhi, A. O. (2020). Challenges of Tuberculosis Control in Lagos State, Nigeria: A Qualitative Study of Health-Care Providers' Perspectives. *Nigerian Medical Journal*, 61(1), 37–41.

Adelekan, I. (2009). Vulnerability of Poor Urban Coastal Communities to Climate Change in Lagos, Nigeria. *Environment and Urbanization*, 22, 433–450.

Adeoye, G., Osayemi, C., Oteniya, O., & Onyemekeihia, S. (2007). Epidemiological Studies of Intestinal Helminthes and Malaria among Children in Lagos, Nigeria. *Pakistan Journal of Biological Sciences*, 10, 2208–2212.

Adeshokan, O. (2020). How Makoko, Nigeria's Floating Slum Went Digital with New Mapping Project. https://www.cnn.com/2020/02/26/africa/nigeria-makoko-mapping-intl/index.html.

Akinwale, O. (2018). Urban Slums in Nigeria: Ensuring Healthy Living Conditions. *Urbanet*. https://www.urbanet.info/nigeria-lagos-slums-urban-health/.

Alcazaren, P., Ferrer, L., Icamina, B., & Oshima, N. (2011). *Lungsod Iskwater: The Evolution of Informality as a Dominant Pattern in Philippine Cities*. Anvil Publishing.

Alibudbud, R. (2021). The Philippine HIV Crisis and the COVID-19 Pandemic: A Worsening Crisis. *Public Health*, *200*, e1. https://doi.org/10.1016/j.puhe.2021.09.008.

Aliu, I., Akoteyon, L., & Soladoye, O. (2021). Living on the Margins: Socio-Spatial Characterization of Residential and Water Deprivations in Lagos Informal Settlements, Nigeria. *Habitat International*, *107*. https://doi.org/10.1016/j.habitatint.2020.102293.

Arcellana, A. E., & Jimeno, C. (2020). Challenges and Opportunities for Diabetes Care in the Philippines in the Time of the COVID-19 Pandemic. *Journal of the ASEAN Federation of Endocrine Societies*, *35*(1), 55.

Asian Development Bank. (2004). *The Garbage Book: Solid Waste Management in Metro Manila*.

Attah, N. (2013). The Historical Conjuncture of Neo-Colonialism and Underdevelopment in Nigeria. *Journal of African Studies and Development*, *5*(5), 70–79.

Bakare, T. (2020). Neglected and Unmapped. https://guardian.ng/stories/makoko-neglected-and-unmapped/.

Baker, J. L. e. (2012). *Climate Change, Disaster Risk and the Urban Poor: Cities Building Resilience for a Changing World*.

Bedock, D., Lassen, P. B., Mathian, A., Moreau, P., Couffignal, J., Ciangura, C., Poitou-Bernert, C., Jeannin, A.-C., Mosbah, H., Fadlallah, J., Amoura, Z., Oppert, J.-M., & Faucher, P. (2020). Prevalence and Severity of Malnutrition in Hospitalized COVID-19 Patients. *Clinical Nutrition ESPEN*, *40*, 214–219.

Bernardo, M. N. G., Alberto, I. R. I., Alberto, N. R. I., Eala, M. A. B., & Roa, C. C. J. (2022). The Way Forward for Drug-Resistant Tuberculosis in the Philippines. *The Lancet*, *22*(June), 760.

Biello, K. B., Colby, D., Closson, E., & Mimiaga, M. J. (2014). The Syndemic Condition of Psychosocial Problems and HIV Risk among Male Sex Workers in Ho Chi Minh City, Vietnam. *AIDS and Behavior*, *18*(7), 1264–1271.

Bouchet, M., Liu, S., Parilla, J., & Kabbani, N. (2018). *Global Metro Monitor 2018*. Brookings. Retrieved December 1 from https://www.brookings.edu/research/global-metro-monitor-2018/.

Cai, Q., Chen, F., Wang, T., Luo, F., Liu, X., Wu, Q., He, Q., Wang, Z., Liu, Y., Liu, L., Chen, J., & Xu, L. (2020). Obesity and COVID-19 Severity in a Designated Hospital in Shenzhen, China. *Diabetes Care*, *43*(7), 1392–1398. https://doi.org/10.2337/dc20-0576.

Casqueiro, J., Casqueiro, J., & Alves, C. (2012). Infections in Patients with Diabetes Mellitus: A Review of Pathogenesis. *Indian Journal of Endocrinology and Metabolism*, *16*(Sup 1), S27–S36. https://doi.org/10.4103/2230-8210.94253.

CDC. (2021). *Treating TB in a Time of COVID* (Global Health – Stories, Issue). https://www.cdc.gov/globalhealth/stories/2020/tb-covid.html.

Clapano, J. (2013, 21 June). P3.2-B Housing Set for Estero Settlers. *The Philippine Star*.

Dayrit, M., Lagrada, L., & Picazo, O. (2018). Pons MC, Villaverde MC. *The Philippines Health System Review*. New Delhi: World Health Organization.

Delamaire, M., Maugendre, D., Moreno, M., LeGoff, M., Allannic, H., & Genetet, B. (1997). Impaired leucocyte Functions in Diabetic Patients. *Diabetic Medicine*, *14*(1), 29–34.

https://doi.org/10.1002/(SICI)1096-9136(199701)14:1<29::AID-DIA300>3.0.
CO;2-V.

Dow, K., Berkhout, F., Preston, B., Klein, R., Midgley, G., & Shaw, M. R. (2013). Limits to Adaptation. *Nature Climate Change*, 3, 305–307.

Du, R., Liang, L., Yang, C., Wang, W., Cao, T., Li, M., Guo, G., Du, J., Zheng, C., Zhu, Q., Hu, M., Li, X., Peng, P., & Shi, H. (2020). Predictors of Mortality for Patients with COVID-19 Pneumonia Caused by SARS-CoV-2. *European Respiratory Journal*, 56(3). https://doi.org/10.1183/13993003.02961-2020.

Ellis, G., Grant, M., Brown, C., Caiaffa, W. T., Shenton, F., Lindsay, S., Dora, C., Nguendo-Yongsih, H. B., & Morgan, S. (2021). The Urban Syndemic of COVID-19: Insights, Reflections and Implications: Cities, Health and COVID-19: Editorial for the Special Issue. *Cities and Health*. https://doi.org/10.1080/23748834.2021.1894843.

Espiritu, A. I., Chiu, H. H. C., Sy, M. C. C., Anlacan, V. M. M., Macalintal, C. M. S. A., Robles, J. B., Cataniag, P. L., Flores, M. K. C., Tangcuangco-Trinidad, N. J. C., Juangco, D. N. A., Paas, G. R. G., Chua, A. M. U., Estrada, V. S., Mejia, P. R. P., Reyes, T. F. B., Cañete, M. T. A., Zapata, F. R. A., Castillo, F. E. B., Esagunde, R. U., … The Philippine, C. S. G. (2021). The Outcomes of Patients with Diabetes Mellitus in The Philippine CORONA Study. *Scientific Reports*, 11(1), 24436. https://doi.org/10.1038/s41598-021-03898-1.

Ewang, A., Wormington, J., & Maki, A. (2021). *Between Hunger and the Virus: The Impact of the Covid-19 Pandemic on People Living in Poverty in Lagos, Nigeria*. https://www.hrw.org/report/2021/07/28/between-hunger-and-virus/impact-covid-19-pandemic-people-living-poverty-lagos#.

Feinstein, A. (1970). The Pre-therapeutic Classification of Co-morbidity in Chronic Disease. *Journal of Chronic Diseases*, 23, 455–468.

Few, R. (2003). Flooding, Vulnerability and Coping Strategies: Local Responses to a Global Threat. *Progress in Development Studies*, 3(1), 43–58.

Flies, E., Mavoa, S., Zosky, G., Mantzioris, E., Williams, C., Eri, R., Brook, B., & Buettel, J. (2019). Urban-Associated Diseases: Candidate Diseases, Environmental Risk Factors, and a Path Forward. *Environment International*, 133(Pt A), 105187. https://doi.org/10.1016/j.envint.2019.105187.

Florentino, J. L., Arao, R. M. L., Garfin, A. M. C., Gaviola, D. M. G., Tan, C. R., Yadav, R. P., Hiatt, T., Morishita, F., Siroka, A., Yamanaka, T., & Nishikiori, N. (2022). Expansion of Social Protection Is Necessary towards Zero Catastrophic Costs Due to TB: The First National TB Patient Cost Survey in the Philippines. *PLOS ONE*, 17(2), e0264689. https://doi.org/10.1371/journal.pone.0264689.

Gangcuangco, L. M. A. (2019). HIV Crisis in the Philippines: Urgent Actions Needed. *The Lancet Public Health*, 4(2), e84.

Gould, W. (1998). African Mortality and the New 'Urban Penalty'. *Health Place*, 4, 171–181.

Grasselli, G., Zangrillo, A., Zanella, A., Antonelli, M., Cabrini, L., Castelli, A., Cereda, D., Coluccello, A., Foti, G., Fumagalli, R., Iotti, G., Latronico, N., Lorini, L., Merler, S., Natalini, G., Piatti, A., Ranieri, M., Scandroglio, A., Storti, E., … Network, C.-L. I. (2020). Baseline Characteristics and Outcomes of 1591 Patients Infected With SARS-CoV-2 Admitted to ICUs of the Lombardy Region, Italy. *JAMA*, 323(16), 1574–1581. https://doi.org/10.1001/jama.2020.5394.

Hapal, K. (2021). The Philippines' COVID-19 Response: Securitising the Pandemic and Disciplining the Pasaway. *Journal of Current Southeast Asian Affairs*, 40(2), 224–244. https://doi.org/10.1177/1868103421994261.

Harpham, T., & Molyneux, C. (2001). Urban Health in Developing Countries: A Review. *Progress in Development Studies*, 1(2), 113–137.

Heckert, C. (2019). Syndemics in Symbiotic Cities: Pathogenic Policy and the Production of Health Inequity Across Borders. *Journal of Borderlands Studies*. https://doi.org/10.1080/08865655.2019.1700823.

Hill, M., Mantzoros, C., & Sowers, J. (2020). Commentary: COVID-19 in Patients with Diabetes. *Metabolism*, 107, 154217. https://doi.org/10.1016/j.metabol.2020.154217.

Hill, M., Sowers, J., & Mantzoros, C. (2021). Commentary: COVID-19 and Obesity Pandemics Converge into a Syndemic Requiring Urgent and Multidisciplinary Action. *Metabolism*, 114, 154408. https://doi.org/10.1016/j.metabol.2020.154408.

Holdoway, A. (2020). Nutritional Management of Patients during and after COVID-19 Illness. *British Journal of Community Nursing*, 25(Sup 8), S6–S10.

Illangasekare, S., Burke, J., Chander, G., & Gielen, A. (2013). The Syndemic Effects of Intimate Partner Violence, HIV/AIDS, and Substance Abuse on Depression among Low-Income Urban Women. *Journal of Urban Health*, 90(5), 934–947. https://doi.org/10.1007/s11524-013-9797-8.

Inyang, A., & Bassey, M. E. (2014). Imperial Treaties and the Origins of British Colonial Rule in Southern Nigeria, 1860–1890. *Mediterranean Journal of Social Sciences*, 5(20), 1946–1953.

Israel Center for Disease Control. (2017). *Israel National Health Interview Survey INHIS-3, 2013–2015, Selected Findings. Publication No.: 374.*

Jensen, S., Hapal, K., & Modvig, J. (2013). *Violence in Bagong Silang: A Research Report Prepared in Collaboration between DIGNITY and Balay.* DIGNITY-Danish Institute against Torture.

JTA, & Staff, T. (2021). 1 in 73 Ultra-Orthodox Israelis over 65 Has Died of COVID, Report Says (February 10, 2021). https://www.timesofisrael.com/1-in-73-ultra-orthodox-israelis-over-65-has-died-of-covid-report-says/.

Kahl, C. H. (2006). *States, Scarcity, and Civil Strife in the Developing World.* Princeton University Press.

Khitam, M., Na'aminh, W., Lapidot, Y., Goren, S., Amir, Y., Perlman, S., Green, M., Chodick, G., & Cohen, D. (2021). A Nationwide Analysis of Population Group Differences in the COVID-19 Epidemic in Israel, February 2020-February 2021. *The Lancet.* https://doi.org/https://doi.org/10.1016/j.lanepe.2021.100130.

King, G., Flisher, A., Mallett, R., Graham, J., Lombard, C., Rawson, T., Morojele, N., & Muller, M. (2003). Smoking in Cape Town: Community Influences on Adolescent Tobacco Use. *Preventive Medicine*, 36(1), 114–123. https://doi.org/10.1006/pmed.2002.1128.

Kurtz, A., Grant, K., Marano, R., Arrieta, A., Grant Jr, K., Feaster, W., Steele, C., & Ehwerhemuepha, L. (2021). Long-Term Effects of Malnutrition on Severity of COVID-19. *Scientific Reports*, 11, 14974.

Kwarteng, K. (2012). Nigeria's Current Troubles and Its British Colonial Roots. https://www.theglobalist.com/nigerias-current-troubles-and-its-british-colonial-roots/.

Leiter, E., Finkelstein, A., Greenberg, K., Keidar, O., Donchin, M., & Zwas, D. (2019). Barriers and Facilitators of Health Behavior Engagement in Ultra-Orthodox Jewish Women in Israel. *European Journal of Public Health*, 29(S4), ckz186.455.

Leiter, E., Greenberg, K. L., Donchina, M., Keidara, O., Siemiatyckic, S., Zwasa, D. R., & Joy, L. (2020). Cardiovascular Disease Risk Factors and Health Behaviors of Ultra-Orthodox Jewish Women in Israel: A Comparison Study. *Ethnicity and Health*. https://doi.org/10.1080/13557858.2020.1849567.

Levkovich, I., Rodin, D., Altman, S., Alperin, M., & Stein, H. (2021). Perceptions among Diabetic Patients in the Ultra-Orthodox Jewish Community Regarding Medication Adherence: A Qualitative Study. *BMC Public Health*, *21*, 1559. https://doi.org/10.1186/s12889-021-11619-6.

Malach, G., & Cahaner, L. (2021). Ultra-Orthodox Population. Statistical Report on Ultra-Orthodox Society in Israel. https://en.idi.org.il/haredi/2020/?chapter=34272.

Maru, D. (2020). F as in Falfak': PH Gov't Getting Failing Marks in Covid-19 Response from These Experts. *ABS-CBN News*, 22.

Mayah, E., Mariotti, C., Mere, E., & Odo, C. O. (2017). *Inequality in Nigeria: Exploring the Drivers*. https://www.oxfam.org/en/research/inequality-nigeria-exploring-drivers.

Mayol, A., Israel, D., & Semilla, N. (2020). *Cebu City Cries Out: 'We Need More Docs, Nurses'*. Retrieved June 26 from https://newsinfo.inquirer.net/1297630/cebu-city-cries-out-we-need-more-docs-nurses.

Mendenhall, E. (2014). Syndemic Suffering in Soweto: Violence and Inequality at the Nexus of Health Transition in South Africa. *Annals of Anthropological Practice*, *38*(2), 300–316. https://doi.org/10.1111/napa.12058.

Mendenhall, E., Omondi, G., Bosire, E., Isaiah, G., Musau, A., Ndetei, D., & Mutiso, V. (2015). Stress, Diabetes, and Infection: Syndemic Suffering at an Urban Kenyan Hospital. *Social Science & Medicine*, *146*, 11–20. https://doi.org/10.1016/j.socscimed.2015.10.015.

Mendiola, E. (1983). Urban Land Reform in the Philippines. In S. Angel, R. Archer, S. Tanphipat, & E. Wegelin (Eds.), *Land for Housing the Poor* (pp. 473–499). Select Books.

Metz, H. (1991). *Nigeria: A Country Study*. Washington, D.C.: Federal Research Division, Library of Congress.

Miller, J. (2001). The Control of Mosquito-Borne Diseases in New York City. *Journal of Urban Health*, *78*(2), 359–366. https://doi.org/10.1093/jurban/78.2.359.

Mimmi, L. M., & Ecer, S. (2010). An Econometric Study of Illegal Electricity Connections in the Urban Favelas of Belo Horizonte, Brazil. *Energy Policy*, *38*(9), 5081–5097.

Moen, M., German, D., Storr, C., Friedmann, E., Flynn, C., & Johantgen, M. (2020). Social Stability Relates Social Conditions to the Syndemic of Sex, Drugs, and Violence. *Journal of Urban Health*, *97*(3), 395–405. https://doi.org/10.1007/s11524-020-00431-z.

Morin, V. M., Ahmad, M. M., & Warnitchai, P. (2016). Vulnerability to Typhoon Hazards in the Coastal Informal Settlements of Metro Manila, the Philippines. *Disasters*, *40*(4), 693–719. https://doi.org/10.1111/disa.12174.

Mwangi, T., Bethony, J., & Brooker, S. (2006). Malaria and Helminth Interaction in Humans: An Epidemiological Viewpoint. *Annuals of Tropical Medicine and Parasitology*, *100*, 551–570.

National Tuberculosis Control Program. (2020). *End TB App Suite*. Republic of Philippines, Department of Health. Retrieved November 30 from https://ntp.doh.gov.ph/resources/downloads/endtb-appsuite/.

NEDA. (2011). *Philippine Development Plan 2011–2016*.

Nigeria Premium Times. (2021). Lagos Reports 700,000 Malaria Cases Annually – Commissioner. https://www.premiumtimesng.com/regional/ssouth-west/457484-lagos-reports-700000-malaria-cases-annually-commissioner.html.

Ofreneo, R. (2013). Precarious Philippines: Expanding Informal Sector, "Flexibilizing" Labor Market. *American Behavioral Scientist, 57*(4), 420–443.

Ogbera, A., Kapur, A., Razzaq, H. A., Harries, A., Ramaiya, K., Adeleye, O., & Kuku, S. (2015). Clinical Profile of Diabetes Mellitus in Tuberculosis. *BMJ Open Diabetes Research and Care, 3*, e000112.

Onder, G., Rezza, G., & Brusaferro, S. (2020). Case-Fatality Rate and Characteristics of Patients Dying in Relation to COVID-19 in Italy. *JAMA, 323*(18), 1775–1776. https://doi.org/10.1001/jama.2020.4683.

One News PH. (2020). *23,660 Quarantine Violations Logged since August 1.* Retrieved August 11 from https://www.youtube.com/watch?v=9ZkLUIqSM1M.

Osae-Brown, A., & Sguazzin, A. (2021). Covid-19 Surges in Africa's Biggest City as Doctors Strike. https://www.bloomberg.com/news/articles/2021-08-02/covid-19-cases-in-lagos-africa-s-biggest-city-surge.

Philippine Daily Inquirer. (2020). Pasaway. Retrieved July 5, 2020 from https://opinion.inquirer.net/131454/pasaway.

Philippine Statistics Authority. (2021). *Causes of Deaths in the Philippines (Preliminary): January to December 2020.*

piMetrics. (2017). *Prescriptions Research Brief: A Look at Urban Health Inequalities in the Philippines.*

Pitpitan, E., Smith, L., Goodman-Meza, D., Torres, K., Semple, S., Strathdee, S., & Patterson, T. (2016). "Outness" as a Moderator of the Association between Syndemic Conditions and HIV Risk-Taking Behavior among Men Who Have Sex with Men in Tijuana, Mexico. *AIDS Behav, 20*(2), 431–438. https://doi.org/10.1007/s10461-015-1172-1.

Porio, E. (2011). Vulnerability, Adaptation, and Resilience to Floods and Climate Change-Related Risks among Marginal, Riverine Communities in Metro Manila. *Asian Journal of Social Science, 39*(4), 425–445.

Presidential Communications Operations Office. (2020). *Talk to the People of President Rodrigo Roa Duterte on Coronavirus Disease 2019 (Covid-19).* Retrieved April 16 from https://pcoo.gov.ph/presidential-speech/talk-to-the-people-of-president-rodrigo-roa-duterte-on-coronavirus-disease-2019-covid-19-2/.

Princewill, N. (2021). Africa's Most Populous City Is Battling Floods and Rising Seas. It May Soon Be Unlivable, Experts Warn. https://www.cnn.com/2021/08/01/africa/lagos-sinking-floods-climate-change-intl-cmd/index.html.

Quinto, C. J. E., Pamittan, J. M. L., Paraguison, C. A. R., Peralta, M. J. B., Perdido, H. M. B., & Ponciano, F. E. (2021). Challenges Faced By Patients in Undergoing Diabetes Care and Management in the Philippines during the Course of the Covid-19 Pandemic. *International Journal of Progressive Research in Science and Engineering, 2*(9), 1–21.

Reyes, K., & Amores, J. C. (2014). *Barriers of Early TB Diagnosis among the Poor in Highly Urbanized Areas in the Philippines* (Discussion Paper Series No. 2014–18, Issue).

Robredo, J. P. G., & Cembrano, D. L. D. (2022). Out on a Limb: Living with Diabetes in the Philippines during the Pandemic. *The Lancet Diabetes & Endocrinology, 10*(11), 771–772. https://doi.org/10.1016/S2213-8587(22)00275-3.

Ross, M. (2015). What Have We Learned about the Resource Curse? *Annual Review of Political Science, 18*, 239–259.

Schaible, U., & Kaufmann, S. (2007). Malnutrition and Infection: Complex Mechanisms and Global Impacts. *PLoS Medicine, 4*(5), e115.

Schlebusch, C. M., Gattepaille, L. M., Engstrom, K., Vahter, M., Jakobsson, M., & Broberg, K. (2015). Human Adaptation to Arsenic-Rich Environments. *Molecular Biology and Evolution*, 32(6), 1544–1555. https://doi.org/10.1093/molbev/msv046.

Sharon, J. (2020). More Than Half of over-65s with COVID Are from the Ultra-Orthodox Community (October 13, 2020). https://www.jpost.com/israel-news/more-than-50-percent-of-over-65s-with-covid-are-from-the-ultra-orthodox-community-645531.

Shatkin, G. (2004). Planning to Forget: Informal Settlements as "Forgotten Places" in Globalising Metro Manila. *Urban Studies*, 41(12), 2469–2484.

Sherwood, S., & Huber, M. (2010). An Adaptability Limit to Climate Change Due to Heat Stress. *Proceedings of the National Academy of Sciences of the United States of America*, 107(21), 9552–9555. https://doi.org/10.1073/pnas.0913352107.

Shimazaki, T., Marte, S. D., Saludar, N. R., Dimaano, E. M., Salva, E. P., Ariyoshi, K., Villarama, J. B., & Suzuki, M. (2013). Risk Factors for Death among Hospitalised Tuberculosis Patients in Poor Urban Areas in Manila, The Philippines. *International Journal of Tuberculosis and Lung Disease*, 17(11), 1420–1426. https://doi.org/10.5588/ijtld.12.0848.

Siegel, B. (1970). Defensive Structuring and Environmental Stress. *American Journal of Sociology*, 76(1), 11–32.

Singer, M. (1982). Life in a Defensive Society: The Black Hebrew Israelites. In J. Wagner (Ed.), *Sex Roles in Contemporary American Communes* (pp. 45–81). Indiana University Press.

Singer, M. (1996). A Dose of Drugs, a Touch of Violence, a Case of AIDS: Conceptualizing the SAVA Syndemic. *Free Inquiry in Creative Sociology*, 24(2), 99–110.

Singer, M. (2013). Development, Coinfection, and the Syndemics of Pregnancy in Sub-Saharan Africa. *Infectious Diseases of Poverty*, 2, 26.

Singer, M., Erickson, P., Badiane, L., Diaz, R., Ortiz, D., Abraham, T., & Nicolaysen, A. (2006). Syndemics, Sex and the City: Understanding Sexually Transmitted Diseases in Social and Cultural Context. *Social Science & Medicine*, 63(8), 2010–2021. https://doi.org/10.1016/j.socscimed.2006.05.012.

Soyemi, T. (2021). Neglect of Common Infectious Disease Outbreaks during the COVID-19 Pandemic: An Impending Crisis in Nigeria? *African Journal of Clinical and Experimental Microbiology*, 22(2), 113–116.

Stein-Zamir, C., Zentner, G., Abramson, N., Shoob, H., Aboudy, Y., Shulman, L., & Mendelson, E. (2008). Measles Outbreaks Affecting Children in Jewish Ultra-Orthodox Communities in Jerusalem. *Epidemiology & Infection*, 136, 207–214.

Strassmann, W., Blunt, A., & Tomas, R. (1994). Land Prices and Housing in Manila. *Urban Studies*, 31(2), 267–285.

Susser, I. (2021). Urban Precarity: The Destructiveness of Neoliberalism and Possibilities for Transformation. *City & Society*, 33(2), 403–412.

Tan, G. H. (2015). Diabetes Care in the Philippines. *Annals of Global Health*, 81(6), 863–869. https://doi.org/10.1016/j.aogh.2015.10.004.

The Times of Israel. (2020). 92% of Israel's COVID-19 Fatalities Had Existing Chronic Diseases - Report (December 16, 2020). https://www.timesofisrael.com/92-of-israels-covid-19-fatalities-had-existing-chronic-diseases-report/.

Valderas, J., Starfield, B., Sibbald, B., Salisbury, C., & Roland, M. (2009). Defining Comorbidity: Implications for Understanding Health and Health Services. *Annals of Family Medicine*, 7(4), 357–363. https://doi.org/10.1370/afm.983.

van Crevel, R., Koesoemadinata, R., Hill, P., & Harries, A. (2018). Clinical Management of Combined Tuberculosis and Diabetes. *International Journal of Tuberculosis and Lung Disease*, 22(12), 1404–1410.

Villegas-Florencio, M. Q. (2021). Diabetes and COVID-19. *The Medical City*. https://www.themedicalcity.com/news/diabetes-and-covid-19#:~:text=Data%20from%20the%20DOST%2DFNRI,Filipinos%20have%20abnormal%20glucose%20levels.

Vlahov, D., & Galea, S. (2003). Urban Health: A New Discipline. *Lancet*, 362(9390), 1091–1092. https://doi.org/10.1016/S0140-6736(03)14499-6.

von Einsiedel, N. D. (2020). Colonization's Impact on Manila. *Positively Filipino*, 2022(December 5). http://www.positivelyfilipino.com/magazine/colonizations-impact-on-manila.

Waitzberg, R., Davidovitch, N., Leibner, G., Penn, N., & Brammli-Greenberg, S. (2020). Israel's Response to the COVID-19 Pandemic: Tailoring Measures for Vulnerable Cultural Minority Populations. *International Journal for Equity in Health*, 19, 71.

Weiler, G. A. (2019). *It's Time to End TB in the Philippines*. World Health Organization. Retrieved November 30 from https://www.who.int/philippines/news/commentaries/detail/it-s-time-to-end-tb-in-the-philippines.

WHO. (2021). *Delivering Patient-Centred Tuberculosis Care during COVID-19 in the Philippines*. World Health Organization. Retrieved November 30 from https://www.who.int/about/accountability/results/who-results-report-2020-mtr/country-story/2021/philippines.

Yazdanbakhsh, M., van der Biggelaar, A., & Maizels, R. (2001). Th2 Responses without Atopy: Immunoregulation in Chronic Helminth Infections and Reduced Allergic Disease. *Trends in Immunolology*, 22, 373–377.

Zaken, D. (2018). Haredim Aren't as Poor as You Think (December 17, 2018). https://en.globes.co.il/en/article-haredim-arent-as-poor-as-you-think-1001265187.

Zhou, F., Yu, T., Du, R., Fan, G., Liu, Y., Liu, Z., Xiang, J., Wang, Y., Song, B., Gu, X., Guan, L., Wei, Y., Li, H., Wu, X., Xu, J., Tu, S., Zhang, Y., Chen, H., & Cao, B. (2020). Clinical Course and Risk Factors for Mortality of Adult Inpatients with COVID-19 in Wuhan, China: A Retrospective Cohort Study. *Lancet*, 395(10229), 1054–1062. https://doi.org/10.1016/S0140-6736(20)30566-3.

Zimmerman, E., Smith, J., Banay, R., Kau, M., & Garfin, A. M. C. G. (2022). Behavioural Barriers and Perceived Trade-Offs to Care-Seeking for Tuberculosis in the Philippines. *Global Public Health*, 17(2), 210–222. https://doi.org/10.1080/17441692.2020.1855460.

Zoleta-Nantes, D. (2002). Differential Impacts of Flood Hazards among the Street Children, the Urban Poor and Residents of Wealthy Neighborhoods in Metro Manila, Philippines. *Mitigation and Adaptation Strategies for Global Change*, 7(3), 239–266.

2 Effects Multiplied

Syndemic Interactions among Structured Disparities, Comorbidities, and COVID-19 in Pakistan

Inayat Ali

The coronavirus disease 2019 (COVID-19) pandemic exhibits several specificities. This is due to the intertwining of local historical, sociocultural, environmental, economic, and political factors, along with structured vulnerabilities. These factors have led to significant differences in the spread and effects of the virus in various countries and regions (Bulled and Singer, 2020; James, 2020; Singer, 2020; Team and Manderson, 2020). The virus has also become entangled with preexisting comorbidities such as chronic kidney disease (CKD) and diabetes. These intersecting factors create a precarious situation, rendering some populations more vulnerable than others, particularly in the Global South. These circumstances reveal forms of structured inequalities and institutionalized violence rooted in politico-economic structures. These countries share similar profiles characterized by inadequate healthcare systems, food scarcity leading to malnutrition, corrupt governance, limited economic resources, overwhelmed populations, distinct sociocultural patterns, and high rates of both communicable and non-communicable diseases. These interplays weaken people's immune systems and overall healthcare systems. Complex relationships exist among pathogen biology, human behavior, viral vectors, and reservoirs, and these, combined with context-specific epidemiological behaviors within sociocultural and politico-economic systems, contribute to the emergence of systematic disparities. These disparities determine the success or failure of structural interventions. Medical anthropologists refer to this entwinement as syndemics (Singer and Clair, 2003). Bulled and Singer (2020: 1240) argued that "COVID-19 syndemics in South Africa are likely to cluster among the economically, politically, and socially marginalized individuals living in densely populated urban areas, where physical distancing and hygiene recommendations are nearly impossible to follow." Similarly, Pakistan exhibits a vulnerable (albeit somewhat different) profile related to sociocultural, political, economic, and healthcare system factors that have created fertile ground for a communicable disease like COVID-19 to have severe effects (Ali and Ali, 2020).

DOI: 10.4324/9781003365358-3

Navigating COVID-19: Pakistan's Strategies, Narratives, and Vaccination

After reporting its first COVID-19 infection on February 26, 2020, Pakistan has stood at a pivotal crossroads from January 3, 2020, to August 16, 2023 (World Health Organization, 2023). Pakistan's response to this unparalleled challenge, marked by 1.58 million confirmed cases and 30,656 lives lost, reveals a panorama of strategies, trials, and triumphs. For containing the virus, Pakistan implemented several "rituals of containment" (Ali, 2021), such as suspending international and national travel, implementing lockdowns and "smart lockdowns," opening quarantine centers, deploying armed forces and police to implement these measures, and invoking Section 188 of the Pakistan Penal Code for violations of these measures (Ali and Ali, 2020). Right at the beginning, the country sent blood samples of people to China and the United States for testing and then imported 1,000 test kits from China and organized a national-level prayer in the Prime Minister House (Ali and Ali, 2020, Ali 2021). The government used "hard" and "soft" power to implement these measures (Ali, 2021), which were appreciated by some people and criticized by others as it exerted pressure and inflicted economic hardships on vulnerable people and groups.

Different competing narratives emerged in the country. People perceived that the pandemic is a "political game" and purportedly the result of "bioengineering," attributed to either the United States, Big Pharma, or Jews (Ali, 2020b; Ali et al., 2021). I have discussed these narratives in detail elsewhere (Ali, 2020b), thus I briefly mention here. Narratives also were about folk remedies, like consuming garlic-infused water, or "directing hot air from a hairdryer into one's nostrils." More specifically, in a Sindh Province's village during the early pandemic, a rumor spread that the government was burning infected individuals to control the virus. Also, another rumor was that shaving heads prevents the virus. More interestingly, a miraculous birth in northern Sindh had an infant convey virus information, suggesting green tea sips for survival before its passing. Similarly, in Azad Jammu and Kashmir, rumors claimed the government was shooting the infected to curb the virus. In Punjab, COVID-19 was linked to divine punishment due to Saudi cinemas and disbelief in the Global North. Faith, not science, was seen as key, factor responsible for the lower infection rate in Pakistan.

Furthermore, Pakistan commenced vaccination rollout in early 2021 to pursue herd immunity as a crucial milestone. By August 2023, around 339.9 million doses have been administered (World Health Organization, 2023). However, challenges in vaccine distribution, supply chain management, hesitancy, natural disasters, and global disparities have affected it (Ali, 2023b; Ali and Hamid, 2022).

Pakistan and Its Vulnerable Profile

First, Pakistan is the fifth most populous country globally, with a total population of approximately 212.82 million (Ali and Ali, 2020). According to one survey conducted by the National Institute of Population Studies with a representative sample (2019), around 10% of households lack access to water, soap, or other cleaning agents for handwashing. Approximately 30% do not have proper sanitation facilities, and only 25% have flush toilets connected to a septic tank. Gender disparities are also prevalent, with 50% of women lacking education compared to 34% of men. The school attendance ratio is relatively low, with 59% at the primary level and 38% at the middle/ secondary level.

Second, Pakistan's healthcare system has encountered persistent difficulties in providing adequate and appropriate services. It was significantly overwhelmed during the pandemic. The country has approximately 1,300 public sector hospitals, 5,530 Basic Health Units (BHUs), 700 Rural Health Centers (RHCs), and 5,680 dispensaries (Ali and Ali 2020). However, there is an imbalance between rural and urban areas, with urban areas having better healthcare facilities, which is why Akbar Zaidi (1985) calls this imbalance the "urban bias."

Third, Pakistan experiences economic disparities. In contrast to the 25% reported in 2020 (Ali and Ali, 2020), the proportion of individuals residing below the poverty threshold has experienced a noteworthy rise, reaching approximately 38% in the year 2023 (Meyer, 2023). However, some perceive it to have more impact than these numbers suggest. Gender and geographical differences further exacerbate these inequalities, with women and rural populations being disproportionately affected. The country ranks 133rd on the Gender Inequality Index (GII) (Ali and Ali, 2020). Corruption is also pervasive, as Pakistan stood at 140th out of 180 countries in Transparency International's (2022) Corruption Perception Index for 2022. This endemic corruption hampers economic growth and weakens the country's ability to effectively respond to challenges and emergencies.

Fourth, sociocultural factors play significant roles in shaping healthcare practices in Pakistan (Ali, 2023a). Many people attribute health and illness to acts of God, leading to a reduced emphasis on preventive measures such as hand hygiene during the COVID-19 pandemic. Cultural norms, particularly living together in extended families, contribute to increased contact and potential disease transmission. The average household size is relatively large, with urban households averaging 6.3 individuals and rural households averaging 6.8 (Ali, 2023a). Animals often share living spaces with humans, especially in rural areas where economically marginalized individuals rely on livestock for their livelihoods. Animals are considered important and even sacred, but they can serve as sources of zoonotic diseases (Ali, 2023a).

Cultural norms like eating with one's hands and close physical contacts, such as handshaking and hugging, are deeply ingrained but also contribute to disease transmission (Ali, 2023a). Misinformation and conspiracy theories, particularly regarding vaccination programs, prevail in the country, leading to vaccine hesitancy and skepticism (Ali, 2020b). These rumors range from suspicions of hidden agendas to false claims about vaccine side effects. Unknown and untraceable sources disseminate competing narratives, primarily in rural areas, complicating efforts to address public health challenges.

Pakistan's demographic characteristics, healthcare system limitations, economic inequalities, corruption, and sociocultural factors have contributed significantly to various communicable and non-communicable diseases. For example, the country is attracting global attention due to several infectious diseases such as human immunodeficiency virus infection/acquired immune deficiency syndrome (HIV/AIDS), hepatitis, measles, and polio. The country has experienced multiple HIV outbreaks since 2003 and is considered the second fastest-growing HIV country in Asia (Ali and Ali, 2020). Hepatitis is also a significant concern, with around 18 million people infected. Some local people consider hepatitis as "silent killer" as many young adults (in their 30s) have died of it. This prevalence makes Pakistan the second highest contributor, just behind Egypt, to the global rate of hepatitis. According to National Institute of Health (2023) in terms of tuberculosis (TB), Pakistan ranks 5th amongst the high burden countries globally. Pakistan ranks among the top ten countries in terms of neglected tropical diseases (NTDs); infections like dengue, malaria, and trachoma cause high morbidity and mortality rates. The same is the case with CKDs, and diabetes, which are the focus of this chapter. Malnutrition is a pressing issue particularly in the economically poor population of Pakistan. This is most common in children located in low-resource settings. One survey (2019) has reported alarming figures: 38% of children are stunted, 7% wasted, and 3% overweight. Another vulnerable social group for malnutrition is women, as many of them do not have sufficient nutritious food that creates critical complications during their pregnancy and delivery (Iqbal et al., 2020). The prevalence of malnutrition, food insecurity, and hunger is higher in rural areas, particularly in the Thar Desert of Sindh Province, compared to the cities. The biosocial interactions highlighted above establish a scenario where individuals become highly susceptible to contracting and being impacted by COVID-19.

Moreover, Pakistan's recent and older political and geo-political disruptive events, such as British colonization and Talibanization, have shaped biosocial interaction. For example, *loot-mar* (lit. stealing and punishment) of British individuals and creation of the Taliban to fight against the USSR in the 1980s are still well preserved in "societal memory" in Pakistan (Ali, 2020a, 2023a). These occurrences are cited by some people as a justification to refuse and resist vaccination, suggesting that the "Western world" have had ulterior motives (Ali, 2023a; Ali et al., 2021). Regarding British colonization, Akbar Zaidi (1988), a political economist, has demonstrated that colonizers adversely impacted the prevailing Indigenous healthcare system, specifically during their time in control (from 1858 to 1947) and even continued thereafter particularly through the creation of "Brown Englishmen." This new category, from Zaidi's perspective, are those who were "brown" in their color but were trained in an English way which is to divide, control, and exploit. The Brown Englishmen became a dominant class in the healthcare sector and established specific societal structures to keep this in an English way.

To study these interactions, I use the syndemics lens as it allows me to reveal critical biosocial health events involving the harmful interactions of a few diseases that are considerably shaped by sociocultural patterns, environmental conditions, economic factors, and political systems. Syndemics refers to the interactions between two or more diseases that exacerbate each other's negative effects and contribute to a higher cumulative health burden (Singer, 2020). I focus on the interactions among COVID-19, CKD, and diabetes from a syndemic perspective. Considering COVID-19, CKDs, and diabetes as a syndemic enables us to acknowledge the interrelatedness and interplay among these health concerns. This perspective helps to identify shared risk factors, common vulnerabilities, and underlying social determinants of health. Instead of treating them as separate problems, a syndemic perspective recognizes that addressing one condition in isolation may not be sufficient and may lead to partial understanding.

Diabetes and CKD at a Glance

The prevalence of diabetes has been rapidly increasing worldwide, making it a significant global health challenge. According to the International Diabetes Federation (2020), the number of adults living with diabetes increased from 151 million in 2000 to 285 million in 2009, representing an 88% increase. Currently, under half a billion people are living with diabetes globally, which is projected to increase by 25% in 2030 and 51% in 2045 (Saeedi et al., 2019). Little and colleagues (2017) conducted a study in India, which revealed that shifting dietary patterns were considered the primary cause of the diabetes epidemic. Participants emphasized the impact of the Public Distribution System (PDS), which provides subsidized rice, sugar, and cooking oil, on their consumption habits. The commercialization of agriculture led to a decrease in the availability of traditional staples and increased reliance on external food sources. Furthermore, the expansion of the food processing sector and rural marketing resulted in a rise in the consumption of unhealthy packaged and processed foods. The study also highlighted economic poverty as a significant factor in the onset and management of diabetes as financial difficulties created tension and posed challenges to proper diabetes care due to the high costs of medical check-ups, medication, and dietary control (Little et al. 2017). In contrast, managing diabetes often exacerbated economic poverty as individuals resorted to selling their possessions or seeking loans to afford treatment, particularly affecting marginalized populations.

As a direct consequence of the rising global rates of diabetes, CKD is rapidly becoming a serious health issue (Naghavi et al., 2015). At the scale of the Global Burden of Disease (GBD), CKD moved from the 27th position in the 1990s to the 18th in 2010 for causing global deaths (Jha et al., 2013). Mortality rate caused by it has increased by over 134% compared to 1990 (Naghavi et al., 2015). Certain countries, particularly those with lower incomes, experience a higher prevalence of CKD, resulting in a greater number of fatalities (Stanifer et al., 2016). Of approximately 500 million people having CKD worldwide, around 80% of them live in low- and middle-income countries (LMICs) (Stanifer et al., 2016). In LMICs, the significant reasons for CKD include diabetes mellitus (DM), hypertension (HTN), obesity, and cardiovascular disease (Imtiaz et al., 2020; Imtiaz et al., 2018). CKD is rapidly growing in Asian countries as several behavioral, socioeconomic, and urbanization factors contribute to the prevalence of CKD (Duan et al., 2020; Jessani et al., 2014; Naghavi et al., 2015).

Diabetes and CKD in Pakistan: Two Interrelated and Growing Health Epidemics in Pakistan

Pakistan has a particularly high burden of diabetes, with approximately 19.4 million people living with the condition (Basit, 2020). The prevalence of diabetes in the country can be attributed to various factors, such as environmental and emotional changes, sedentary lifestyle, internet and TV usage, and caloric rich diets leading to increasing obesity (Basit et al., 2019). Traditional dietary patterns and physical activity levels have been replaced by sedentary lifestyles and the consumption of processed foods along with little to no physical activity (Azeem et al., 2022). Consequently, the rise in obesity rates has contributed to the increasing number of diabetes cases. Also, many people are choosing to live in cities owing to availability of facilities (e.g., health, education), and employment opportunities. This process of urbanization is changing lifestyle factors, such as increased consumption of processed food and less physical exercise, which is why incidence of diabetes is higher in urban areas (15.1%) than rural areas (1.6%) (Azeem et al., 2022). Although consuming wheat bread or rice as staple food is a historic tradition, drinking sugary drinks (e.g., coca cola) and eating fast food (such as McDonald's and KFC, especially in urban areas) are a consequence of the capitalist penetration and the global food economy, especially in the cities.

Economic factors such as poverty, income inequality, and limited access to healthcare services impact the burden of diabetes. Individuals from lower socioeconomic backgrounds often lack the necessary resources to maintain a healthy lifestyle, access medical care, or afford the medications required for effective diabetes management. Likewise, inadequate and inappropriate access to healthcare facilities, particularly in rural areas, lead to undiagnosed and improperly managed diabetes cases. As mentioned earlier, healthcare facilities are insufficient in Pakistan; yet, the allocated budget never crosses 2% of the country's gross domestic product (GDP) (Ali, 2023a).

Additionally, in Pakistan, diabetes and hypertension significantly contribute to CKD or end-stage kidney disease (ESKD). These conditions contribute to the development and progression of CKD in the following ways. Diabetes is a prevalent cause of CKD worldwide, and Pakistan is no exception to this trend. When diabetes is not effectively managed over an extended period, it can lead to damage in the kidneys' blood vessels and filtration units. The kidneys, affected by high blood sugar levels, start filtering an excessive amount of blood, resulting in strain and eventual kidney damage. Consequently, individuals with diabetes are at a higher risk of developing CKD or progressing to end-stage kidney disease (ESKD). Hypertension, also known as high blood pressure, is another significant contributor to CKD in Pakistan. Prolonged and uncontrolled high blood pressure can cause damage to the blood vessels in the kidneys, impairing their ability to efficiently filter waste from the bloodstream. This gradual damage can ultimately lead to the development of CKD or the progression to ESKD. It is worth noting that diabetes and hypertension often coexist, creating a particularly high risk for developing CKD (Webster et al., 2017). When these two conditions are present simultaneously, they can accelerate kidney damage and increase the likelihood of reaching ESKD.

Moreover, both diabetes and hypertension are syndemically influenced by sociocultural and economic factors, which exacerbate the impact of diabetes and hypertension on CKD. Unhealthy dietary patterns, limited healthcare resources, and inadequate management of these conditions contribute to the overall burden of CKD in the country. In addition, growing urbanization exposes around 180 million people to chronic diseases, such as diabetes and hypertension (Jessani et al., 2014). In March 2020, Pakistan's *Dawn* (2020) newspaper reported that over 17 million people were suffering from kidney diseases in Pakistan, ranking the country eighth globally in terms of kidney diseases.

Due to reporting issues, it is difficult to estimate the number of people suffering from end-stage renal disease and needing renal replacement therapy (Jha, 2013). Kidney transplantation, though the optimal long-term solution, substantially lags in execution due to insufficient funding and lack of organized deceased donor programs, leading to demand surpassing supply. Most implants come from living donors. Inadequate organ procurement networks, lack of facilities to supply potential donors, and inadequate public awareness result in the exploitation of deceased as well as living donors that led the Pakistani government to pass laws in 2007 and 2009 mandating that donating kidneys should be transparent as many people started selling their kidneys due to economic poverty to earn some money and meet their needs (Jha, 2013). According to media outlets and social discourse, this phenomenon also gave rise to a "black market" for kidney donors and recipients, with incidents of murders and instances of bodies being found without their kidneys, primarily in major urban areas such as Karachi.

Moreover, my current ethnographic research on a dialysis ward in rural Sindh shows a different form of "corruption" of healthcare providers, mainly of attendants (those who are technicians, nurses), which I call *moral corruption* (Ali, n.d.). It is practiced in the dialysis ward in different ways. For example, patients are often neglected by healthcare providers (HCPs) for extended periods as they are left unattended for hours, with excuses like the requirement of a doctor's receipt to initiate dialysis. In rural areas where healthcare services are scarce, especially at night, patients are left with no choice but to pay a bribe or endure excruciating pain. Although HCPs do not explicitly demand money, they readily accept it when offered, exploiting the desperation of CKD patients and undermining their right to timely and adequate healthcare. Another prevalent form of corruption in the dialysis ward is the direct exploitation of patients and their companions. HCPs utilize them for unpaid labor, such as transporting medicines, performing tasks, and using patients' vehicles, such as motorbikes, for personal work. Patients and their companions are unable to refuse these demands due to the potential additional suffering for the patients. This direct corruption not only violates the rights of CKD patients but also exploits their vulnerability for the personal gain of the HCPs.

The carelessness displayed by HCPs in the dialysis ward exacerbates the suffering of CKD patients. Delays in initiating dialysis and neglecting proper cleaning of dialysis machines prolong the patients' pain and compromise their health. Each act of negligence or oversight by HCPs leads to additional suffering for these vulnerable individuals. It is important to recognize that corruption and bribery occur on both sides: HCPs perpetuate corruption, while patients are forced to bribe their way to receiving essential care.

Understanding the corruption in the dialysis ward requires placing it within the broader context of Pakistan's economic and political disparities. The inadequacies of the healthcare system and the prevalence of corruption can be attributed, in part, to systemic issues at the national level. Structural corruption and disparities perpetuated by those in power have a trickle-down effect, disproportionately affecting vulnerable populations in rural areas. Addressing corruption within the healthcare sector necessitates addressing the systemic issues that fuel it. The dialysis ward in rural Sindh exemplifies the corruption and exploitation prevalent within Pakistan's healthcare system.

The Syndemics of Diabetes, CKD, and COVID-19

There is association between and among the abovementioned biosocial events. Studies have shown how various comorbidities and prevailing conditions have affected the outcomes of COVID-19 worldwide (Emami et al., 2020; Guan et al., 2020; Richardson et al., 2020). To illustrate the intricate relationship between diabetes and COVID-19, for example, Singer (2020) found that numerous factors contribute to the heightened vulnerability of individuals with diabetes to COVID-19. The viral infection itself is known to trigger elevated stress levels, which subsequently lead to the release of hyperglycemic hormones and to an increase in blood glucose levels (Chen et al., 2020a). Nandy and colleagues (2020) conducted a systematic review and meta-analysis that revealed the substantial impact of diabetes mellitus on the mortality rate among COVID-19 patients. One study of around 45,000 COVID-19-infected people in China reported an overall case fatality rate (CFR) of 2.3%, which was higher among people with underlying health conditions, such as 10.5% for people with cardiovascular disease and 7.3% for those with diabetes (Zhu et al., 2020). Similarly, another study in China, involving around 1,600 infected individuals, demonstrated that those with diabetes were more prone to developing critical COVID-19 infections (Zhu et al., 2020).

In England, Barron and colleagues (2020) claim to cover almost England's entire population and nearly the entire population diagnosed with type 1 and type 2 diabetes and found both types had greater odds of in-hospital death with COVID-19 than people without a diagnosis of diabetes. In the United States, Muniyappa and Gubbi (2020) show that individuals with diabetes mellitus (DM), hypertension, and severe obesity are at a significant risk to be infected and develop severe complications, including death, from COVID-19. In Italy, Onder and colleagues (2020) studied 355 people who died due to COVID-19, and of that, 35% (126) had diabetes. Likewise, Huang and colleagues (2020b) found that diabetes was significantly associated with severity, mortality, and acute respiratory distress syndrome in COVID-19. In India, Hussain, and colleagues (2020) demonstrate that people with diabetes were at a higher risk of mortality and ICU admission. In Pakistan, diabetes was among the considerable comorbidities in people infected with COVID-19 in Karachi and Rawalpindi (Asghar et al., 2020; Nasir et al., 2020; Zeb et al., 2020).

Akhtar and colleagues (2021) found in their retrospective observation study of 1,812 people in Pakistan that patients lacking any known comorbidities displayed minimal requirements for ICU admission, occurrences of ventilator assistance, and instances of mortality. In stark contrast, patients with two or more comorbidities exhibited these proportions at a magnitude approximately ten times higher. About 50% of individuals with any type of comorbidity, such as CKD and diabetes, necessitated ICU admission, with or without ventilator support, and a considerable number met a fatal outcome. Similarly, in another study from Pakistan it was found that most patients who recovered had no pre-morbidities, whereas majority of those who died had underlying chronic medical conditions (Toori et al., 2022).

The interaction of CKD and COVID-19 has been documented as resulting in severe complications, including deaths. Ssentongo and colleagues (2020) showed that people having preexisting diseases such as cardiovascular disease, hypertension, diabetes, and CKD were at a considerable risk of mortality after being infected with COVID-19 compared to those who do not have these comorbidities. In their sample of around 800 people, Chen and colleagues (2020b) found that 28% of those who died due to COVID-19 had CKD. Another study from China found that 42% of 701 people infected with COVID-19 had comorbidities in which CKD appeared as decisive risk factor (Cheng et al., 2020). In England, CKD and diabetes were among the significant preexisting comorbidities that increase the risks of COVID-19 infection and of developing critical complications, including death (Atkins et al., 2020). Three other studies showed a substantial relationship between CKD and critical COVID-19 complications (Dorjee et al., 2020; Richardson et al., 2020; Singh et al., 2020). In contrast, Yin and colleagues (2021) found that although people with chronic obstructive pulmonary disease (COPD) and CKD seem to be at a low risk of contracting COVID-19, they face critical effects once they are infected.

The studies mentioned above reveal several important findings regarding the relationships among diabetes, CKD, and COVID-19. Multiple studies have highlighted the fact that individuals with diabetes are more vulnerable to COVID-19. They have a higher risk of severe infections, critical complications, and increased mortality rates compared to those without diabetes. Research has demonstrated that individuals with CKD, along with other comorbidities such as cardiovascular disease, hypertension, and diabetes, face a significantly higher risk of mortality if infected with COVID-19. CKD is identified as a decisive risk factor for severe complications and death. The presence of both diabetes and CKD increases the risk of COVID-19 infection and the development of critical complications, including mortality. However, and as previously noted, individuals with COPD and CKD have a low risk of contracting COVID-19 but may experience severe effects if infected. This suggests that while these individuals might not be as susceptible to initial infection, their existing health conditions could make them more vulnerable to experiencing more severe symptoms and complications should they contract COVID-19.

It is important to discuss the underlying reasons, especially the sociocultural and economic aspects, that cause diabetes and support COVID-19 infections. For example, people with diabetes often experience compromised immune function, which can make it more difficult for their bodies to fight off infections, including COVID-19. Hyperglycemia, or high blood sugar levels, can lead to a weakened immune response, affecting the body's ability to control viral replication and the inflammatory response. This impaired immune function may increase the severity and complications of COVID-19 in individuals with diabetes (Guo et al., 2020; Yang et al., 2006). Several behavioral factors related to diabetes management and lifestyle can influence the risk of COVID-19 infection. People with diabetes often need to visit healthcare facilities frequently for check-ups and treatments, which can increase their exposure to the virus. Additionally, individuals with diabetes may face challenges in maintaining a healthy lifestyle during the pandemic. Limited access to nutritious food, reduced opportunities for physical activity, and increased stress levels can all contribute to worsened diabetes control and to an increased risk of COVID-19 complications (Huang et al., 2020a). Likewise, the impact of socioeconomic factors is considerable in determining the vulnerability of individuals with diabetes to contracting COVID-19 and experiencing severe health outcomes. People from lower socioeconomic backgrounds may encounter barriers to healthcare access, including difficulties in accessing regular check-ups, medications, and proper diabetes management. Limited access to healthcare services can result in suboptimal diabetes control and increase the risk of severe COVID-19 outcomes in this population (Huang et al., 2020a; Ssentongo et al., 2021). Individuals living in low-income settings may reside in overcrowded housing conditions, making it challenging to practice physical distancing and maintain proper hygiene, further increasing the risk of viral transmission (Kumar et al., 2020).

Conclusion

Biosocial worlds interact with and mutually influence each other. In this chapter, I have focused on examining the intricate relationships among diabetes, chronic kidney disease (CKD), and COVID-19, along with their interconnectedness with various sociocultural, economic, and political factors in Pakistan. These relationships underscore the heightened vulnerability of individuals with preexisting comorbidities and critical health conditions to severe COVID-19 outcomes, including mortality. Pal and Bhadada (2020) referred to the coexistence of diabetes and COVID-19 as an "unholy situation," accentuating the detrimental synergy between these two health conditions. Notably, CKD can also be included in this "unholy" relationship, exacerbating the severity of these effects. It is worth noting that while proper documentation regarding the morbidity and mortality resulting from these interactions is lacking in Pakistan, an estimated 36.5 million people in the country were at a heightened risk of developing severe COVID-19 infections and related adverse outcomes. Pakistan's susceptibility extends beyond the syndemic involving these three diseases and encompasses a range of sociocultural, economic, and geo-political factors. Furthermore, various communicable and non-communicable diseases, as well as historical and structural factors, contribute to the vulnerability of the population. The intricate interplay among these factors, however, remains complex. To comprehend and effectively address these syndemics, comprehensive efforts are imperative. Such efforts must extend beyond the confines of healthcare and encompass interventions at multiple levels to mitigate the adverse consequences experienced by vulnerable populations.

Practical Suggestions

Both the pandemic and syndemics have served as reminders to a country like Pakistan of the imperative need to devise and implement effective and appropriate policies to address these vulnerabilities, which result in critical biosocial events. The nation urgently requires swift and substantial changes to elevate the level of formal education, enhance healthcare services and their accessibility, reduce the escalating poverty rates, bridge the gender gap, narrow the disparities between rural and urban areas, eliminate malnutrition, curb the country's contributions to the Climate Crisis, and aptly manage the challenges posed by its rapidly growing population. Failure to do so will perpetuate the structural vulnerabilities that allow communicable and noncommunicable diseases to afflict millions of people syndemically.

It is essential to recognize that these factors are intricately interconnected, and thus, they can mutually influence each other. Tackling the high burden of diabetes in Pakistan demands a comprehensive approach that encompasses the enhancement of healthcare infrastructure, the promotion of healthy lifestyle choices, heightened awareness, and the implementation of effective policies to combat the disease. Achieving these objectives is undoubtedly challenging, but a steadfast commitment to such an initiative constitutes the essential first step in the process. History underscores that genuine change often originates at the grassroots level; thus, it is precisely there that we must seek the initial stirrings of a movement for change.

References

Akhtar, Hashaam, Khalid, Sundas, Rahman, Fazal Ur, Umar, Muhammad, Ali, Sabahat, Afridi, Maham, ... Khan, Muhammad Mujeeb. (2021). Presenting characteristics, comorbidities, and outcomes among patients with COVID-19 hospitalized in Pakistan: Retrospective observational study. *JMIR Public Health and Surveillance,* 7(12), e32203.

Ali, Inayat. (2020a). *Constructing and negotiating measles: The case of Sindh Province of Pakistan.* Vienna: University of Vienna.

Ali, Inayat. (2020b). Impacts of rumors and conspiracy theories surrounding COVID-19 on preparedness programs. *Disaster Medicine and Public Health Preparedness,* 1–6. doi:10.1017/dmp.2020.149.

Ali, Inayat. (2021). Rituals of containment: Many pandemics, body politics, and social dramas during COVID-19 in Pakistan. *Frontiers in Sociology,* 6, 648149.

Ali, Inayat. (2023a). *Contesting measles and vaccination in Pakistan: Cultural beliefs, structured vulnerabilities, mistrust, and geo-politics.* London: Routledge.

Ali, Inayat. (2023b). Culture of vaccine acceptability or resistance: The curious case of Chile's COVID-19 vaccine rollout and anthropology's role in increasing vaccination uptake. *Vaccine: X, 13,* 100272.

Ali, Inayat, & Ali, Shahbaz. (2020). Why may COVID-19 overwhelm low-income countries like Pakistan? *Disaster Medicine and Public Health Preparedness.* doi:10.1017/dmp.2020.149.

Ali, Inayat, & Hamid, Saima. (2022). Implications of COVID-19 and "super floods" for routine vaccination in Pakistan: The reemergence of vaccine preventable-diseases such as polio and measles. *Human Vaccines & Immunotherapeutics, 18*(7), 2154099.

Ali, Inayat, Saddique, Salma, & Ali, Shahbaz. (2021). Local perceptions of COVID-19 in Pakistan's Sindh Province: "Political game", supernatural test, or Western conspiracy? *Disaster Medicine and Public Health Preparedness,* 16(6), 2577–2582.

Ali, Inayat, Sadique, Salma, & Ali, Shahbaz. (2021). COVID-19 and vaccination campaigns as "Western plots" in Pakistan: Government policies, (geo-) politics, local perceptions, and beliefs. *Frontiers in Sociology,* 6, 82. doi:10.3389/fsoc.2021.608979.

Asghar, Muhammad Sohaib, Haider Kazmi, Syed Jawad, Ahmed Khan, Noman, Akram, Mohammed, Ahmed Khan, Salman, Rasheed, Uzma, … Memon, Gul Muhammad. (2020). Clinical profiles, characteristics, and outcomes of the first 100 admitted COVID-19 patients in Pakistan: A single-center retrospective study in a Tertiary Care Hospital of Karachi. *Cureus, 12*(6), e8712. doi:10.7759/cureus.8712.

Atkins, Janice L., Masoli, Jane A. H., Delgado, Joao, Pilling, Luke C., Kuo, Chia-Ling, Kuchel, George A., & Melzer, David. (2020). Preexisting comorbidities predicting COVID-19 and mortality in the UK Biobank community cohort. *The Journals of Gerontology: Series A, 75*(11), 2224–2230. doi:10.1093/gerona/glaa183.

Azeem, Saleha, Khan, Ubaid, & Liaquat, Ayesha. (2022). The increasing rate of diabetes in Pakistan: A silent killer. *Annals of Medicine and Surgery, 79*, 103901.

Barron, Emma, Bakhai, Chirag, Kar, Partha, Weaver, Andy, Bradley, Dominique, Ismail, Hassan, … Sattar, Naveed. (2020). Associations of type 1 and type 2 diabetes with COVID-19-related mortality in England: A whole-population study. *The Lancet Diabetes & Endocrinology, 8*(10), 813–822.

Basit, Abdul. (2020). The diabetic foot worldwide. In Andrew J. M. Boulton, Gerry Rayman, & Dane K. Wukich (Eds.), *The foot in diabetes* (pp. 47–49). New Delhi: John Wiley & Sons.

Basit, Abdul, Fawwad, Asher, & Baqa, Kulsoom. (2019). Pakistan and diabetes—A country on the edge. *Diabetes Research and Clinical Practice, 147*, 166–168.

Bulled, Nicola, & Singer, Merrill. (2020). In the shadow of HIV & TB: A commentary on the COVID epidemic in South Africa. *Global Public Health, 15*(8), 1231–1243. doi:10.1080/17441692.2020.1775275.

Chen, Nanshan, Zhou, Min, Dong, Xuan, Qu, Jieming, Gong, Fengyun, Han, Yang, … Zhang, Li. (2020a). Epidemiological and clinical characteristics of 99 cases of 2019 novel coronavirus pneumonia in Wuhan, China: A descriptive study. *The Lancet, 395*(10223), 507–513. doi:10.1016/S0140–6736(20)30211-7.

Chen, Tao, Wu, Di, Chen, Huilong, Yan, Weiming, Yang, Danlei, Chen, Guang, … Wang, Hongwu. (2020b). Clinical characteristics of 113 deceased patients with coronavirus disease 2019: Retrospective study. *Bmj, 368*, 1–12.

Cheng, Yichun, Luo, Ran, Wang, Kun, Zhang, Meng, Wang, Zhixiang, Dong, Lei, … Xu, Gang. (2020). Kidney disease is associated with in-hospital death of patients with COVID-19. *Kidney International, 97*(5), 829–838. doi:10.1016/j.kint.2020.03.005.

Dawn. (2020, 12 March). World Kidney Day. Editorial *Dawn*. Retrieved from https://www.dawn.com/news/1540263/world-kidney-day.

Dorjee, Kunchok, Kim, Hyunju, Bonomo, Elizabeth, & Dolma, Rinchen. (2020). Prevalence and predictors of death and severe disease in patients hospitalized due to COVID-19: A comprehensive systematic review and meta-analysis of 77 studies and 38,000 patients. *PloS one, 15*(12), e0243191.

Duan, Jia-Yu, Duan, Guang-Cai, Wang, Chong-Jian, Liu, Dong-Wei, Qiao, Ying-Jin, Pan, Shao-Kang, … Liang, Lu-Lu. (2020). Prevalence and risk factors of chronic kidney disease and diabetic kidney disease in a central Chinese urban population: a cross-sectional survey. *BMC Nephrology, 21*, 1–13.

Emami, Amir, Javanmardi, Fatemeh, Pirbonyeh, Neda, & Akbari, Ali. (2020). Prevalence of underlying diseases in hospitalized patients with COVID-19: A systematic review and meta-analysis. *Archives of Academic Emergency Medicine, 8*(1), e35.

Guan, Wei-jie, Liang, Wen-hua, Zhao, Yi, Liang, Heng-rui, Chen, Zi-sheng, Li, Yi-min, … He, Jian-xing. (2020). Comorbidity and its impact on 1590 patients with COVID-19 in China: A nationwide analysis. *European Respiratory Journal, 55*(5), 2000547. doi:10.1183/13993003.00547-2020.

Guo, Weina, Li, Mingyue, Dong, Yalan, Zhou, Haifeng, Zhang, Zili, Tian, Chunxia, … Du, Keye. (2020). Diabetes is a risk factor for the progression and prognosis of COVID-19. *Diabetes/Metabolism Research and Reviews, 36*(7), e3319.

Huang, Ian, Lim, Michael Anthonius, & Pranata, Raymond. (2020a). Diabetes mellitus is associated with increased mortality and severity of disease in COVID-19 pneumonia–A systematic review, meta-analysis, and meta-regression. *Diabetes & Metabolic Syndrome: Clinical Research & Reviews, 14*(4), 395–403.

Huang, Ian, Lim, Michael Anthonius, & Pranata, Raymond. (2020b). Diabetes mellitus is associated with increased mortality and severity of disease in COVID-19 pneumonia – A systematic review, meta-analysis, and meta-regression. *Diabetes & Metabolic Syndrome: Clinical Research & Reviews, 14*(4), 395–403. doi:10.1016/j.dsx.2020.04.018.

Hussain, Salman, Baxi, Harveen, Chand Jamali, Mohammad, Nisar, Nazima, & Hussain, Md Sarfaraj. (2020). Burden of diabetes mellitus and its impact on COVID-19 patients: A meta-analysis of real-world evidence. *Diabetes & Metabolic Syndrome: Clinical Research & Reviews, 14*(6), 1595–1602. doi:10.1016/j.dsx.2020.08.014.

Imtiaz, Salman, Alam, Ashar, & Salman, Beena. (2020). The role of the poultry industry on kidney and genitourinary health in Pakistan. *Pakistan Journal of Medical Sciences, 36*(1), S67–S74. doi:10.12669/pjms.36.ICON-Suppl.1718.

Imtiaz, Salman, Salman, Beena, Qureshi, Ruqaya, Drohlia, Murtaza, & Ahmad, Aasim. (2018). A review of the epidemiology of chronic kidney disease in Pakistan: A global and regional perspective. *Saudi Journal of Kidney Diseases and Transplantation, 29*(6), 1441–1451. doi:10.4103/1319-2442.248307.

International Diabetes Federation. (2020). IDF diabetes atlas 9th edition. Retrieved from https://diabetesatlas.org/en/sections/worldwide-toll-of-diabetes.html.

Iqbal, Sehar, Ali, Inayat, Rust, Petra, Kundi, Michael, & Ekmekcioglu, Cem. (2020). Selenium, zinc, and manganese status in pregnant women and its relation to maternal and child complications. *Nutrients, 12*(3), 725.

James, James J. (2020). From COVID-19 to COVID-20: One virus, two diseases. *Disaster Medicine and Public Health Preparedness, 14*(6), e18–e20.

Jessani, Saleem, Bux, Rasool, & Jafar, Tazeen H. (2014). Prevalence, determinants, and management of chronic kidney disease in Karachi, Pakistan - A community based cross-sectional study. *BMC Nephrology, 15*(1), 90. doi:10.1186/1471-2369-15-90.

Jha, Vivekanand. (2013). Current status of end-stage renal disease care in India and Pakistan. *Kidney International Supplements, 3*(2), 157–160. doi:10.1038/kisup.2013.3.

Jha, Vivekanand, Garcia-Garcia, Guillermo, Iseki, Kunitoshi, Li, Zuo, Naicker, Saraladevi, Plattner, Brett, … Yang, Chih-Wei. (2013). Chronic kidney disease: Global dimension and perspectives. *The Lancet, 382*(9888), 260–272. doi:10.1016/S0140-6736(13)60687-X.

Kumar, Ashish, Arora, Anil, Sharma, Praveen, Anikhindi, Shrihari Anil, Bansal, Naresh, Singla, Vikas, … Srivastava, Abhishyant. (2020). Is diabetes mellitus associated with mortality and severity of COVID-19? A meta-analysis. *Diabetes & Metabolic Syndrome: Clinical Research & Reviews, 14*(4), 535–545.

Little, Matthew, Humphries, Sally, Patel, Kirit, & Dewey, Cate. (2017). Decoding the type 2 diabetes epidemic in rural India. *Medical Anthropology, 36*(2), 96–110.

Meyer, Moritz. (2023). *Poverty & equity brief*. Retrieved from https://databankfiles. worldbank.org/public/ddpext_download/poverty/987B9C90-CB9F-4D93-AE8C-750588BF00QA/current/Global_POVEQ_PAK.pdf.

Muniyappa, Ranganath, & Gubbi, Sriram. (2020). COVID-19 pandemic, coronaviruses, and diabetes mellitus. *American Journal of Physiology-Endocrinology and Metabolism, 318*(5), E736–E741. doi:10.1152/ajpendo.00124.2020.

Naghavi, Mohsen, Wang, Haidong, Lozano, Rafael, Davis, Adrian, Liang, Xiaofeng, Zhou, Maigeng, & Vollset, Stein Emil. (2015). Global, regional, and national age-sex specific all-cause and cause-specific mortality for 240 causes of death, 1990–2013: A systematic analysis for the Global Burden of Disease Study 2013. *The Lancet, 385*(9963), 117–171. doi:10.1016/S0140-6736(14)61682-2.

Nandy, Kunal, Salunke, Abhijeet, Pathak, Subodh Kumar, Pandey, Apurva, Doctor, Chinmay, Puj, Ketul, … Warikoo, Vikas. (2020). Coronavirus disease (COVID-19): A systematic review and meta-analysis to evaluate the impact of various comorbidities on serious events. *Diabetes & Metabolic Syndrome, 14*(5), 1017–1025. doi:10.1016/j.dsx.2020.06.064.

Nasir, Nosheen, Farooqi, Joveria, Mahmood, Syed Faisal, & Jabeen, Kauser. (2020). COVID-19-associated pulmonary aspergillosis (CAPA) in patients admitted with severe COVID-19 pneumonia: An observational study from Pakistan. *Mycoses, 63*(8), 766–770.

National Institute of Health. (2023). Tuberculosis (TB) Control Program. Retrieved from https://www.nih.org.pk/national-tb-control-program#:~:text=Pakistan%20ranks%205th%20amongst%20the,348%2C%20276%20and%2034%20respectively.

National Institute of Population Studies (NIPS) and ICF. (2019). *Pakistan demographic and health survey 2017–18*. Islamabad, Pakistan: National Institute of Population Studies (NIPS), and Rockville, MD, USA.

Onder, Graziano, Rezza, Giovanni, & Brusaferro, Silvio. (2020). Case-fatality rate and characteristics of patients dying in relation to COVID-19 in Italy. *JAMA, 323*(18), 1775–1776. doi:10.1001/jama.2020.4683.

Pal, Rimesh, & Bhadada, Sanjay K. (2020). COVID-19 and diabetes mellitus: An unholy interaction of two pandemics. *Diabetes & Metabolic Syndrome: Clinical Research & Reviews. 14*(4), 513–517.

Richardson, Safiya, Hirsch, Jamie S., Narasimhan, Mangala, Crawford, James M., McGinn, Thomas, Davidson, Karina W., & Consortium, and the Northwell COVID-19 Research. (2020). Presenting characteristics, comorbidities, and outcomes among 5700 patients hospitalized with COVID-19 in the New York City area. *JAMA, 323*(20), 2052–2059. doi:10.1001/jama.2020.6775.

Saeedi, Pouya, Petersohn, Inga, Salpea, Paraskevi, Malanda, Belma, Karuranga, Suvi, Unwin, Nigel, … Ogurtsova, Katherine. (2019). Global and regional diabetes prevalence estimates for 2019 and projections for 2030 and 2045: Results from the International Diabetes Federation Diabetes Atlas. *Diabetes Research and Clinical Practice, 157*, 107843.

Singer, Merill, & Clair, Scott. (2003). Syndemics and public health: Reconceptualizing disease in bio-social context. *Medical Anthropology Quarterly, 17*(4), 423–441.

Singer, Merrill (2020). Deadly companions: COVID-19 and diabetes in Mexico. *Medical Anthropology*, 1–6. doi:10.1080/01459740.2020.1805742.

Singh, Awadhesh K., Gillies, Clare L., Singh, Ritu, Singh, Akriti, Chudasama, Yogini, Coles, Briana, … Khunti, Kamlesh. (2020). Prevalence of co-morbidities and their association with mortality in patients with COVID-19: A systematic review and meta-analysis. *Diabetes, Obesity and Metabolism, 22*(10), 1915–1924.

Ssentongo, Paddy, Heilbrunn, Emily S., Ssentongo, Anna E., Advani, Shailesh, Chinchilli, Vernon M., Nunez, Jonathan J., & Du, Ping. (2021). Epidemiology and outcomes of COVID-19 in HIV-infected individuals: A systematic review and meta-analysis. *Scientific Reports, 11*(1), 6283.

Ssentongo, Paddy, Ssentongo, Anna E., Heilbrunn, Emily S., Ba, Djibril M., & Chinchilli, Vernon M. (2020). Association of cardiovascular disease and 10 other pre-existing comorbidities with COVID-19 mortality: A systematic review and meta-analysis. *PloS one, 15*(8), e0238215.

Stanifer, John W., Muiru, Anthony, Jafar, Tazeen H., & Patel, Uptal D. (2016). Chronic kidney disease in low- and middle-income countries. *Nephrology Dialysis Transplantation, 31*(6), 868–874. doi:10.1093/ndt/gfv466.

Team, Victoria, & Manderson, Lenore. (2020). How COVID-19 reveals structures of vulnerability. *Medical Anthropology*, 1–4. doi:10.1080/01459740.2020.1830281.

Toori, Kaleem Ullah, Qureshi, Muhammad Arsalan, & Chaudhry, Asma. (2022). Pre-morbidity and COVID-19 disease outcomes in Pakistani population: A cross-sectional study. *Pakistan Journal of Medical Sciences, 38*(1), 287.

Transparacny International. (2022). Corruption perceptions index. Retrieved from https://www.transparency.org/en/countries/pakistan.

Webster, Angela C., Nagler, Evi V., Morton, Rachael L., & Masson, Philip. (2017). Chronic kidney disease. *The Lancet, 389*(10075), 1238–1252.

World Health Organization. (2023). Pakistan: WHO coronavirus disease (COVID19) dashboard. Retrieved from https://covid19.who.int/region/emro/country/pk.

Yang, J. K., Feng, Y., Yuan, M. Y., Yuan, S. Y., Fu, H. J., Wu, B. Y., … Wang, L. (2006). Plasma glucose levels and diabetes are independent predictors for mortality and morbidity in patients with SARS. *Diabetic Medicine, 23*(6), 623–628.

Yin, Tingxuan, Li, Yuanjun, Ying, Ying, & Luo, Zhijun. (2021). Prevalence of comorbidity in Chinese patients with COVID-19: Systematic review and meta-analysis of risk factors. *BMC Infectious Diseases, 21*(1), 200. doi:10.1186/s12879-021-05915-0.

Zaidi, S Akbar. (1985). The urban bias in health facilities in Pakistan. *Social Science & Medicine, 20*(5), 473–482.

Zaidi, S Akbar. (1988). *The political economy of healthcare in Pakistan*: Lahore: Vanguard Books.

Zeb, Shazia, Shahid, Rizwana, Umar, Muhammad, Aziz, Qaiser, Akram, Muhammad Omar, Khurram, Muhammad, & Khan, Muhammad Mujeeb. (2020). Analysis of COVID-19 mortality in allied hospitals of Rawalpindi Medical University Pakistan. *Biomedica, 36*, 260–264.

Zhu, Na, Zhang, Dingyu, Wang, Wenling, Li, Xingwang, Yang, Bo, Song, Jingdong, … Tan, Wenjie. (2020). A novel coronavirus from patients with pneumonia in China, 2019. *New England Journal of Medicine, 382*(8), 727–733. doi:10.1056/NEJMoa2001017.

3 Deadly Companions

The Diabetes/COVID-19 (DiaCOVID-19) Syndemic in Mexico and the U.S. Mexican Diaspora

Merrill Singer and Jennifer A. Cook

"We heard they weren't accepting any more patients in the hospital near where we live, so we decided to bring our brother here" to the 1,200-bed General Hospital in central Mexico City explained Blanca Díaz, age 30 (McDonnell & Sanchez, 2020). She and her two sisters, Maria and Sarai, then joined relatives of other patients waiting for updates. Family visits to coronavirus patients were banned to prevent infection. With hospital staff too busy with a rising number of COVID-19 patients to speak with families, the task frequently fell to guards. The sisters became alarmed when their brother, Julio Cesar Díaz, a 43-year-old with diabetes began having trouble breathing. They traveled from Iztapalapa, one of the economically poorest neighborhoods of the city, noted for its high crime rate, poor access to education, and an unclean water supply, that had become a coronavirus hotspot. Residents there live in crowded quarters, and many were forced by their fragile economic situation to continue working despite the spread of COVID-19. Julio Díaz died the day after he was hospitalized. Doctors told the family that he had succumbed to complications from the coronavirus. Despite firm objections from hospital staff, the Diaz sisters demanded that they be allowed to see their brother's body. The sisters had heard on social media about hospitals misidentifying bodies. In the end, a brother-in-law was allowed to enter the hospital and he sadly confirmed that it was Julio who had died. "My brother went into the hospital, and suddenly he was gone, and we couldn't even see him, embrace him, say farewell...There is now a very profound sadness," Blanca lamented (McDonnell & Sanchez, 2020).

Armando Torres, a 67-year-old father of four from rural Chiapas where he spent most of his life working in coffee production, faced a similar health crisis. In mid-August 2020, Armando woke up feeling nauseous. As the day wore on, he felt feverish and began vomiting. His first thought was that he was suffering from an intestinal infection caused by something he had eaten. One thing was clear to him, his distress did not feel like the usual ill effects of his diabetes. Soon he began coughing and felt exhausted after talking or walking in his house. Then his legs shook as he attempted to stand up from his chair. "I can't remember anything after that, until I woke up later that

DOI: 10.4324/9781003365358-4

night in the hospital... I was in a wheelchair and the doctors were bringing an oxygen concentrator to me. I felt so lost" (Partners in Health, 2020). While family members had been hesitant to take Armando to the hospital – because of rumors that hospitals were killing people – it was at the Compañeros En Salud (Partners in Health, 2020) Respiratory Disease Center in Jaltenango where his symptoms were diagnosed as COVID-19 and treatment began.

Mexicans across the border in the U.S. have faced their own set of COVID-19-related challenges. Overwhelmingly employed in "essential" industries like agriculture, Mexicans found themselves at once overly exposed and largely unprotected by the U.S. public health response to the pandemic. Twin narratives emerged around immigrant workers forced by the imminent threat of poverty to continue working in restaurants, factories, and fields around the country. One focused on the "heroic" nature of immigrant workers' sacrifices, and another focused on the extreme vulnerability these workers faced. "Don't call immigrant farmworkers heroes," argued a piece in the San Francisco Chronicle "call them what they really are – victims" (Sánchez, 2020). Regardless of one's preferred narrative, presence in the richest country in the world did little to protect Mexicans from COVID-19-driven illness and death. Rather, Mexicans in the U.S. have faced some of the highest rates of morbidity and mortality of any demographic subgroup in the U.S.

In this chapter, we examine COVID-19 in Mexico and in the Mexican diaspora using a syndemics framework. Syndemics are defined as significant biosocial health events involving the deleterious interaction of two or more diseases or other health conditions (e.g., malnutrition) that is promoted or facilitated by political economic and unjust social relationships (e.g., inequality, structurally imposed poverty) and/or anthropogenic environmental conditions (Everett & Wieland, 2013; Singer et al., 2017). Syndemics researchers explore how and why two or more diseases cluster together in a population or population subgroup (based on gender, social class, ethnicity, location, etc.), how this clustering leads to adverse disease interactions, how this interaction as well as vulnerability to disease is driven in society, and the pathways of biological and/or biopsychological and social interaction that increase disease burden (Carlson & Mendenhall, 2019). The goal of research and application using this approach is to change the political-economic forces that promote syndemic structural vulnerabilities in oppressed and marginalized populations (Quesada et al., 2011; Team & Manderson, 2020) while improving health care for people already enduring syndemic suffering (Mendenhall, 2012).

Specifically, we assess the adverse syndemic interactions between COVID-19 and diabetes mellitus, a complex biosocial phenomenon we label diaCOVID-19. Mexico now has one of the highest rates of diabetes in the world and faced a burdensome COVID-19 caseload. Mexicans in the U.S. also have endured disproportionate morbidity and mortality during the

COVID-19 pandemic, which began amidst rising diabetes rates in the population. We examine the social structural causes and health consequences of diabetes and the diaCOVID-19 syndemic in Mexico and the U.S. Mexican diaspora, the subpopulations at the highest risk, pathways of disease interaction, and the evolving impact of the syndemic. In bringing together a discussion of the diaCOVID-19 syndemic impacting Mexicans both in Mexico and in the U.S. diaspora, we hope to highlight "the malleable nature of national borders that are meaningless to pathogens, illness, and disease" (Houston et al., 2022, p. 12).

The Coming of the Diabetes Crisis in Mexico

The first health condition of concern here is type-2 diabetes (diabetes mellitus), the most common type of diabetes. Diabetes is a chronic disease involving abnormally high and dangerous levels of sugar (glucose) circulating in the bloodstream. Absence or insufficient production of insulin or an inability of the body to correctly use insulin causes diabetes which can lead to an array of disorders of the body's circulatory, nervous, and immune systems. Insulin is a hormone produced by a cluster of cells within the pancreas known as the islets of Langerhans.

United Nations General Ban Ki-moon once called diabetes a "public health crises in slow motion" (Elwes, 2011), a description that ill fits the pace of diabetes in Mexico. Diabetes was once mainly a problem for wealthy countries but since the turn of the 21st century, prevalence has been rising faster in low- and middle-income countries than in high-income ones. Consequently, today in Mexico, a middle-income country, diabetes is both more widespread and accounts for more of the country's mortality than in a high-income country like its northern neighbor the U.S.

Mexico, in fact, has one of the highest rates of death linked to diabetes (almost 15% of all deaths) in the world (Singer, 2020). Although 7% of people in Mexico had diabetes in 2006, one decade later this had risen to 10.4% (Meza et al., 2015; WHO, 2016). Presently, approximately 14% of adults in the country of 120 million people suffer from the disease (Beaubien, 2017). Based on a longitudinal study, among Mexican aged 45–84 years living in Mexico City, diabetes prevalence increased from 26% in the period from 1998–2004 to 35% by 2015–2019 (Aguilar-Ramirez et al., 2021). This trend is seen as well in Mexico's statistics on diabetes-related mortality. In 1992, diabetes was the fifth most important cause of death in the Mexican population (Phillips & Salmerón, 1992). According to the Pan American Health Organization (2012), diabetes has now become the second leading cause of death in Mexico, only trailing heart disease. Longitudinal research by Alegre-Díaz and colleagues (2016) found that approximately three-quarters of the deaths among Mexicans with diabetes among individuals between the ages of 35 and 74 years were directly or indirectly due to their diabetes. Patients with diabetes had about twice the mortality rate of the general population.

As the authors of this study emphasize, diabetes is "associated with a far worse prognosis than that seen in high-income countries" (Alegre-Díaz et al., 2016). The disease takes almost 87,000 lives every year in Mexico (World Health Organization, 2016) and 20% of the preventable deaths that occur in Mexico are caused by diabetes or related metabolic diseases (Bello-Chavolla et al., 2017). Age-specific mortality rates correlated with the duration of having diabetes, meaning that the lifetime hazard of death due to diabetes is greater for people who developed diabetes in early adult life rather than in later adult life.

Moreover, by 2004, diabetes in Mexico had become the first cause of adult non-obstetrical hospital admissions and hospital mortality (Jiménez-Cruz & Bacardi-Gascon 2004). A cross-sectional analysis of probabilistic household survey findings with an analytic sample of over 40,000 Mexican households found that 24% had at least one member who had been diagnosed with diabetes, hypertension, or both. Healthcare expenditures in these households were 25–34% higher than in those in which these health conditions were not present (Gutierrez et al., 2018). Diabetes has become a significant national healthcare burden in Mexico. Annual average costs per diabetes patient in Mexico have been estimated to range from 700 to 3,200 USD (Rodriguez et al., 2010). In 2013, diabetes costs in Mexico were over 700 million USD for outpatient treatment, over 200 million USD for inpatient care, and over 175 million USD for indirect costs (Barquera et al., 2013). Reports Jason Beaubin (2017), "Diabetes poses an increasing challenge for the nation's hospitals and clinics. The dramatic surge in diabetes threatens the very stability of Mexico's public health care system."

Distribution of Diabetes, Overweight, and Obesity

Diabetes rates in Mexico vary across regions, age groups, social classes, and ethnicities, producing intersecting patterns and experiences with the disease (e.g., poor, rural, and indigenous identity). Describing income inequality in Mexico, Moreno-Altamirano and colleagues (2015, p. 335) report that "In 2010, more than 56% of the income was concentrated in 20% of the richest households, whereas 20% of the poorest households concentrated barely 4.9% of the income." Additionally, the country is geographically diverse and cultural identities and consumption patterns vary greatly across the landscape. Mexico is home to the largest indigenous population in Latin America, estimated in 2000 to comprise over 12% of the population (Bush, 2005). Mexico's indigenous population is quite diverse, consisting of people speaking 60 different languages. Further, as Batalla (1996) notes, despite a dominant cultural ideology of racial democracy and mestizaje, racial mixture is unequal across class and ethnic social strata, a fact that underlies the continuation of inequality in Mexico. As Sue (2013, p. 6) described in her ethnography, "A remnant from Mexico's colonial past, Mexico is a pigmentocracy in which light-skinned individuals with European features dominate the top positions of society and dark-skinned individuals of indigenous or African descent are over-represented at the bottom rungs of society." Colonialism in Mexico began a legacy of "subjugating some groups and elevating others along lines of ethnicity and class. The most deeply affected were the indigenous populations, which is apparent from their present social, health, and financial problems" (Montesi, 2018, p. 4). Juárez-Ramírez and colleagues (2014) report that 79% of indigenous language speakers in Mexico live in poverty or extreme poverty, and more than 80% have no social health insurance.

These patterns of socio-economic and ethno-racial inequality shape the distribution of diabetes across Mexico's population. Rates of diabetes are generally higher in urban areas (CCD Factsheet, 2017; ENSANUT-MC, 2016; Jimenez-Corona et al., 2019; Soto-Estrada et al., 2018). The capital, Mexico City, has an estimated 2.3 million people suffering from diabetes (CCD Factsheet, 2017). However, diabetes rates are climbing at much higher rates in some of Mexico's least developed regions. In the southern states of Campeche, Chiapas, Guerrero, Oaxaca, Puebla, Tlaxcala, Quintana Roo, Tabasco, Veracruz, and Yucatán, the death rate from diabetes rose 128% between 1980 and 2000, while in the north there was an increase of 32.5% (ENSANUT-MC, 2016; Soto-Estrada et al., 2018). These results confirm findings from the 2000 National Health Survey and the Mexican Family Life Surveys 2002 and 2005 which indicate an association between lower socioeconomic status and diabetes among Mexican adults aged 20–69 (Nava-Ledezma, 2011). Inequities in healthcare coverage, access, and quality are likely sources of the differences in the distribution and impact of diabetes across Mexican states. Residents of states with the highest rates of diabetes have limited access to medical care. Although 60% of diabetes mortality is concentrated in poorer states, these regions have the lowest concentration of health resources, including clinics, doctors, nurses, and medical equipment (Dávila-Cervantes & Agudelo-Botero, 2019).

While there is limited research on diabetes in Mexico's indigenous populations, the Comitan Study, a population-based examination of diabetes and prediabetes-based blood glucose measures in southeastern Mexico, found that the prevalence of both conditions was significantly lower in indigenous (based on self-report of ethnicity) than in non-indigenous participants (Jimenez-Corona et al., 2019). However, according to Juárez-Ramírez and colleagues (2014), the principal causes of death among elderly indigenous people are chronic conditions such as diabetes and undernourishment. Lower levels of diabetes among indigenous people, especially in rural parts of the country, may be tied to less access to imported energy-dense foods and sedentary employment and pastimes. Simultaneously, cultural values may reinforce the consumption of diets that are higher in complex carbohydrates, fiber, and vegetable proteins and lower in fats than those found in the dominant society (Stoddard et al., 2011).

Alongside troubling diabetes rates, Mexico has one of the highest rates of overweight and obesity in the world (Barquera et al., 2013; Özcan et al.,

2004). Over 70% of the Mexican population is now overweight (Gurría, 2020), compared to 20% in 1996. In addition, 34% of obese in Mexico are morbidly obese, which is the highest level of obesity. According to OECD projections, overweight-related diseases will reduce life expectancy in Mexico by more than four years over the next three decades. At the same time, Gurría reported that child obesity doubled from 7.5% in 1996 to 15% in 2016. The combined prevalence of overweight and obesity is almost 17% in preschool children, 26% in school children, and 31% in adolescents. For adults, the prevalence of overweight and obesity is 40% and 30%, respectively (Barquera et al., 2010).

These findings point to an important cause of the diabetes epidemic in Mexico, a process that has been called the modern "nutritional transition." On the one hand, this entails a significant increase in the consumption of cheap, calorie-filled diets that are high in oils, animal fat, sugar, and processed foods. On the other hand, it involves a drop in calorie-burning activities associated with less active daily life patterns.

Social and Political Economic Drivers

In no small part, Mexico's particular diabetes health burden relates directly to its position in the Global South, especially its physical and asymmetrical political-economic relations with a powerhouse of the Global North, the U.S. The dramatic changes in diet and activity that have contributed to diabetes and overweight-related health crises in Mexico and elsewhere are driven by several interlinked factors, including urbanization, neoliberal governance, and integration into the global food system.

Neoliberal Governance

Implementation of neoliberal policies and resulting economic restructuring have transformed the Mexican state from a provider of public welfare and backer of the social safety net into an ardent promoter of market-based access to needed resources including food and health care. The neoliberal ascension facilitated the movement of foreign investment capital (from wealthier countries) into Mexico and the outflow of profits to multinational corporations.

Amidst the 1979 global financial crisis, Mexico borrowed large amounts of money from U.S. investment banks to avoid bankruptcy driven by the decline in demand for Mexican products and oil. However, the strategy failed, and Mexico was forced to declare bankruptcy in 1983. In response, under pressure from the International Monetary Fund, the U.S. treasury, and the World Bank, the county's elite agreed to a two-part demand for the implementation of structural and fiscal reforms that led to a dramatic redistribution of the nation's wealth between affluent individuals and corporations (rising from 48% to 64%) and working people (dropping from 42% to 29%). This involved a 30–40% decrease in wages and salaries, and a rapid rise in unemployment and job precariousness (Laurell, 1992), a change Harvey (2004) refers to as elite "accumulation by dispossession." One such reform was the 1992 Agrarian Law in Mexico, which created a market for land and fostered the transition to capitalist relations of production in rural Mexico. Small farmers were pushed off the land and became a cheap workforce in expanding cities. Neoliberalization of the agricultural sector and food policy during the presidencies of Salinas de Gortari (1988–1994) and Ernesto Zedillo (1994–2000) further concentrated poverty in rural areas, as employment in the agricultural sector, diminished and commodity prices for farm products declined (Nevin, 2007). Amidst these economic upheavals, migration to the U.S. expanded dramatically.

Another key contributor to this process was the North American Free Trade Agreement (NAFTA) between Canada, the U.S., and Mexico (Laurell, 2015). NAFTA was framed as a plan to decrease poverty in Mexico by increasing the number of middle-class jobs. However, while NAFTA produced some limited economic growth (compared to that seen in Brazil, Chile, and Peru during the same period), it did not yield higher wages or reduce inequality. NAFTA ushered in a huge influx of cheap corn from the U.S., pushing small-scale Mexican farmers, especially corn producers, into direct competition for the Mexican market with heavily subsidized U.S. agriculture (Chatzky et al., 2020). A World Bank study (Salas et al., 2006) estimated over 1 million jobs were lost in corn production between 1991 and 2000, while research led by economist Mark Weisbrot estimated that almost 2 million Mexican farmers were pushed out of a livelihood by NAFTA, many of whom opted to cross the northern border in search of a new source of livelihood.

Increases in foreign direct investment and the expansion of employment in border town manufacturing companies (maquiladoras) precipitated by NAFTA increased internal migration from rural areas of the country (Polaski, 2004). The U.S. manufacturing sector (garments, automobiles, electronics, appliances, heavy equipment, and others) quickly abandoned U.S. production to exploit Mexico's relatively inexpensive labor pool. Mexican workers were not paid enough to afford the cars, televisions, computers, and other goods their labor produced. The deterioration of the rural agricultural sector and eventual decline of Mexico's maquila sector (in favor of even cheaper labor sources elsewhere) also drove dramatic increases in international migration to the U.S. From 1994 to 2000, the estimated annual number of immigrants from Mexico to the U.S. rose by 79% (Weisbrot et al., 2017).

NAFTA provided a windfall for the corporate sector (Public Citizen, 2019), distributing new income upwards, not to the poor and working classes as promised (Cypher, 2011). Mexico's poverty rate of 55.1% was higher in 2014 than in 1994. This means that there were about 20.5 million more Mexicans living below the poverty line compared to 1994 (Weisbrot et al., 2017). As the impacts of NAFTA and similar trade agreements hit home, attitudes among the Mexican working class have generally become very critical. In December 2002, for example, a group of Mexican farmers broke down the door of the lower house of the Mexican Congress to denounce NAFTA.

In subsequent demonstrations that erupted throughout the country, farmers were joined by teachers, utility workers, and others in closing bridges and highways and taking over government offices (Faux, 2003).

Health infrastructure has also deteriorated (Laurell, 2015). Limited spending on the nation's health under neoliberal governance resulted in Mexico having low numbers of medical facilities, most of which are poorly equipped and understaffed. In 2019, for example, the U.S. had 8.8 nurses, 3.5 doctors, and 4.7 hospital beds per 1,000 population, while its Southern neighbor had 2.9 nurses, 2.4 doctors, and 1.4 beds per 1,000 population (Institute for Global Sciences, 2021). An even bigger problem for Mexico is the highly unequal distribution of health resources. Wealthier localities such as Mexico City or the state of Nuevo Leon have three to four times the average number of doctors in poorer locations. This disparity is especially notable regarding the kinds of specially trained doctors needed to respond to COVID-19, such as certified pneumologists or critical care doctors and nurses. Because of cuts in health care, Mexico has had to face its health problems with a fragmented and weakened health system. This decline has continued in recent years and have been characterized by a substantial number of layoffs of health workers and a further drop in Mexico's emergency health response. As a result, by 2020, the health budget per capita accumulated a 26.4% loss in real terms relative to its 2015 maximum, regressing to levels seen a decade before. Cuts have disproportionately affected spending on health for the informal poor who lack social security (Institute for Global Sciences, 2021, p. 144).

The overall social impact of neoliberal austerity policies in Mexico has been destructive, causing falling wages, increased employment uncertainty, and rising inequality in Mexico, especially in rural areas (Eakin, 2005). Health conditions and diseases like diabetes that are associated with chronic stress and unhealthy dietary patterns have become widespread (Laurell, 2015). Furthermore, neoliberal governance and economic restructuring have pushed Mexico to become what Megan Crowley-Matoka (2016) calls a "slippery state." By this term, she means a nation in which citizens see their government institutions as both unreliable and as a needed source of life-sustaining resources like health care. Lacking other avenues, people must depend on what the government offers but lack trust that the government will deliver on its promises. It is under these slippery conditions, with a woefully underfunded public health system, that Mexico was hit by a diaCOVID-19 syndemic.

Urbanization

Another important socio-political factor shaping disease outcomes in Mexico is urbanization. In part due to the ascension of neoliberal economic policy in Mexico, rapid urbanization has occurred in Mexico since the 1960s, and over 75% of Mexicans now live in urban areas. There are 38 cities in the country with populations between 300,000 and 1 million people, and another 16 with populations of more than 1 million. Two of the latter are megacities with more than 5 million residents. Mexico City, the capital, is among the five largest cities in the world. Three of the country's largest cities, Mexico City, Guadalajara, and Monterrey, contain a quarter of Mexico's total population (Kamiya, 2018).

There are several forces at work pushing rural-to-urban migration in Mexico, including climate change (Hunter et al., 2013). Analysis of 2000 and 2010 Mexican census and high-resolution climate data reveals that droughts caused by anthropogenic climate change are promoting rural-urban migration. For instance, an increase in cumulative exposure to drought months is a significant predictor of rural-to-urban migration, with every drought month increasing the odds of migration by 3.6% (Nawrotzki et al., 2017). Most cultivated land in Mexico is rainfed and very susceptible to both short- and long-term changing weather and climate patterns (Conde et al., 2006). Rural Mexicans, who are especially dependent upon farming, are particularly vulnerable to weather stress and climate shocks. Appendini and Liverman (1994) estimate that droughts are the cause of more than 90% of all crop losses in Mexico. Flooding also increases "livelihood insecurity and can lead to elevated migration probabilities from rural areas" in Mexico (Nawrotzki et al., 2015).

Urbanization impacts diet and daily life in Mexico in several ways, including a reduction in physical activity compared to country life. Moreover, urban areas provide physical proximity to supermarkets and the types of highly processed and packaged foods they commonly stock. In 1990, across Latin America, no more than 20% of food purchases were from grocery stores. Ten years later, 50–60% of food was bought in supermarkets (Reardon & Berdegué, 2002).

The Global Food System and Food Marketing

Changes in diet in Mexico are also being shaped by the global food system. In the mid-1970s, Mexico produced most of its own staple foodstuffs. However, since NAFTA, that is no longer the case. Instead "rising agricultural prices [in the global market], combined with growing import dependence, have driven Mexico's food import bill over $20 billion USD per year and increased its agricultural deficit" (Turrent et al., 2012, p. 2). Mexico, now the seventh largest food importer worldwide, imports 45% of the food its residents consume. Much of the food that is imported into Mexico comes from the U.S., although the constituent ingredients are sourced globally by multinational food corporations. Other exporters of food to Mexico include Canada, Spain, the United Kingdom, and China.

Dietary changes are also being promoted through mass media and other advertising (Gálvez, 2018). Despite bans on advertising junk food to children, for example, research in the Mexican cities of Cuernavaca and Guadalajara (Barquera et al., 2018) found that the number of junk food advertisements (e.g., printed posters showing mostly sugar-sweetened beverages, sweet breads, candies, and bottled water) was significantly more common in the areas around public schools than around private schools. Enticing promotions, such as special prices and gifts, were included on 30% of printed posters hung near schools. This difference may contribute to the finding that lower-income populations in Mexico consume a greater proportion of less-healthy beverages than wealthier groups (López-Olmedo et al., 2018).

A study of consumption in Mexico in the years 1961–2013 found an average daily increase from 2,316 to 3,209 calories per person (Soto-Estrada et al., 2018). In this transition in the nutritional landscape, the consumption of cereals and legumes decreased by 12.9% and 3.1%, respectively. By contrast, consumption of sugars, meat, animal fats, and vegetable oils increased substantially (by 3.0%, 7.4%, 1.5%, and 4.0%, respectively). An increase in fat consumption is notable. In the 11-year period between 1988 and 1999, the percentage of total energy from fat went from 23.5% to 30.3% (Rivera et al., 2004). Additionally, there was an explosion of soft drink consumption in Mexico (Maupomé-Carvantes et al., 1995).

A survey of soft drink consumption among 2,000 people over ten years of age in Mexico City in 1993 found that 82.5% drank soft drinks daily. Although high consumption was frequent in all age groups, it was highest in younger age groups. The mean number of soft drinks ingested per week was 9.3 per week (Maupomé-Carvantes et al., 1995). Reports Agren (2020):

> Mexicans drink more soda per capita than any other country – about 163 liters per year. Bottlers such as Coca-Cola deliver products to the remote corners of the country – where potable water is scant, and soda is often sold for less than water.

In the food retail segment, the food market in Mexico is dominated by major U.S. companies like Costco and Walmart, with a share of over 50% of the market. In 2017, Mexico imported almost 6 billion USD worth of processed foods from the U.S., an increase of 2% from the previous year. The items imported included syrups and sweeteners, fats and oils, soft drinks, and snack foods, all of which have the lowest ranking for a healthy diabetic diet. Major food retailers, in turn, have developed increasingly sophisticated distribution systems for the products and have allocated more shelf space to them. There has also been a rapid growth in Mexico of convenience stores, an outlet sector that sells a high volume of junk foods and snacks.

The multiply determined restructuring of consumption has rendered the Mexican population highly vulnerable during the COVID-19 pandemic, while providing a significant driver of the pandemic in the country. Urbanization, urban poverty and crowding, and poor diet quality all helped to promote the spread of COVID-19. Moreover, Mexico never implemented a full shutdown, and, as many Mexicans live in poverty, they must rely on daily work (and potential daily COVID-19 exposure) to survive.

Chronology of an Epidemic: The Evolving Spread of COVID-19

Like elsewhere, COVID-19 hit Mexico in waves with periods of rising and falling caseloads, hospitalizations, and mortality rates. During periods of decline in new cases, COVID-19 does not go away but continues to infect people, if at a slower pace. Over time, the appearance and spread of viral variants changed and complicated the COVID-19 story, as did the encumbered arrival of vaccines. Over the course of this history, it came to be recognized that diaCOVID-19 was not a unidirectional syndemic (with diabetes worsening COVID-19 infection), but a bidirectional syndemic (in which COVID-19 was also triggering the onset of diabetes). Signaling the arrival of the first wave, the first case of COVID-19 in Mexico, confirmed on February 27, 2020, was a 35-year-old man in Mexico City who had recently traveled to northern Italy (Harrup, 2020). By the end of April, a mere 64 days after this first diagnosis, the number of patients with COVID-19 had jumped to over 19,000 with 1,859 (9.67% of cases) deaths (Suárez et al., 2020). While the initial cases appear to have been imported (i.e., occurring among individuals who had recently traveled outside of the country), cases of local transmission were soon recorded.

Mexico's President Andrés Manuel López Obrador initially downplayed the seriousness of the COVID-19 virus, asserting, "it isn't even equivalent to flu... I repeat, according to the available information, it is not something terrible, fatal" (Associated Press, 2020). Concurrently, López Obrador vowed to mount a swift response to the COVID-19 outbreak. He stressed that there would not be a repeat of what happened when H1B1 influenza (swine flu) broke out in Mexico in 2009 and resulted in almost 400 deaths. Despite such promises, he had already dismantled the pandemic preparedness measures implemented after 2009. Critics accused the Mexican government at the time of being too slow in reacting to the outbreak. By late May 2020, Mexico was burdened with a surging COVID-19 epidemic. One sign of the impact of the disease is that Mexico City issued over 8,000 more death certificates than usual in the period between January 1 and May 20, 2020. On June 2, 2020, there were 1,002 deaths from COVID-19, Mexico's highest daily tally of COVID-19 deaths, a number greater than the U.S. COVID-19 fatalities that day (Sheridan, 2020). At the peak of the first wave, in early July 2020, Mexico became the country with the third highest number of fatalities globally, behind the U.S. and Brazil (46,688) and sixth place in the total number of confirmed cases (424,637) (Marca, 2020). In mid-August 2020, José Luis Alomía, director of Epidemiology of the Secretariat of Health, announced that for the third week in a row, the total number of new cases in a week was in decline and, for the first time, the number of recovered cases in a week was greater than the number of newly confirmed cases, marking the end of the first wave (Infobae, 2020). The decline in cases reflected the implementation of masking, social distancing, and lockdowns at the state and local levels. During the first wave, the federal government, President López Obrador, as well as the Ministry of Health, were criticized for poorly communicated and inconsistent messaging and a lack of clear prevention guidelines (e.g., Ibarra-Nava et al., 2020).

Optimism that the pandemic was ending evaporated as cases and fatalities began to rise again in November 2020. Mexico passed 1 million confirmed cases by mid-month along with over 100,000 COVID-19 deaths, the fourth country to reach this grim milestone (Choi, 2020; NBC News, 2020). A record 10,000 new cases reported on a single day were recorded a week later. On January 5, Mexico passed 150,000 total deaths due to COVID-19 (Infobae, 2021). The signs of the arrival of a second wave of COVID-19 were by now undeniable. Soon hospitals in Mexico City and some states were again overwhelmed with COVID-19 patients.

On December 11, 2020, Hugo López-Gatell, the deputy secretary of Prevention and Health Promotion, reported that the average age of death due to COVID-19 in Mexico was 55, compared to 75 in Europe. The difference, he explained, was the high rates of obesity and diabetes in Mexico (ABC News, 2020). The first doses of the Pfizer vaccine arrived in Mexico City in early January, destined for frontline health workers, a group that had been especially hard hit by viral infection because of poor working conditions. Despite initial vaccinations, Mexico's mortality rate of 59 deaths per million people became the highest in Latin America in February 2021, surpassing Panama and Peru. However, by late January, rates of new cases began to decline once more marking the beginning of the end of the second wave.

Having reached a low point in May 2021, COVID-19 cases began to rise yet again in July. The Mexican Health Ministry reported 940 new COVID-19 deaths bringing the total of viral fatalities to well over 250,000. Daily deaths rose above 900 for the first time in over five months, signaling the beginning of a third wave of infection. Almost all the COVID-19 deaths (95%) in 2021 were among the unvaccinated, including among younger people who were not yet eligible for vaccines. By mid-August, Mexico had vaccinated 61% of adults with at least one dose, with a little more than half having received complete vaccination (Orozco, 2021). New COVID-19 cases in Mexico soon approached the highest levels seen during the second wave.

Before long, there were close to 22,000 cases daily, mostly in younger people and other unvaccinated people. Three variants of the virus – alpha, gamma, and delta – were spreading across the country (Valle & Knaul, 2021). In the assessment of Valle and Knaul (2021):

the Mexican government response... has not followed a robust, evidence-based public health approach to its pandemic management. Lockdowns were late and partial. Testing, contact tracing, quarantines and isolation programs – essential elements in managing outbreaks to avoid resorting to painful and costly national shutdowns – have been minimal.

While some states have implemented renewed public health measures, others have not. Despite its noted failures in responding to COVID-19, by September 2021, there were some signs that the third wave was plateauing and even declining (Sherman, 2021).

Analyses of the distribution of COVID-19 since the beginning of the pandemic find that COVID-19 fatality is higher among indigenous than among non-indigenous populations and that fatality rates are higher among both non-indigenous and indigenous outpatients that are male, older, and suffering from comorbidities (e.g., hypertension, diabetes, obesity) (Argoty-Pantoja et al., 2021).

The U.S. Mexican Diaspora

Mexican immigrants and Mexican Americans in the U.S. face myriad social and political-economic factors, which may intersect with diabetes and COVID-19. Historical patterns of exclusion from legal immigration pathways, labor rights, protections, and healthcare benefits, as well as racist anti-immigrant sentiment and immigrant scapegoating subject Mexicans in the U.S. to intense structural vulnerability (Plascensia, 2009). Mexicans have comparatively higher levels of poverty and lower levels of education than their non-Hispanic white counterparts (Morales et al., 2002). Mexicans in the U.S. are also particularly impacted by precarious immigration status and restrictive immigration enforcement which contribute to poor health outcomes. Undocumented immigrants in the U.S. are more likely to be uninsured, live in poverty, and experience food insecurity. In Texas, for example, nearly a third of undocumented immigrants live below the poverty line, and close to two-thirds are uninsured (Clark et al., 2020).

Mexicans in the U.S. are at elevated risk for several adverse health outcomes which increase the risk of severe illness and death associated with COVID-19, including overweight/obesity, type 2 diabetes, and nonalcoholic fatty liver disease (Castillo et al., 2021). A recent CDC (2020) report indicates that Mexicans have the highest diabetes prevalence compared to other Hispanic groups (14.4%, compared to 11.9% for the white "non-Hispanic" population). Data from the 2018 National Health Interview Survey (NHIS) indicate that 35.5% of the Mexican-origin population had obesity or extreme obesity, and 17% of the Mexican and Mexican American population had been diagnosed with hypertension (Alarcón & Ramirez-Garcia, 2022). Mexicans who have lived longer in the U.S. have higher rates of diabetes – those who have been in the U.S. for more than ten years have the highest rate compared to other subgroups, suggesting that "sociocultural and structural forces such as poverty and discrimination that act with time" (Starosta, 2016, p. 1) are influential in producing this disparity.

Especially in the early days of the pandemic, U.S. Hispanics bore a disproportionate burden of COVID-19 morbidity and mortality (Pinheiro et al., 2021). A study of Florida's Hispanic populations found that Mexicans had the highest age-adjusted mortality rate of any country-of-origin group (170.7), and the youngest mean age at death (63.6 years), including when compared to U.S.-born and foreign-born Blacks. Somewhat surprisingly, the same study found that Mexicans had the fewest mean comorbidities of any group, suggesting that social and political barriers to access to care driven by precarious immigration status likely play a key role in shaping COVID-19 disease outcomes for this population by posing "significant impediments for accessing and utilizing COVID-19 testing and care services" (Pinheiro et al., 2021, p. 7). Immigrant detention may exacerbate diabetes-related health complications, and some 25% of U.S. Immigration and Customs Enforcement (ICE) detainees may suffer from diabetes and/or hypertension (Houston et al., 2022). Immigrants being held in ICE detention centers, of which a significant proportion are Mexican nationals, face food deprivation and provision of spoiled food, lack of access to or inadequate medical care, and stress related to deprivation, family separation, and abuse (Houston et al., 2022). Houston and colleagues (2022, p. 2) argue that the overcrowded and unsanitary conditions in detention centers contribute to "the transmission and deleterious interaction of multiple biological conditions" including COVID-19, tuberculosis, and type 2 diabetes. These patterns have concrete impacts on population demographics; life expectancy for the broader U.S. population declined by one year in 2020; for U.S. Hispanics it declined by two years (Vilar-Compte et al., 2022).

Mexicans are disproportionately represented in lower-skilled, often dangerous, and poorly compensated occupations. During the pandemic, many Mexican immigrants and Mexican Americans were designated as "essential critical infrastructure" workers (CISA, 2021). According to the analysis of 2020 labor force participation data, 70% of undocumented workers, 70% of Mexican immigrant workers, and 58.2% of Mexican American workers, respectively, were employed in positions deemed "essential" (Alarcón & Ramirez-Garcia, 2022, p. 120). These high rates of participation in essential labor amidst the pandemic create a greater risk of COVID-19 infection for Mexican immigrants.

Agricultural workers, for instance, were deemed "essential" workers. The nature of agricultural labor makes it nearly impossible to engage in appropriate physical distancing, and farmworkers often live in cramped housing with shared bathrooms, kitchens, and sleeping areas. Furthermore, farmworkers have historically been excluded from health and labor protections. A significant proportion of farmworkers are undocumented, increasing their vulnerability and decreasing their access to health care (Xiuhtecutli & Annie, 2021). Close to half (45%) of Mexican-born agricultural workers lack any type of health insurance (Alarcón & Ramirez-Garcia, 2022).

Farmworkers face high rates of food insecurity despite their crucial role in ensuring the U.S. food supply (Castillo et al., 2021). As of 2018, 11.45% of farmworkers surveyed in the National Agricultural Workers Survey, of whom a substantial proportion are Mexican-born, had diabetes, a 785%

change from the year 2000, and 13.5% had high blood pressure and/or heart problems (Fan & Pena, 2021). A 2022 study of primarily Mexican farmworkers in Central Florida found that 11% were pre-diabetic, 3% had diabetes, 47% were obese, and an additional 36% were overweight. The study also found that 50% of workers had elevated or high blood pressure. Close to 70% of the participants had at least one major risk factor (obesity, elevated blood pressure, or prediabetes) associated with severe COVID-19 illness and mortality (Chicas et al., 2022). Farmworkers also have an elevated risk of acute kidney injury and chronic kidney disease due to heat stress and strain and dietary constraints (Castillo et al., 2021; Horton, 2016).

One model estimated that farmworkers are about two times more likely to become infected with COVID-19, compared to the overall population of the country (Xiuhtecutli & Annie, 2021). Agricultural workers in Monterey County, California, had COVID-19 positivity rates three times higher than those of workers in other categories (Alarcón & Ramirez-Garcia, 2022). Another study found that food and agricultural workers in California had the third-highest excess mortality rate (75 per 100,000). Excess mortality for Hispanic/Latino workers in food and agriculture was even worse (97 per 100,000). Ninety-five percent of COVID-19 deaths among California's farmworker population were Hispanic/Latino individuals, and immigrants made up 85% of farmworker deaths in the state (Keeney et al., 2022).

Mexican residents of the borderlands are another sub-population of special concern. Diabetes and obesity rates in borderlands are "amongst the highest in the world" (Soto et al., 2022, p. 2). In Texas's Rio Grande Valley, one-quarter of the Latino population is diabetic, and the proportion is probably even higher when considering individuals with undiagnosed diabetes (Blackburn & Sierra, 2021). Immigrants born in Mexico and Mexican Americans are both more likely than white Americans to experience complications or even to die, from undiagnosed or untreated diabetes (Blackburn & Sierra, 2021). The predominantly Hispanic (of Mexican origin) population of the Rio Grande Valley of Texas bore a disproportionate burden of COVID-19 deaths, accounting for 9% of the state's COVID-19 mortality with just 3% of the state's overall population. In the early days of the pandemic, the region had "one of the highest per capita infection rates in the United States" (Blackburn & Sierra, 2021, p. 50) and "case fatality rates... were double or triple the case fatality rates in Texas's largest cities" (Blackburn & Sierra, 2021, p. 54). Anti-immigrant rhetoric and changes to the public charge rule contributed to the uneven distribution of COVID-19 in the Rio Grande Valley, undocumented immigrants and immigrants with legal status embedded in mixed-status families feared the repercussions of accessing healthcare resources (Blackburn & Sierra, 2021). More than half of the region's children have at least one immigrant parent, and half of the children of immigrants have at least one non-citizen parent. The Rio Grande Valley also has some of the highest poverty rates in the U.S., as well as a large uninsured population (Blackburn & Sierra, 2021).

Stress produced by structural vulnerability is also a key factor with likely syndemogenic repercussions. A study by Keeney and colleagues (2022, p. 9) found that around 40% of mostly Mexican-born and Mexican American Hispanic/Latino farmworkers surveyed in Imperial County, California, reported very high stress levels that "pose significant mental health risks." The stressors they reported were primarily related to their status as Latinx im/migrants working as marginalized agricultural workers, including lack of sleep, family separation, work in bad weather, lack of access to medical care, long working hours, inadequate standards of living, and language barriers. Imperial County reported the highest COVID-19 mortality rate in California – more than twice the rate of the next-highest county (Keeney et al., 2022). Fear of deportation has also been linked to increased inflammation (measured via levels of proinflammatory cytokines in the saliva) in members of families with at least one Mexican-origin immigrant family member, across both mixed-status and non-mixed-status families (Martínez et al., 2018). Fear of deportation has been linked to anxiety and depression, indicators of overweight and obesity, and a higher pulse pressure (Castillo et al., 2021), all of which exacerbate diabetes and COVID-19 disease outcomes.

The DiaCOVID-19 Syndemic

The World Health Organization (WHO) (2004) has determined that diabetes onset and development are closely associated with overweight and obesity. This relationship has been called the 'diabesity' epidemic (Golay & Ybarra, 2005). Along with diabetes, obesity constitutes a negative health component in many cases of critical COVID-19 outcomes (Caussy et al., 2020).

Diabetes and sustained high glucose blood levels have been reported as significant predictors of severity and death during several previous pandemics, including the 2009 pandemic influenza (H1N1), and both the severe acute respiratory syndrome (SARS) and Middle East respiratory syndrome (MERS) coronavirus pandemics (Schoen et al., 2019; Yang et al., 2006). The co-presence of diabetes and COVID-19 has been referred to as "an unholy situation wherein one disease entity tends to complement the other" (Pal & Bhadada, 2020) forming a bidirectional syndemic. Because it has many diabetes patients, Mexico has been called "a petri dish for COVID-19" (San Diego Union Tribune, 2020).

Several studies have found that having diabetes is associated with poor COVID-19 prognosis in patients, however, this has not been confirmed in all such research (e.g., Lippi & Plebani, 2020; Zhang et al., 2020). In a study of almost 45,000 COVID-19 cases in China, Wu and McGoogan (2020) reported an overall case-fatality rate (CFR) of 2.3%. CFR was elevated among patients with pre-existing comorbid conditions: 10.5% for patients with cardiovascular disease, 7.3% for diabetes, 6.3% for chronic respiratory disease, 6.0% for hypertension, and 5.6% for cancers. In a Wuhan, China study, Yang and colleagues (2020) found that among the 32 non-survivors from a group of 52 COVID-19 intensive care unit patients, the most distinctive pre-existing non-communicable comorbidities were cerebrovascular diseases (22%) and diabetes (22%). Of the 1,099 confirmed patients with COVID-19 reported by Guan and colleagues (2020), those with severe infection had a higher prevalence of diabetes compared to those without severe infection. Additionally, Bhatraju and colleageus (2020) reported that diabetes was associated with 58% of patients with COVID-19 in a small U.S. study, while diabetes was present in 20.3% of the patients with COVID-19 who died in Italy (Onder et al., 2020). A comparison of intensive care and non-intensive care COVID-19 patients found a twofold increase in the incidence of patients in intensive care having diabetes, while mortality appeared to be about threefold higher in people with diabetes compared with the general mortality of COVID-19 patients (Ruan et al., 2020; Yang et al., 2020). Research in Mexico and South Korea (Jang et al., 2020) confirms that having diabetes has a significant association with complications and lethality attributable to COVID-19 (Bello-Chavolla, 2020). A systematic review of the literature concludes that "diabetes should be considered as a risk factor not only for increased susceptibility to infection but also for a rapid progression and bad prognosis of COVID-19" (Corrao et al., 2021).

The adverse relationship between diabetes and COVID-19 is complex but several intertwined pathways of interaction have been suggested. One possibility is that SARS-CoV-2 sets off higher stress levels in the body, causing both a greater release of hyperglycemic hormones (e.g., glucocorticoids and catecholamines) and increased blood glucose levels (Wang et al., 2020). Approximately, one in 10 people afflicted with both diabetes and COVID-19 have been found to suffer at least one episode of hypoglycemia (Zhou & Tan, 2020). There is a well-established link between diabetes and atherosclerotic cardiovascular disease (Haffner et al., 1998) and hypoglycemia is recognized as both activating pro-inflammatory white blood cells and increasing platelet reactivity, factors that contribute to heart-related mortality in patients with diabetes (Iqbal et al., 2019). This suggests that people with both diabetes and COVID-19 "are more susceptible to an inflammatory cytokine storm eventually leading to ARDS [Acute respiratory distress syndrome], shock, and rapid deterioration of COVID-19" (Pal & Bhadada, 2020). Also, diabetes is linked to reduced expression of angiotensin-converting enzyme 2 (ACE2). This enzyme is a critical component of the biochemical pathway that regulates blood pressure and wound healing. Additionally, in the lungs, this enzyme plays potent anti-inflammatory and anti-oxidant roles and ACE2 is known to be protective against lethal avian influenza A H5N1 infection (Zou et al., 2014). Lowered ACE2 expression in diabetes might help explain the increased incidence of serious lung injury and ARDS with COVID-19 (Batah & Fabro, 2021; Tikellis & Thomas, 2012). Also of note, COVID-19 binds with and enters cells through ACE2 receptors on the surfaces of target cells. Once entry is achieved, viral RNA replication begins. The host cell responds by releasing an enzyme that eliminates all the remaining ACE2 receptors on its surface, thereby blocking the production of molecules required for maintaining the functioning of the lungs, heart, and other vital organs.

A number of comorbidities associated with the worst COVID-19 outcomes, including diabetes, chronic lung diseases, cardiovascular diseases, and obesity, are characterized by systemic hyperinflammation. The body's anti-inflammatory process may constitute the key mechanism that puts people suffering with diabetes at risk, but also those experiencing periods of hyperglycemia and obesity are at heightened risk for infection. While inflammation is a component of the immune system and helps fight acute infection, chronic inflammation hyperinflammation can weaken innate and adaptive immunity, enabling accelerated viral uptake and reduced pathogen clearance capacity (Azar et al., 2020). A systematic review and meta-analysis of the research on the association between diabetes and infections (Abu-Ashour et al., 2017) showed that diabetes is associated with a heightened occurrence of infection, especially of the skin, respiratory system, and blood. Additionally, patients with diabetes tend to be hospitalized for the treatment of infections more frequently than those without diabetes (Shah & Hux, 2003). Some of the studies that were reviewed by Abu-Ashour and colleageus (2017) also suggest that people with diabetes are at an increased risk of infection-related mortality (Bertoni et al., 2001; Rao Kondapally Seshasai et al., 2011). The specific relationship between infection and the "pathophysiology of lung abnormalities in patients who have diabetes is believed to involve microangiopathic changes in the basement membrane of pulmonary blood vessels and respiratory epithelium, as well as non-enzymatic glycosylation of tissue protein" (Abu-Ashour et al., 2017, p. 9). Poorly controlled diabetes has been linked to impaired functioning of important immune system components, including macrophages and neutrophils (Knapp, 2013). In the case of influenza virus infection and replication, for example, laboratory studies have shown that when the epithelial cells that line the lungs are exposed to high glucose concentrations pathogen growth quickens, suggesting that hyperglycemia enhances viral replication (Kohio & Adamson, 2013). It is also known that elevated blood glucose can increase glucose concentrations in airway secretions, and, in the case of influenza, expose lung cells to elevated glucose, significantly increasing viral infection (Hill et al., 2020). A comparison study of patients with diabetes and healthy volunteers found that there was a significant negative correlation between fasting glucose level and the ability of immune cells to perform phagocytosis, the immune system process by which a cell uses its plasma membrane to engulf and remove pathogens and cell debris (Lecube et al., 2011). Furthermore, high blood glucose levels may prevent a normal respiratory burst, the process by which immune cells kill invasive pathogens by releasing toxic oxidative chemicals (Jafar et al., 2016).

In the blood of people with diabetes and COVID-19, important immune T cells like CD4+ and CD8+ that coordinate the immune response are decreased in concentration. SARS-CoV-2 may infect circulating immune cells and cause increased cell death leading to low lymphocyte levels, a condition associated with greater COVID-19 severity (Muniyappa & Gubbi, 2020). The death of CD4+ and CD8+ T cells causes a powerful release of inflammatory cytokines. Through these changes, COVID-19 triggers an inept and aggressive immune response in people with diabetes that causes intense damage to organs. More-over, suggests Means (2020), it is "possible that pancreatic damage from the virus and resultant impairment in beta-cell insulin secretion could worsen pre-existing diabetes or even predispose to new cases of diabetes in non-diabetic subjects." Conversely, enzymes that break down proteins are gener-ally elevated in people with diabetes, and this may facilitate SARS-CoV-2 entry into human cells, hastening the production of new viruses (Muniyappa & Gubbi, 2020). While there is much to be learned about the complex ways that COVID-19 exacerbates or even causes diabetes, as well as the ways dia-betes magnifies body damage from COVID-19, there is a growing body of studies that affirm the existence of a dangerous diaCOVID-19 syndemic that unfolds across multiple pathways of interaction, including research described in this volume (see Chapters 1, 2, 7, and 9).

While diabetes has been found to have deleterious interactions with COVID-19 in studies from multiple countries, including other countries of the Global South (Ali, 2021, Barone et al., 2020), the specific contours of the diaCOVID-19 syndemic in Mexico and in the U.S. Mexican diaspora affirm that there are no global syndemics (Singer et al., 2022). Even in our highly interconnected world in which infectious agents, commodities, and people cross borders incessantly, local biosocial factors shape differing local disease and death profiles even when infectious diseases achieve global diffusion.

Conclusion

As Manderson and Wahlberg (2020) point out, "until 2020, global health agendas had been mobilizing around what the WHO and other public health institutions called the 'global chronic disease pandemic,'" which includes diseases like diabetes. Then COVID-19 arrived, and these institutions neces-sarily shifted their focus toward the immediate spread of a lethal infectious disease and its impact on health care. But, as COVID-19 and other recent infectious disease pandemics have demonstrated, the most severe impact of these lethal health events is the syndemic interaction of infectious diseases and chronic health conditions. In Mexico, diabetes, which is particularly com-mon, is a significant pre-existing condition shaping the impact of COVID-19. This interaction reflects what Martínez and Leal (2003) describe as Mexico's "double burden" of disease involving both high rates of infectious diseases and high rates of chronic diseases. Structural factors enabling this dangerous interaction lie in the country's history of global governance and economic restructuring ushered in by Mexico's dominant social class and international lenders, the intrusion of foreign capital, and the environmental effects of anthropogenic climate change. These factors have reshaped Mexican diets, work and living patterns, healthcare institutions, and health. In the U.S. context, Mexicans face a decades-long history of xenophobic immigration policy, exclusion from access to adequate medical care through the U.S. privatized healthcare system, limited access to the social determinants of good health like adequate nutrition due to food insecurity, and heightened exposure to the deadly COVID-19 virus as designated "essential" workers.

It is for these reasons that Amy Moran-Thomas (2019) calls diabetes a "para-communicable" condition. It is materially transmitted as bodies, political economies, and ecologies intimately shape each other over time. Effectively addressing the diaCOVID-19 syndemic, and the likely occurrence of future devastating infectious/chronic disease syndemics, necessitates overcoming these deep structural problems. This requires prioritizing public health and the welfare of the masses over private profit for the few. Mexican economist Gerardo Esquivel Hernandez (2015, p. 37) maintains there is a need for the establishment of social state structures that implement a "shift to a rights-based approach to social policy" that includes the right to an adequate and healthy diet, housing, employment, education, and health care. Achieving this goal will not be easy because of the resistance of the rich who benefit most from existing structures of inequality. As activist/scholar Laurence Cox (2018, p. 173), author of *Why Social Movements Matter*, has said, in a time of neoliberal decline "What gives … hope …is a consistent focus on struggles from below and what they have achieved," as well as what they can achieve in the future.

References

ABC News. (2020). Mexico's COVID-19 deaths average 55 years vs. 75 in Europe. https://abcnews.go.com/International/wireStory/mexicos-covid-19-deaths-average-5-years-75-74664370.

Abu-Ashour, W., Twells, L., Valcour, J., Randell, A., Donnan, J.H., Howse, P., & Gamble, J.M. (2017). The association between diabetes mellitus and incident infections: a systematic review and meta-analysis of observational studies. *BMJ Open Diabetes Research and Care*, 5, e000336. https://doi.org/10.1136/bmjdrc-2016-000336.

Agren, D. (2020). Soda or 'bottled poison'? Mexico finds a COVID-19 villain in sugary drinks. *USA Today*. https://www.usatoday.com/story/news/world/2020/08/23/coca-cola-bottled-poison-mexico-finds-covid-19-villain-soda/5607741002/.

Aguilar-Ramirez, D., Alegre-Díaz, J., Gnatiuc, L., Ramirez-Reyes, R., Wade, R., Hill, M., Collins, R., Peto, R., Emberson, J., Herrington, W., Kuri-Morales, P., & Tapia-Conyer, R. (2021). Changes in the diagnosis and management of diabetes in Mexico City between 1998–2004 and 2015–2019. *Diabetes Care*, 44(4), 944–951.

Alarcón, R., & Ramírez-García, T. (2022). Esenciales pero vulnerables. *Mexican Studies/Estudios Mexicanos*, 38(1), 114–139.

Alegre-Díaz, J., Herrington, W., López-Cervantes, M., Gnatiuc, L., Ramirez, R., Alegre-Díaz, J., Herrington, W., López-Cervantes, M., Gnatiuc, L., Ramirez, R.,

Hill, M., Baigent, C., McCarthy, M., Lewington, S., Collins, R., Whitlock, G., Tapia-Conyer, R., Peto, R., Kuri-Morales, P., Emberson, J. (2016). Diabetes and cause-specific mortality in Mexico City. *New England Journal of Medicine*. https://doi.org/10.1056/NEJMoa1605368.

Ali, I. (2021). Syndemics at play: chronic kidney disease, diabetes and COVID-19 in Pakistan. *Annals of Medicine*, 3(1), 581–586.

Appendini, K., & Liverman, D. (1994). Agricultural policy, climate change, and food security in Mexico. *Food Policy*, 19(2), 149–164.

Argoty-Pantoja, A., Robles-Rivera, K., Rivera-Paredez, B., & Salmeron, J. (2021). COVID-19 fatality in Mexico's indigenous populations. *Public Health*, 193, 69–75.

Associated Press. (2020). Mexico confirms first 2 cases of coronavirus. https://apnews.com/a7d2aaac19fc3022ba686ba91e7d4395.

Azar, W., Njeim, R., Fares, A., Azar, N., Azar, S., El Sayed, M., & Eid, A. (2020). COVID-19 and diabetes mellitus: how one pandemic worsens the other. *Reviews in Endocrine and Metabolic Disorders*, 21, 451–463.

Barone, M., Harnik, S.B., de Luca, P.V., de Souza Lima, B.L., Wieselberg, R.J.P., Ngongo, B., Pedrosa, H.C., Pimazoni-Netto, A., Franco, D.R., de Souza, M.F.M., Malta, D.C., & Giampaoli, V. (2020). The impact of COVID-19 on people with diabetes in Brazil. *Diabetes Research and Clinical Practice*, 166, 108304. https://doi.org/10.1016/j.diabres.2020.108304.

Barquera, S., Campirano, F., Bonvecchio, A., Hernández-Barrera, L., Rivera, J., Popkin, B. 2010. Caloric beverage consumption patterns in Mexican children. *Nutrition Journal*, 9, 47. https://doi.org/10.1186/1475-2891-9-47.

Barquera, S., Campos-Nonato, I., Aguilar-Salinas, C., Lopez, R., Arredondo, A., & Rivera-Dommarco, J. (2013). Diabetes in Mexico: cost and management of diabetes and its complications and challenges for health policy. *Globalization & Health*, 9(3). https://doi.org/10.1186/1744-8603-9-3.

Barquera, S., Hernández-Barrera, L., Rothenberg, S., & Cifuentes, E. (2018). The obesogenic environment around elementary schools: food and beverage marketing to children in two Mexican cities. *BMC Public Health*, 18, 461. https://doi.org/10.1186/s12889-018-5374-0.

Batah, S., & Fabro, A. (2021). Pulmonary pathology of ARDS in COVID-19: a pathological review for clinicians. *Respiratory Medicine*, 176. https://doi.org/10.1016/j.rmed.2020.106239.

Batalla, B. (1996). *México Profundo: Reclaiming a Civilization*. Austin: University of Texas Press.

Beaubin, J. (2017) Pork tacos topped with fries: Fuel for Mexico's diabetes epidemic. NPR. https://www.npr.org/transcripts/522184483?storyId=522184483

Beaubien, J. (2017). How diabetes got to be the no. 1 killer in Mexico. *Goats and Soda*. National Public Radio. https://www.npr.org/sections/goatsandsoda/2017/04/05/522038318/how-diabetes-got-to-be-the-no-1-killer-in-mexico.

Bello-Chavolla, O.Y., Bahena-López, J.P., Antonio-Villa, N.E., Vargas-Vázquez, A., González-Díaz, A., Márquez-Salinas, A., Fermín-Martínez, C.A., Naveja, J.J., & Aguilar-Salinas, C.A. (2020). Predicting mortality due to SARS-CoV-2: a mechanistic score relating obesity and diabetes to COVID-19 outcomes in Mexico. *Journal of Clinical Endocrinology and Metabolism*, 105(8), dgaa346. https://doi.org/10.1210/clinem/dgaa346.

Bello-Chavolla, O.Y., Rojas-Martinez, R., Aguilar-Salinas, C.A., & Hernández-Avila, M. (2017). Epidemiology of diabetes mellitus in Mexico. *Nutrition Reviews*, 75(suppl 1), 4–12. https://doi.org/10.1093/nutrit/nuw030.

Bertoni, A., Saydah, S., & Brancati, F. (2001). Diabetes and the risk of infection-related mortality in the US. *Diabetes*, 24(6), 1044–1049.

Bhatraju, P., Ghassemieh, B., Nichols, M., Kim R., Jerome, K., & Nalla, A. (2020). Covid-19 in critically ill patients in the Seattle region—case series. *New England Journal of Medicine*, 382(21), 2012–2022. https://doi.org/10.1056/NEJMoa2004500.

Blackburn, C. & Sierra, L. (2021). Anti-immigrant rhetoric, deteriorating health access, and COVID-19 in the Rio Grande Valley, Texas. *Health Security*, 19(1). https://doi.org/10.1089/hs.2021.0005

Bush, P. (2005). *Proyecciones de indígenas de México y de las entidades federativas 2000-2010*. Mexico City: Consejo Nacional de Población.

Carlson, C., & Mendenhall, E. (2019). Preparing for emerging infections means expecting new syndemics. *The Lancet*, 394(10195), 297. https://doi.org/10.1016/S0140-6736(19)31237-1.

Castillo, F., Mora, A.M., Kayser, G.L., Vanos, J., Hyland, C., Yang, A.R., & Eskenazi, B. (2021). Environmental health threats to Latino migrant farmworkers. *Annual Review of Public Health*, 42, 257–276. https://doi.org/10.1146/annurev-publhealth-012420-105014.

Caussy, C., Pattou, F., Wallet, F., Simon, C., Chalopin, S., Telliam, C., Mathieu, D., Subtil, F., Frobert, E., Alligier, M., Delaunay, D., Caussy, C., Pattou, F., Wallet, F., Simon, C., Chalopin, S., Telliam, C., Mathieu, D., Subtil, F., Frobert, E., Alligier, M., Delaunay, D., Vahhems, P., Laville, M., Jourdain, M., Disse, E. (2020). Prevalence of obesity among adult inpatients with COVID-19 in France. *The Lancet: Diabetes & Endocrinology*, 8(7), 562–564. https://doi.org/10.1016/S2213-8587(20)30160-1.

CCD Factsheet. (2017). Cities changing diabetes. Diabetes projection model, Mexico City. https://www.citieschangingdiabetes.com/content/dam/nnsites/ccd/en/network/mexico-city/pdfs/CCD%20factsheet_MEXICO%20CITY_Q12019_Screen.pdf.

CDC. (2020). National diabetes statistics report, 2020, estimates of diabetes and its burden in the United States. Centers for Disease Control, Atlanta, GA. https://www.cdc.gov/diabetes/pdfs/data/statistics/national-diabetes-statistics-report.pdf.

Chatzky, A., McBride, J., & Sergie, M. (2020). NAFTA and the USMCA: weighing the impact of North American trade agreement. Council on Foreign Relations. https://www.cfr.org/backgrounder/naftas-economic-impact#:~:text=NAFTA%20and%20the%20USMCA%3A%20Weighing%20the%20Impact%20of%20North%20American%20Trade,-President%20Trump%20reached&text=It%20contributed%20to%20an%20explosion,to%20job%20losses%20and%20outsourcing.

Chicas, R., Xiuhtecutli, N., Houser, M., Glastra, S., Elon, L., Sands, J.M., McCauley, L., & Hertzberg, V. (2022). COVID-19 and agricultural workers: a descriptive study. *Journal of Immigrant and Minority Health*, 24(1), 58–64. https://doi.org/10.1007/s10903-021-01290-9.

Choi, J. (2020). Mexico surpasses grim milestone: 1 million coronavirus cases. *The Hill*. https://thehill.com/homenews/news/526055-mexico-surpasses-grim-milestone-1-million-coronavirus-cases.

CISA. (2021). Guidance on the essential critical infrastructure workforce. CISA. https://www.cisa.gov/resources-tools/resources/guidance-essential-critical-infrastructure-workforce.

Clark, E., Fredricks, K., Woc-Colburn, L., Bottazzi, M.E., & Weatherhead, J. (2020). Disproportionate impact of the COVID-19 pandemic on immigrant communities in the United States. *PLOS Neglected Tropical Diseases*, 14(7), e0008484. https://doi.org/10.1371/journal.pntd.0008484.

Conde, C., Ferrer, R., & Orozco, S. (2006). Climate change and climate variability impacts on rainfed agricultural activities and possible adaptation measures. A Mexican case study. *Atmosfera*, 19(3), 181–194.

Corrao, S., Pinelli, K., Vacca, M., Raspanti, M., & Argano, C. (2021). Type 2 diabetes mellitus and COVID-19: a narrative review. *Frontiers in Endocrinology*, 12, 609470. https://doi.org/10.3389/fendo.2021.609470.

Cox, L. (2018). Struggles from below in the twilight of neoliberalism. *Counterfutures*, 6, 150–173.

Crowley-Matoka, M. (2016). *Domesticating Organ Transplant: Familial Sacrifice and National Aspiration in Mexico*. Durham: Duke University Press.

Cypher, J. (2011). Mexico since NAFTA. *New Labor Forum*, 20(3), 61–69.

Dávila-Cervantes, C., & Agudelo-Botero, M. (2019). Sex disparities in the epidemic of type 2 diabetes in Mexico: national and state level results based on the Global Burden of Disease Study, 1990–2017. *Diabetes, Metabolic Syndrome and Obesity: Targets and Therapy*, 12, 1023–1033.

Eakin, H. (2005). Institutional change, climate risk, and rural vulnerability: cases from central Mexico. *World Development*, 33(11), 1923–1938.

Elwes, J. 2011. Health emergency in slow motion. Prospect. https://www.prospectmagazine.co.uk/ideas/technology/49594/health-emergency-in-slow-motion

Everett, M., & Wieland, J. (2013). Diabetes among Oaxaca's transitional population: an emerging syndemic. *Annals of Anthropological Practice*, 36(2), 295–311.

Fan, M., & Pena, A.A. (2021). How vulnerable are U.S. crop workers?: evidence from representative worker data and implications for COVID-19. *Journal of Agromedicine*, 26(2), 256–265.

Faux, J. (2003). How NAFTA failed Mexico. *The American Prospect*. https://prospect.org/features/nafta-failed-mexico/.

Gálvez, A. (2018). *Eating NAFTA: Trade, Food Policies, and the Destruction of Mexico*. Berkeley: University of California Press.

Golay, A., & Ybarra, J. (2005). Link between obesity and type 2 diabetes. *Best Practice & Research Clinical Endocrinology & Metabolism*, 19(4), 649–663.

Guan, W.-j., Ni, Z.y., Hu, Y., Liang, H.-h., Ou, C.-q., He, J.-x., Liu, L., Shan, H., Lei, C.-l., Hui, D., Du, B., Li, L.-j., Zeng, G., Yuen, K.-y., Chen, R.-c., Tang, C.-l., Wang, T., Chen, P.-y., Xiang, J., Li, S.-y., Wang, J.-l., Liang, Z.-j., Peng, Y.-x., Wei, L., Liu, Y., Hu, Y.h., Peng, P., Wang, J.-m., Liu, J.-y., Chen, Z., Li, G., Qiu, S.-q., Luo, J., Ye, C.-jD., Zhu, S.-y., Zhong, N.-s. (2020). Clinical characteristics of coronavirus disease 2019 in China. *New England Journal of Medicine*, 382, 1708–1720. https://doi.org/10.1056/NEJMoa2002032

Gurría, A. (2020). Launch of the study: "the heavy burden of obesity: the economics of prevention." OECD. https://www.oecd.org/about/secretary-general/heavy-burden-of-obesity-mexico-january-2020.htm.

Gutierrez, J., Garcia-Saiso, S., & Aracena, B. (2018). Mexico's household health expenditure on diabetes and hypertension: what is the additional financial burden? *PLOS One*, 13(7), e0201333. https://doi.org/10.1371/journal.pone.0201333.

Haffner, S., Lehto, S., Rönnemaa, T., Pyörälä, K., & Laakso, M. (1998). Mortality from coronary heart disease in subjects with type 2 diabetes and in nondiabetic subjects with and without prior myocardial infarction. *New England Journal of Medicine*, 339(4), 229–234.

Harrup, A. (2020). Mexico confirms first case of coronavirus. *The Wall Street Journal*. https://www.wsj.com/articles/mexico-confirms-first-case-of-coronavir-11582898181.

Hernandez, G. (2015). Extreme inequality in Mexico: Concentration of economic and political power. Inequality Oxfam. https://www.scribd.com/document/665058870/inequality-oxfam

Hill, M., Mantzoros, C., & Sowers, J. (2020). Commentary: COVID-19 in patients with diabetes. *Metabolism*, 107, 154217. https://doi.org/10.1016/j.metabol.2020.154217.

Horton, S.B. (2016). *They Leave Their Kidneys in the Fields: Illness, Injury, and Illegality among U.S. Farmworkers*. Oakland: University of California Press.

Houston, A.R., Lynch, K., Ostrach, B., Isaacs, Y.S., Nvé Díaz San Francisco, C., Lee, J.M., Emard, N., & Proctor, D.A. (2022). United States immigration detention amplifies disease interaction risk: a model for a transnational ICE-TB-DM2 syndemic. *Global Public Health*, 17(7), 1152–1171. https://doi.org/10.1080/17441692.2021.1919737.

Hunter, L., Murray, S., & Riosmena, F. (2013). Rainfall patterns and U.S. migration from rural Mexico. *International Migration Review*, 47(4), 874–909.

Ibarra-Nava, I., Cardenas-de la Garza, J., Ruiz-Lozano, R., & Salazar-Montalvo, R. (2020). Mexico and the COVID-19 response. *Disaster Medicine and Public Health Preparedness*, 1–3. https://doi.org/10.1017/dmp.2022.177.

Infobae. (2020). Mapa del coronavirus en México 17 de agosto: el país registra la tercera semana con descenso en contagios totals. https://www.infobae.com/america/mexico/2020/08/17/mapa-del-oronavirus-en-mexico-17-de-agosto-el-pais-registra-la-tercera-semana-con-descenso-en-contagios-totales/.

Infobae. (2021). México supera las 150,000 muertes por COVID-19. https://www.infobae.com/america/agencias/2021/01/26/mexico-supera-las-150000-muertes-por-covid-19-3/.

Institute for Global Sciences. (2021). Mexico's response to COVID-19: a case study. University of California, San Francisco. https://globalhealthsciences.ucsf.edu/news/mexicos-response-covid-19-case-study.

Iqbal, A., Prince, L.R., Novodvorsky, P., Bernjak, A., Thomas, M.R., Birch, L., Lambert, D., Kay, L.J., Wright, F.J., Macdonald, I.A., Jacques, R.M., Storey, R.F., McCrimmon, R.J., Francis, S., Heller, S.R., & Sabroe, I. (2019). Effect of hypoglycemia on inflammatory responses and the response to low-dose endotoxemia in humans. *Journal of Clinical Endocrinology and Metabolism*, 104(4), 1187–1199. https://doi.org/10.1210/jc.2018-01168.

Jafar, N., Edriss, H., & Nugent, K. (2016). The effect of short-term hyperglycemia on the innate immune system. *American Journal of the Medical Sciences*, 351(2), 201–211.

Jang, J., Hur, J., Choi, E., Hong, K., Lee, W., & Ahan, J. (2020). Prognostic factors for severe coronavirus disease 2019 in Daegu, Korea. *Journal of Korean Medical Science*, 35(23), e209. https://doi.org/10.3346/jkms.2020.35.e209.

Jimenez-Corona, A., Nelson, R.G., Jimenez-Corona, M.E., Franks, P.W., Aguilar-Salinas, C.A., Graue-Hernandez, E.O., Hernandez-Jimenez, S., & Hernandez-Avila, M. (2019). Disparities in prediabetes and type 2 diabetes prevalence between indigenous and nonindigenous populations from Southeastern Mexico: the Comitan study. *Journal of Clinical & Translational Endocrinology*, 16, 100191. https://doi.org/10.1016/j.jcte.2019.100191.

Jiménez-Cruz, A., & Bacardi-Gascon, M. (2004). The fattening burden of type 2 diabetes on Mexicans. *Diabetes Care*, 27(5), 1213–1215.

Juárez-Ramírez, C., Márquez-Serrano, M., de Snyder, N.S., Pelcastre-Villafuerte, B.E., Ruelas-González, M.G., & Reyes-Morales, H. (2014). La desigualdad en salud de grupos vulnerables de México: Adultos mayores, indígenas y migrantes. *Revista Panamericana de Salud Pública*, 35(4), 284–290.

Kamiya, M. (2018). Infographics: urbanisation and urban development in Mexico. Urbanet. https://www.urbanet.info/urbanisation-and-urban-development-in-mexico/.

Keeney, A.J., Quandt, A., Villaseñor, M.D., Flores, D., & Flores, L. (2022). Occupational stressors and access to COVID-19 resources among commuting and residential Hispanic/Latino farmworkers in a US-Mexico border region. *International Journal of Environmental Research and Public Health*, 19(2), 763.

Knapp, S. (2013). Diabetes and infection: is there a link? A mini-review. *Gerontology*, 59(2), 99–104.

Kohio, H., & Adamson, A. (2013). Glycolytic control of vacuolar-type ATPase activity: a mechanism to regulate influenza viral infection. *Virology*, 444(1–2), 301–309. https://doi.org/10.1016/j.virol.2013.06.026.

Laurell, A. (1992). Mexico's pseudo-democracy. *New Left Review*, 194, 33–53.

Laurell, A. (2015). Three decades of neoliberalism in Mexico: the destruction of society. *International Journal of Health Services*, 45(2), 246–264.

Lecube, A., Pachón, G., Petriz, J., Hernández, C., & Simó, R. (2011). Phagocytic activity is impaired in type 2 diabetes mellitus and increases after metabolic improvement. *PLoS One*, 6(8), e23366. https://doi.org/10.1371/journal.pone.0023366.

Lippi, G., & Plebani, M. (2020). Laboratory abnormalities in patients with COVID-2019 infection. *Clinical Chemistry and Laboratory Medicine*, 58(7), 1131–1134. https://doi.org/10.1515/cclm-2020-0198.

López-Olmedo, N., Popkin, B., & Taillie, L. (2018). The socioeconomic disparities in intakes and purchases of less-healthy foods and beverages have changed over time in urban Mexico. *Journal of Nutrition*, 148(1), 109–116.

Manderson, L., Wahlberg, A. (2020). Chronic living in a communicable world. *Medical Anthropology*, 39(5), 428–439. https://doi.org/10.1080/01459740.2020.1761352

Marca, C. (2020). Coronavirus México 31 de julio; resumen de las últimas noticias, contagios y muertes. https://www.marca.com/claro-mx/trending/coronavirus/2020/07/31/5f23b678ca4741fb1a8b4607.html.

Martínez, A.D., Ruelas, L., & Granger, D.A. (2018). Household fear of deportation in relation to chronic stressors and salivary proinflammatory cytokines in Mexican-origin families Post-SB 1070. *Social Science & Medicine-Population Health*, 5, 188–200.

Martínez, C., & Leal, G. (2003). Epidemiological transition: model or illusion? A look at the problem of health in Mexico. *Social Science & Medicine*, 57(3), 539–550.

McDonnell, P., & Sanchez, C. (2020). Mexico's fragile health system running out of room for coronavirus patients. *The Los Angeles Times*. https://www.latimes.com/world-nation/story/2020-05-04/mexican-hospitals-brace-for-coronavirus-crunch.

Maupomé-Carvantes, G., Sánchez-Reyes, V., Laguna-Ortega, S., Andrade-Delgado, L., & Diez de Bonilla-Calderón, J. (1995). Patron de Consumo de Refrescos en una Poblacion Mexicana. *Salud Publica de México*, 37(4), 323–328.

Means, C. (2020). Mechanisms of increased morbidity and mortality of SARS-CoV-2 infection in individuals with diabetes: what this means for an effective management strategy. *Metabolism*, 154254. https://doi.org/10.1016/j.metabol.2020.154254.

Mendenhall, E. (2012). *Syndemic Suffering: Social Distress, Depression, and Diabetes among Mexican Immigrant Women.* New York: Routledge.

Meza, R., Barrientos-Gutierrez, T., Rojas-Martinez, R., Reynoso-Noverón, N., Palacio-Mejia, L.S., Lazcano-Ponce, E., & Hernández-Ávila, M. (2015). Burden of type 2 diabetes in Mexico: past, current and future prevalence and incidence rates. *Preventive Medicine*, 81, 445–450. https://doi.org/10.1016/j.ypmed.2015.10.015.

Montesi, L. (2018). Diabetes, alcohol abuse, and inequality in southern Mexico: a synergistic interaction. *Medicine Anthropology Theory*, 5(1). https://doi.org/10.17157/mat.5.1.541.

Morales, L.S., Lara, M., Kington, R.S., Valdez, R.O., & Escarce, J.J. (2002). Socioeconomic, cultural, and behavioral factors affecting Hispanic health outcomes. *Journal of Health Care for the Poor and Underserved*, 13(4), 477–503. https://doi.org/10.1177/104920802237532.

Moran-Thomas, A. (2019). *Traveling with Sugar Chronicles of a Global Epidemic.* Berkeley: University of California Press.

Moreno-Altamirano, L., Silberman, M., & Hernández-Montoya, D. (2015). Type 2 diabetes and dietary patterns 1961 to 2009: some social determinants in Mexico. *Gaceta Medica de Mexico*, 151, 330–343.

Muniyappa, R., & Gubbi, S. (2020). COVID-19 pandemic, coronaviruses, and diabetes mellitus. *American Journal of Physiology. Endocrinology and Metabolism*, 318(5), E736–E741. https://doi.org/10.1152/ajpendo.00124.2020.

Nava-Ledezma, I. (2011). Socioeconomic status and diabetes among Mexican adults. Doctoral Thesis. School of Social Sciences, University of Southampton.

Nawrotzki, R., DeWaard, J., Bakhtsiyarava, M., & Ha, J. (2017). Climate shocks and rural-urban migration in Mexico: exploring nonlinearities and thresholds. *Climate Change*, 40(2), 243–258.

Nawrotzki, R., Hunter, L., Runfola, D., & Riosmena, F. (2015). Climate change as a migration driver from rural and urban Mexico. *Environmental Research Letters*, 10(11), 114023.

NBC News. (2020). Mexico is fourth country to top over 100,000 Covid deaths. https://www.nbcnews.com/news/latino/mexico-fourth-country-top-over-100-000-covid-deaths-n1248408?cid=sm_npd_ms_fb_lw&fbclid=IwAR2pXF9bdjkebp5Qz c46E7Yxzw--eHnLL7CmLmIIJ0jvnCZ83BVSR_VoKak.

Onder, G., Rezza, G., & Brusaferro, S. (2020). Case-fatality rate and characteristics of patients dying in relation to COVID-19 in Italy. *JAMA*, 323(18), 1775–1776. https://doi.org/10.1001/jama.2020.4683.

Orozco, J. (2021). Mexico covid cases rise by record 28,953 amid third wave. *Bloomberg*. https://www.bloomberg.com/news/articles/2021-08-18/mexico-covid-cases-rise-by-daily-record-28-953-amid-third-wave.

Özcan, U., Cao, Q., Yilmaz, E., Lee, A.H., Iwakoshi, N., Özdelen, E., Tuncman, G., Gorgun, C., Glimcher, L., & Hotamisligil, G. (2004). Endoplasmic reticulum stress links obesity, insulin action, and type 2 diabetes. *Science*, 306, 457–461.

Pal, R., & Bhadada, S.K. (2020). COVID-19 and diabetes mellitus: an unholy interaction of two pandemics. *Diabetes & Metabolic Syndrome*, 14(4), 513–517. https://doi.org/10.1016/j.dsx.2020.04.049.

Pan American Health Organization. (2012). *Health in the Americas, 2012 Edition: Country Volume, Mexico.* Washington, DC: PAHO.

Partners in Health. (2020). In Mexico, COVID-19 patient recovers after seeking care at hospital. https://www.pih.org/article/mexico-covid-19-patient-recovers-after-seekingcare-hospital.

Pinheiro, P.S., Medina, H.N., Espinel, Z., Kobetz, E.N., & Shultz, J.M. (2021). New insights into the burden of COVID-19 mortality for U.S. Hispanics and Blacks when examined by country/region of origin: an observational study. *Lancet Regional Health. Americas, 5,* 100090. https://doi.org/10.1016/j.lana.2021.100090.

Phillips, M., & Salmerón, J. (1992). Diabetes in Mexico--a serious and growing problem. *World Health Statistics Quarterly. Rapport trimestriel de statistiques sanitaires mondiales, 45*(4), 338–346.

Plascencia, L.F. (2009). The "undocumented" Mexican migrant question: re-examining the framing of law and illegalization in the United States. *Urban Anthropology and Studies of Cultural Systems and World Economic Development, 38*(2-4), 375–434.

Polaski, S. (2004). Mexican employment, productivity and income a decade after NAFTA. Carnegie Endowment for International Peace. https://carnegieendowment.org/2004/02/25/mexican-employment-productivity-and-income-decade-after-nafta-pub-1473

Public Citizen. (2019). Fact sheet: NAFTA's legacy: lost jobs, lower wages, increased inequality. https://www.citizen.org/article/fact-sheet-naftas-legacy-lost-jobs-lower-wages-increased-inequality/.

Quesada, J., Hart, L.K., & Bourgois, P. (2011). Structural vulnerability and health: Latino migrant laborers in the United States. *Medical Anthropology, 30*(4), 339–362.

Reardon, T., & Berdegué, J. (2002). The rapid rise of supermarkets in Latin America: challenges and opportunities for development. *Development Policy Review.* https://doi.org/10.1111/1467-7679.00183.

Rivera, J.A., Barquera, S., González-Cossío, T., Olaiz, G., & Sepúlveda, J. (2004). Nutrition transition in Mexico and in other Latin American countries. *Nutrition Reviews, 62*(7 Pt 2), S149–S157. https://doi.org/10.1111/j.1753-4887.2004.tb00086.x.

Rodríguez, L., Reynales, L., Jiménez, A., Juárez, S., Hernández, M. (2010). Direct costs of medical care for patients with type 2 diabetes mellitus in Mexico microcosting analysis]. *Revista Panamerica de Salud Public.* 28(6), 412–420.

Ruan, Q., Yang, K., Wang, W., Jiang, L., & Song, J. (2020). Clinical predictors of mortality due to COVID-19 based on an analysis of data of 150 patients from Wuhan, China. *Intensive Care Medicine, 46*(5), 846–848. https://doi.org/10.1007/s00134-020-05991-x.

Salas, C., Scott, R., & Faux, J. (2006). Revisiting NAFTA still not working for America's workers. Economic Policy Institute. Briefing Paper #173. https://www.epi.org/publication/bp173/.

Sánchez, C.A. (2020). Don't call immigrant farmworkers heroes, they are underappreciated essential workers. *San Francisco Chronicle.* https://www.sfchronicle.com/bayarea/article/Don-t-call-immigrant-farmworkers-heroes-they-15677053.php.

San Diego Union Tribune. (2020). Coronavirus could hit Mexico's high obesity, diabetes rates. https://www.sandiegouniontribune.com/news/nation-world/story/2020-03-25/coronavirus-could-hit-mexicos-high-obesity-diabetes-rates.

Schoen, K., Horvat, N., Guerreiro, N., de Castro, I., & de Giassi, K. (2019). Spectrum of clinical and radiographic findings in patients with diagnosis of H1N1 and correlation with clinical severity. *BMC Infectious Diseases*, 19(1), 964. https://bmcinfectdis.biomedcentral.com/articles/10.1186/s12879-019-4592-0.

Rao Kondapally Seshasai, S., Kaptoge, S., Thompson, A., Di Angelantonio, E., Gao, P., Sarwar, N., Whincup, P.H., Mukamal, K.J., Rao Kondapally Seshasai, S., Kaptoge, S., Thompson, A., Di Angelantonio, E., Gao, P., Sarwar, N., Whincup, P.H., Mukamal, K., Gillum R., Holme, I., Njølstad, I., Fletcher, A., Nilsson, P., Lewington, S., Collins, R., Gudnason, V., Thompson, S., Sattar, N., Selvin, E., Hu, F., Danesh, J. (2011). Diabetes mellitus, fasting glucose, and risk of cause-specific death. *New England Journal of Medicine*, 364(9), 829–841. https://doi.org/10.1056/NEJMoa1008862.

Shah, B., & Hux, J. (2003). Quantifying the risk of infectious diseases for people with diabetes. *Diabetes Care*, 226, 510–513.

Sheridan, M. (2020). Mexico issues highest daily tally of coronavirus deaths, more than 1,000. *New York Times*. https://www.washingtonpost.com/world/the_americas/mexico-issues-highest-daily-tally-of-coronavirus-deaths-more-than-1000/2020/06/04/3cca0ba6-a623-11ea-898e-b21b9a83f792_story.html.

Sherman, C. (2021). Mexico sees easing in its third wave of COVID-19 cases. *US News*. https://www.usnews.com/news/world/articles/2021-09-01/mexico-sees-easing-of-third-covid-19-wave.

Singer, M. (2020). Deadly companions: diabetes and COVID-19 in Mexico. *Medical Anthropology*, 39(8), 660–665. https://doi.org/10.1080/01459740.2020.1805742.

Singer, M., Bulled, N., & Leatherman, T. (2022). Are there global syndemics? *Medical Anthropology*, 41(1), 4–18. https://doi.org/10.1080/01459740.2021.2007907.

Singer, M., Bulled, N., Ostrach, B., & Mendenhall, E. (2017). Syndemics and the biosocial conception of health. *Lancet*, 389(10072), 941–950. https://doi.org/10.1016/S0140-6736(17)30003-X.

Soto, S., Yoder, A.M., Nuño, T., Aceves, B., Sepulveda, R., & Rosales, C.B. (2022). Health conditions among farmworkers in the Southwest: an analysis of the National Agricultural Workers Survey. *Frontiers in Public Health*, 10, 962085. https://doi.org/10.3389/fpubh.2022.962085.

Soto-Estrada, G., Altamirano, L., Garcia-García, J., Moreno, I., & Silberman, M. (2018). Trends in frequency of type 2 diabetes in Mexico and its relationship to dietary patterns and contextual factors. *Gaceta Sanitaria*, 32(3), 283–290.

Starosta, A. (2016). Diabetes: health inequity of Mexican immigrants in the United States. *The Yale Global Health Review*. https://yaleglobalhealthreview.com/2016/07/08/diabetes-health-inequit-of-mexican-immigrants-in-the-united-states/#:~:text=Studies%20have%20shown%20that%20Mexicans,any%20subgroup%2C%20at%2010%25.

Stoddard, P., Handley, M., Bustamante, A., & Schillinger, D. (2011). The influence of indigenous status and community indigenous composition on obesity and diabetes among Mexican adults. *Social Science & Medicine*, 73(11), 1635–1643.

Suárez, V., Quezada Suarez, M., Oros Ruiz, S., & Ronquillo De Jesús, E. (2020). Epidemiology of COVID-19 in Mexico: from the 27th of February to the 30th of April 2020. *Revista Clínica Española*, 220(8), 463–471.

Sue, C. (2013). *Land of the Cosmic Race: Race Mixture, Racism, and Blackness in Mexico*. New York: Oxford University Press.

Team, V., & Manderson, L. (2020). How COVID-19 reveals structures of vulnerability. *Medical Anthropology*, 39(8), 671–674. https://doi.org/10.1080/01459740. 2020.1830281.

Tikellis, C., & Thomas, M.C. (2012). Angiotensin-converting enzyme 2 (ACE2) is a key modulator of the renin angiotensin system in health and disease. *International Journal of Peptides*, 2012, 256294. https://doi.org/10.1155/2012/256294.

Turrent, A., Wise, T., & Garvey, E. (2012). Achieving Mexico's maize potential. *US: Global Development and Environment Institute*, Working Paper No. 12-03. https:// pdfs.semanticscholar.org/8833/f3aa207605109e298357a72e3ba9ae59a14f. pdf?_ga=2.33723369.997543249.1590968948-1107409701.1589328837.

Valle, A., & Knaul, F. (2021). Mexico, facing its third COVID-19 wave, shows the dangers of weak federal coordination. *The Conversation*. https://theconversation. com/mexico-facing-its-third-covid-19-wave-shows-the-dangers-of-weak-federal-coordination-164995.

Vilar-Compte, M., Gaitán-Rossi, P., Félix-Beltrán, L., & Bustamante, A.V. (2022). Pre-COVID-19 social determinants of health among Mexican migrants in Los Angeles and New York City and their increased vulnerability to unfavorable health outcomes during the COVID-19 pandemic. *Journal of Immigrant and Minority Health*, 24(1), 65–77. https://doi.org/10.1007/s10903-021-01283-8.

Wang, A., Zhao, W., Xu, Z., & Gu, J. (2020). Timely blood glucose management for the outbreak of 2019 novel coronavirus disease (COVID-19) is urgently needed. *Diabetes Research and Clinical Practice*, 162, 108118. https://doi.org/10.1016/j. diabres.2020.108118.

Weisbrot, M., Merling, L., Mello, V., Lefebvre, S., & Sammut, J. (2017). Did NAFTA help Mexico? An update after 23 years. The Sanders Institute. https://www. sandersinstitute.org/blog/did-nafta-help-mexico-an-update-after-23-years.

World Health Organization. (2004). Obesity and overweight. Facts. Geneva: World Health Organization. http://www.who.int/dietphysicalactivity/media/en/gsfs_obesity. pdf.

World Health Organization. (2016). Diabetes country profiles, 2016. https://www. who.int/teams/noncommunicable-diseases/surveillance/data/diabetes-profiles.

Wu, Z., McGoogan, J. (2020). Characteristics of and important lessons from the Coronavirus Disease 2019 (COVID-19) outbreak in China: Summary of a report of 72 314 cases from the Chinese Center for Disease Control and Prevention. *JAMA*, 323(13): 1239–1242. https://doi.org/10.1001/jama.2020.2648.

Xiuhtecutli, N., & Annie, S. (2021). Crisis politics and US farm labor: health justice and Florida farmworkers amid a pandemic. *Journal of Peasant Studies*, 48(1), 73–98.

Yang, J., Feng, Y., Yuan M., Yuan, S., Fu, H., & Wu, B. (2006). Plasma glucose levels and diabetes are independent predictors for mortality and morbidity in patients with SARS. *Diabetic Medicine*, 23(6), 623–628.

Yang, X., Yu, Y., Xu, J., Shu, H., Xia, J., Liu, H., Wu, Y., Zhang, L., Yu, Z., Fang, M., Yu, T., Wang, Y., Pan, S., Zou, X., Yuan, S., & Shang, Y. (2020). Clinical course and outcomes of critically ill patients with SARS-CoV-2 pneumonia in Wuhan, China: a single-centered, retrospective, observational study. *Lancet*. Respiratory Medicine, 8(5), 475–481. https://doi.org/10.1016/S2213-2600(20)30079-5.

Zhang, J.J., Dong, X., Cao, Y.Y., Yuan, Y.D., Yang, Y.B., Yan, Y.Q., Akdis, C.A., & Gao, Y.D. (2020). Clinical characteristics of 140 patients infected with SARS-CoV-2 in Wuhan, China. *Allergy*, 75(7), 1730–1741. https://doi.org/10.1111/all.14238.

Zhou, J., & Tan, J. (2020). Diabetes patients with COVID-19 need better blood glucose management in Wuhan, China. *Metabolism: Clinical and Experimental*, 107, 154216. https://doi.org/10.1016/j.metabol.2020.154216.

Zou, Z., Yan, Y., Shu, Y., Gao, R., Sun, Y., Li, X., Ju, X., Liang, Z., Liu, Q., Zhao, Y., Guo, F., Bai, T., Zou, Z., Yan, Y., Shu, Y., Gao, R., Sun, Y., Li, X., Ju, X., Liang, Z., Liu, Q., Zhao, Y., Guo, F., Bai, T., Han, Z., Zhu, J., Zhou, H., Huang, F., Li, C., Lu, H., Li, N., Li, D., Jin, N., Penninger, J., Jiang, C. (2014). Angiotensin-converting enzyme 2 protects from lethal avian influenza A H5N1 infections. *Nature Communications*, 5, 3594. https://doi.org/10.1038/ncomms4594.

4 TB-COVID-19 Syndemic in the Philippines

A Double Challenge amidst Public Health Emergency and Social, Political, and Economic Inequalities

Trisha Denise D. Cedeño, Kimberly G. Ramos, Mary Grace A. Pelayo, Princess Rayevy I. Esmillo, and Ian Christopher N. Rocha

Tuberculosis in the Philippines

Every March 24, the World Tuberculosis (TB) Day commemorates the day in 1882 when Dr. Robert Koch discovered the bacterium that causes TB (World Health Organization, 2022a). The WHO declared TB a global emergency in 1993. In the Philippines, August 19 has been proclaimed as National TB Day, which also marks the birth anniversary of former President Manuel L. Quezon, who succumbed to TB (Official Gazette of the Philippines, 1996). TB is ranked second among the leading causes of maternal, neonatal, and nutritional diseases in the country. One in three Filipinos is known to be infected with TB (WHO, 2022a).

For the decade prior to the COVID-19 pandemic, the Philippines ranked fourth in global TB cases and second in regional TB cases for both the Western Pacific Region and the Association of Southeast Asian Nations (ASEAN), contributing to 6% of the total TB global burden (Tanchuco, 2020; Wi, 2021; WHO, 2022a). The Philippines documents approximately 554 cases per 100,000 population, with an estimated incidence rate of 149 TB cases per 100,000 population, and an average death rate of 62 people daily (WHO, 2022a). Alongside six other countries in the Global South (Bangladesh, India, Indonesia, Myanmar, Nigeria, and Pakistan), the Philippines has been known to account for more than 60% of the discrepancy in estimated actual global TB incidence as compared to the number of diagnosed TB cases and those reported to national authorities (WHO, 2022a). The Philippines also belongs to high multi-drug resistant-TB (MDR-TB) burden countries, with an estimated MDR-TB prevalence of 5.3% among new TB cases and 20.6% among previously treated TB cases in 2020 (WHO, 2022a). The Philippines was found to have the highest rates of lost to follow-up TB cases, which have been worsened by rapid migration and urbanization, as well as coexisting

DOI: 10.4324/9781003365358-5

diseases among TB patients such as HIV/AIDS (WHO, 2022a; Wi, 2021). TB cases in the Philippines mostly occur among individuals belonging to the working population, which severely affects the country's socioeconomic status. Hence, the National TB Control Program (NTP) has been implemented to control the disease through the provision of resources and services by local and national government units, together with non-government organizations and the private sector (Wi, 2021).

The NTP Manual of Procedures (MOP) serves as the framework for the TB program control among Directly Observed Therapy-Short Course (DOTS) facilities in the Philippines which provides the basis for diagnosing, treating, and counseling of TB patients (Department of Health, 2023). Additionally, the MOP ensures supportive health systems for the NTP and guides various organizational levels on the monitoring, evaluation, and supervision of programs for TB cases in the country (Department of Health, 2023). Prior to the COVID-19 pandemic, an initial estimate of at least 1.4 million TB cases was expected to be detected and treated within the succeeding 2.5 years (Department of Health, 2020a).

Double Burden of TB and COVID-19 in the Country

Syndemics have affected many countries in the Global South, including the Philippines. The majority of recent syndemic situations are associated with the COVID-19 pandemic. Examples include the mucormycosis and COVID-19 syndemic in India (described in Chapter 8; Rocha et al., 2021), and the arboviral infections and COVID-19 syndemic in Southeast Asia (Wiyono et al., 2021), South Asia (Khatri et al., 2022), and South America (Jain et al., 2021). Meanwhile, in the Philippines, the double burden of COVID-19 and TB has aggravated the current healthcare system. Before this pandemic, TB was already the most common infectious disease worldwide. Although the number of people developing TB has been decreasing in recent years, disruptions caused by COVID-19 have undone years of progress in the fight against TB, as noted in the recent Global TB Report (WHO, 2022a).

During the initial surge of COVID-19, the Philippines desperately engaged in drastic measures to mitigate and flatten the pandemic curve by imposing strict lockdowns. The Philippines was one of the worst-affected countries in the ASEAN and the Western Pacific Region during the pandemic (Miranda et al., 2021; Cedeño et al., 2023). As a result, TB programs were discontinued, TB case finding and supply of TB drugs were disrupted, consultation and visits of symptomatic patients to healthcare facilities were reduced, priority of healthcare services was diverted to COVID-19, and TB contact tracing was curtailed. Disruptions in health services due to the pandemic have severely affected the incidence notification of drug-resistant TB – the Philippines is one of ten countries accounting for 70% of the gap between the estimated global incidence of drug-resistant TB and the number of people enrolled in treatment (Saunders & Evans, 2020). The implementation of quarantine measures and lockdowns has made it more difficult for people with TB to access healthcare services, leading to an increase in TB mortality (Calnan et al., 2022; WHO, 2021a, 2021b, 2022a, 2022b).

The COVID-19 pandemic has had a significant effect on TB control efforts in the Philippines, particularly among marginalized and vulnerable populations, such as refugees and prisoners. A recent study indicates profound disruptions in TB prevention and control due to COVID-19 measures such as: (1) diversion of resources to manage the COVID-19 pandemic; (2) health service, politics, and media focus on the pandemic management and responses; (3) poor quality of healthcare due to stress and anxiety factors among the healthcare personal, self-isolation, and infection; and (4) fear of contracting COVID-19 infection at healthcare facilities, which discouraged visiting TB hubs (Eike et al., 2022). Furthermore, testing, strict enforcement of infection control protocols, and separation of people who have TB concurrent with COVID-19 infection might not be feasible in hospitals due to overcrowding (Eike et al., 2022). Such significant barriers to accessing healthcare services and treatment resulted in poor treatment adherence and outcomes and is likely to increase further community transmission of TB (Florentino et al., 2022). In particular, the pandemic has dramatically hampered the progress of TB treatment in the world. In comparison with the previous year, 1.4 million fewer people in 2020 (approximately 21% reduction) have been estimated to receive complete TB treatment. Furthermore, there are several countries with the most significant relative gaps, such as Indonesia (42%), South Africa (41%), the Philippines (37%), and India (25%) (Caren et al., 2022).

TB and COVID-19 are infectious diseases that can have serious health consequences and cause significant morbidity and mortality. Both are respiratory infections caused by different pathogens. TB is caused by *Mycobacterium tuberculosis*, while COVID-19 is caused by severe acute respiratory syndrome coronavirus 2 (SARS-CoV-2) (WHO, 2021a). Despite the differences in their causative agents, there are several similarities between both infections. One similarity is that both TB and COVID-19 can be transmitted through respiratory droplets, either by coughing or sneezing, and people who are in close proximity to an infected individual are at risk of contracting the infection. Severe respiratory symptoms, such as cough, fever, and difficulty in breathing are also similar for both disease conditions. In such severe cases, both infections can lead to hospitalization and, in some cases, death (Centers for Disease Control and Prevention, 2021; WHO, 2023).

Moreover, TB and COVID-19 both have a higher morbidity and mortality rate among certain population groups, such as older individuals, those with underlying health conditions, and people who are immunocompromised. As for diagnostic methods, both can be diagnosed through a combination of clinical symptoms, radiological findings, and laboratory tests, such as sputum culture and polymerase chain reaction (PCR) tests. In terms of treatment, both can be effectively treated with appropriate medical care. TB is treated with a combination of antibiotics, while COVID-19 can be treated with antiviral medications and supportive care (CDC, 2021; WHO, 2023). The continuum of care during the pandemic includes significant gaps because of the decrease in case notification and the restriction of access to programs for TB (Dychiao et al., 2022). In fact, effects of COVID-19 were expected to result in a 170% rise in TB-related mortality (WHO, 2022a).

In the context of COVID-19, the NTP created a TB adaptable plan. In addition to the traditional DOTS in a clinic, interventions included video-observed treatment, digital adherence technology, and support from other family members for patient treatment adherence. As a result of these interventions, after six months of treatment there was a 75% decrease in loss to follow-up (DOH, 2021). COVID-19 vaccines could serve as another, unanticipated, TB intervention measure as COVID-19 vaccines have been shown to elicit an immune response to TB antigens. Thus, offering a "one-two punch" vaccine that could provide protection against both COVID-19 and TB (Hotez et al., 2021). Meanwhile, a combination of targeted interventions, such as expanding TB screening in high-risk populations, and broader efforts to improve healthcare access and quality could be effective in reducing the burden of TB in the Philippines (Calderon et al., 2022).

Social Inequalities Exacerbating the Impact of Pandemic in TB Services

Zimmerman and colleagues (2021) argued that social determinants of health often overlap in terms of infection and mortality. This is the case for both TB and COVID-19 infection and mortality rates. Common social determinants that aggravate adverse health outcomes for both infectious diseases include the socioeconomic status of individuals, weak political will and health governance or lack thereof, insufficient health financing, physical environments, and demographic factors.

Globally, it was estimated that 150 million people were subjected to economic poverty from the onset of the pandemic until 2021 (Lakner et al., 2021). Since movement restrictions were implemented worldwide, employment and businesses were also hampered. Government funds were eventually heavily burdened as governments continued to spend billions to prevent COVID-19 transmission, morbidity, and mortality. Consequently, people at and below the poverty line were forced into extreme poverty. Governments were also forced to implement austerity measures to lessen government spending. States were subjected to high inflation rates as businesses were heavily affected during the lockdown measures.

For communicable and infectious diseases like HIV/AIDS and TB, attention has been paid to the significance of socioeconomic factors in examining health and its negative effects. According to the Commission on Social Determinants of Health (CSDH) of the WHO, the conditions under which people are born, raised, employed, and age, as well as the procedures put in place to address sickness, result in unequal and unfair distributions of population health. Hargreaves and colleagues (2011) created a paradigm for understanding the socioeconomic determinants of TB based on the WHO-CSDH. In 2010, it was shown that disadvantaged groups, including the underprivileged, the hungry, and indigenous peoples, tend to have larger concentrations of TB cases. TB itself also affects how well people will fare with other illnesses like COVID-19. In their investigation, Zimmerman and colleagues (2021) noted that those who had both a current and a former TB infection considerably increased their chance of COVID-19 death. According to studies in the Philippines, people with TB infection have a greater probability of dying from COVID-19 (TB/COVID-19 Global Study Group, 2022). In order to concurrently restrict the spread and ameliorate the effects of both COVID-19 and TB, it is urgently necessary to create effective interventions that address the health equity gap underlying impediments to universal health coverage (Zimmerman et al., 2021).

Specifically, CSDH characterized structural determinants of health as socially repressive environments. Social stratification leads to an uneven distribution of the social determinants of health. The primary structural determinants of TB include global socioeconomic inequality, high levels of population mobility, rapid urbanization, and population growth (Hargreaves et al., 2011). These factors cause unequal distributions of social determinants of TB, including food insecurity and malnutrition, subpar housing and environmental conditions, and monetary, physical, and cultural barriers to accessing healthcare. These social factors are some of the important TB risk factors. For instance, uninfected people are more likely to get TB infection in homes, workplaces, and communities with poor ventilation and overcrowding. Malnutrition, indigence, and hunger may make people more vulnerable to illness, infection, and worse clinical outcomes. People with TB symptoms, such as persistent cough, frequently encounter significant social and economic obstacles that prevent them from accessing the healthcare systems where an accurate diagnosis could be made. These obstacles include transportation issues to medical facilities, anxiety about being stigmatized if they seek a TB diagnosis, and a lack of social support to seek care when they become ill.

Poverty is a powerful determinant that increases the incidence of TB (WHO, 2022a; 2023). The Philippines has 1.5 times higher prevalence in urban poor communities than in non-poor counterparts (Querri et al., 2017). Living and working conditions that are crowded and inadequately ventilated, which are frequently linked to poverty, are direct risk factors for the spread of TB. The living conditions in the country where nearly 10 million people reside in urban slums, social determinants are major drivers of the endemicity of TB (Saunders & Evans, 2020; WHO, 2020).

Treatment and prevention can greatly benefit from actions taken on the factors that contribute to poor health through "health-in-all-policies" approaches. Therefore, addressing broader determinants such as poverty associated with rapid urbanization and transmission of the disease, exacerbated by the COVID-19 pandemic remains to be one of the challenges in battling TB (Kuddus et al., 2020; United Nations, 2020).

The distribution of socioeconomic variables that impact the four stages of TB pathogenesis – exposure to infection, progression to illness, delayed or ineffective diagnosis and treatment, and poor treatment adherence and success – reflects the distribution of TB in the population. As such, TB and COVID-19 infection can be considered a "cursed duet," diseases that need to be given urgent attention and care especially if patients are coming from underserved communities with disadvantaged socioeconomic backgrounds. In this sense, preventive measures in dealing with both the causation and effects of TB and COVID-19, especially in terms of immunization campaigns, need to be strengthened globally.

Lack of Political Will to Address the TB Epidemic before the COVID-19 Pandemic

According to the Department of Budget and Management (2021), the 2019 national budget was increased by 10.1% compared to the 2018 national budget. Unfortunately, the budget for health was only ranked sixth among the nine top government agencies prior to the COVID-19 pandemic. The priorities of the national government before the pandemic were education and infrastructure. Among the departments, the Department of Health was one of the lowest priorities despite health crises such as TB ongoing in the country. In developing nations like the Philippines where TB is endemic, a disease associated with poverty requires political and medical intervention and attention. The rise of the COVID-19 pandemic has shown how crucial political will is in responding to global crises, specifically in the public health system.

Medical approaches to combat TB are neither sufficient to eradicate nor prevent the spread of the disease as the disease is not only a health concern. Political will plays a critical role in health issues as it dramatically influences policies and regulations of the national programs and public health is a collective effort and not an individual initiative (Oliver, 2006). Thus, fighting TB must extend beyond the health sector.

In the Philippines, about 150,000 TB patients go to the nearest, most accessible hospitals. These hospitals are usually private and charge for services. Patients from economically poor neighborhoods lack the funds accessible to travel to public hospitals where TB services are free. As TB treatment is expensive in private facilities, patients are unable to comply with long-term treatment plans. In addition, around 6–9% of the Filipino people need to undergo chest X-ray every year and 2–3% of this population needs to undergo rapid molecular tests annually (DOH, 2020b). The Department of Health needs to provide parallel support in the medical treatments and diagnostic procedures of poor TB patients, extending to the private sector. If the treatment of TB in poor communities is not funded and supported by the national government, the cases of TB patients will continue to rise.

In the global context, the WHO developed the Stop TB Strategy on World TB Day in 2006 and the End TB Strategy during the 67th World Health Assembly in 2014 to end TB in the world. These strategies aimed to drop the number of people suffering from TB by 90% while decreasing mortality from the disease by 95% and securing families from the adverse effect of the disease (WHO, 2022c). One of the major components includes pursuing high-quality DOTS expansion and enhancement. This involves political commitment with increased and sustained financing, case detection through quality-assured bacteriology, standardized treatment with supervision and patient support, effective drug supply and management, monitoring and evaluation system, and impact measurement. Despite all of these effective initiatives, the Philippines DOH ranked sixth in the 2019 national budget in the pre-pandemic era. TB programs, laboratory testing facilities, supply of medications, and campaign efforts were not supported and funded enough to be mobilized.

As anticipated, the COVID-19 pandemic severely challenged the public health and healthcare systems in the country including the delivery of TB services (WHO, 2022a, 2022b). Political incompetence and the lack of urgency of the Department of Health to act on the rising cases of COVID-19 resulted in a collapsing healthcare system (Chiang et al., 2020). Access to healthcare services was hampered because of the guidelines imposed by the Inter-Agency Task Force for the Management of Emerging Infectious Disease to control the spread of the COVID-19 virus. Some of the guidelines including long lockdowns, suspension of public transportation, and no face-to-face consultation, resulted in delaying the diagnosis and treatment of TB. Case finding of TB was ceased, active TB patients were prevented from visiting health facilities, COVID-19 health services were prioritized, TB contact tracing was restricted, and diagnostic use of GeneXpert in TB was allocated to COVID-19 screening resulting in an abrupt reduction of 71.7% weekly of TB notifications (WHO, 2022a).

Although the Philippines reacted quickly to create an adaptive plan to ensure the continuity of TB services such as assistance including taking home a one-month supply of medications and healthcare workers visiting patients' homes to conduct sputum collection for laboratory follow-ups, the WHO (2022a) reported that there was a significant fall in TB notifications in 2020–2021 that departed from the pre-2020 trends. Despite the effort of the Global Fund to control the negative impact of COVID-19 on TB services, it showed how the case reduction is indirectly proportional to the undiagnosed and untreated patients of TB resulting in an undetected increase in the number of developing TB infections and more deaths. Hence, this event defeats the objective and purpose of NTP of early detection of presumptive TB and rapid diagnosis of TB.

Economic Inequalities Exacerbating the Impact of the Pandemic on TB Services

The COVID-19 pandemic has made it undeniably clear that governance and policy choices in the health sector have come at very high costs to lives and the economy and it posed an unprecedented challenge to every aspect of public health, economic resources, human resources, essential service delivery, food systems, and the employment systems. It is likely to be the defining global health crisis of our generation. In its early days, the disease was described as an "equal opportunity offender" because people from all walks of life could be infected and all countries could suffer huge economic effects (Bainbridge, 2020; Saunders & Evans, 2020). Indeed, the economic and social disruption brought about by the pandemic is devastating, tens of millions of people are at risk of falling into extreme poverty, while the number of undernourished individuals continued to increase throughout the course of the pandemic (Saunders & Evans, 2020). It has become clear that the most economically disadvantaged sectors of society have suffered disproportionately from the consequences of this pandemic. It has caused what Ali (2021) calls "many pandemics."

It is no coincidence that the countries predicted to be most affected by the social and economic consequences of COVID-19 are also those with the highest TB burden. This is because aside from being an infectious disease, TB is also considered a cause and consequence of economic poverty – where poorer, undernourished people living in densely populated areas are at higher risk of TB, and TB entrenches poverty by increasing costs, reducing income, and causing stigma and discrimination (Florentino et al., 2022). In the Philippines, the annual inflation data for November 2022 soared to 8%, which marked the country's fastest inflation in 14 years (Crismundo, 2022).

Although the Philippines has made remarkable progress over the last decade, the COVID-19 pandemic and various measures to contain it (e.g., lockdowns) exacerbated existing inequalities that further posed a heavy financial burden for TB patients. In fact, Florentino and colleagues (2022) found that the overall proportion of costs in TB-affected households in the Philippines was about 42.4%, with the mean total costs of US$ 601.4, which is about 2.4 times the reported household income per month. The occurrence of catastrophic costs due to TB was significantly higher among drug-resistant TB patients (89.7%) than among drug-susceptible TB patients (41.7%). Of the study participants, 40.4% mobilized their savings, sold their household assets, or borrowed money to cope with the economic impacts of TB. The total TB patient costs in the Philippines were largely driven by direct non-medical costs such as expenses for transportation and nutritional supplements and food, and regular meals. Similar situations were observed in five countries including Ghana, Kenya, Uganda, Laos, and Timor-Leste (Eike et al., 2022; Florentino et al., 2022).

The Philippines stepped up its efforts to curb the spread of COVID-19 by implementing lockdown measures and repurposing healthcare personnel (WHO, 2021b; McQuaid et al., 2022). Simultaneously, health authorities collaborated with key stakeholders, including the WHO Office in the Philippines, to ramp up and adopt easy-to-implement solutions to mitigate the economic impact of COVID-19 on TB services (WHO, 2021b, 2022a). The Global Fund provides extensive financial support through a TB enabler package; however, this only catered to drug-resistant TB patients who sought care in public health facilities. As it was limited to drug-resistant TB patients, which accounted for 3.5% of estimated incident cases in the Philippines, the impact of the enabler package to reduce the overall proportion of catastrophic costs was minimal (from 42.4% to 42.0%) (Balisacan & Dela Cruz, 2021; Florentino et al., 2022). Realignment of health and economic policies is necessary to decentralize TB care, as well as to springboard an expansion of the TB enabler package to include all TB patients, especially those living under the poverty line.

Conclusions and Recommendations

TB remains a significant public health challenge in the Philippines, with a high burden of disease and a complex set of factors that contribute to high rates of TB transmission even until recent times. Efforts to prevent and control TB in the country have been hindered by a range of challenges, including insufficient resources, limited access to healthcare, inadequate infrastructure, and most especially, the emergence of the COVID-19 pandemic. Although innovative approaches have been employed, such as expanding TB screening in high-risk populations and improving access to healthcare through initiatives like universal health coverage and telemedicine modalities, progress is yet to be made in addressing the underlying factors that contribute to the persistence and transmission of TB cases that were present even prior to the COVID-19 pandemic.

The syndemic of TB and COVID-19 in the Philippines requires a coordinated and comprehensive social and biomedical response. The socioeconomic determinants of disease can be addressed through urban regeneration, strengthened social protection, and livelihood-strengthening initiatives. People who live in areas with high rates of chronic economic poverty and malnutrition bore a disproportionately high burden of TB and COVID-19. Subsequent TB infection can worsen food insecurity, poverty, and malnutrition. Initiatives for social protection lessen the effects of economic shocks like illness or job loss and assist those who are chronically disabled due to old age, illness, disability, or discrimination in securing basic livelihoods.

Meanwhile, social protection is motivated in part by the fact that poverty limits investments in child health, nutrition, and education, which results in lower income potential in later life and perpetuates intergenerational cycles of poverty. In turn, poor populations among developing nations like the Philippines have recently begun to see social protection only as an option. If the NTP was more actively involved in creating, promoting, and inspiring projects to improve living circumstances in areas where TB is a significant public health problem, TB control could be strengthened even in poverty-stricken communities.

Expanding access to TB prevention, diagnosis, and treatment services, particularly in underserved areas and among high-risk populations is another important step. This involves decentralizing TB services from facilities to community-based or home-based care, as well as realigning health and economic policies to expand the coverage of NTP. Enhancement of the use of digital technology and telemedicine to track and monitor adherence to TB treatment and improve the delivery of care may be facilitated which would include utilizing telephone and internet-based communication tools, such as instant messaging and video conferencing applications, to connect patients with healthcare providers.

Training of more barangay health workers and other allied healthcare professionals should also be considered in active TB case finding, contact assessments, and management. Support should be given to further their efforts in providing home-based treatment methods and in delivering TB medications to patients. This goes hand-in-hand with addressing TB-related stigma through more effective health education campaigns at the barangay level, along with the celebration of National TB Day and World TB Day by every local government unit.

In areas where TB services are currently inaccessible, allocating more facilities may aid in ensuring that all Filipinos have equal access to TB treatment, regardless of social status in both private and public facilities. Likewise, there should be regular conducting of a comprehensive study and analysis before implementing new policies or programs to address TB. Similarly, granting adequate funding to support TB control efforts should be prioritized. Ultimately, addressing the root causes of TB (i.e., poverty and overcrowding) and strengthening the implementation of government health programs to reduce the burden of TB in the Philippines are key strategies that could help to stabilize the country's health sector efforts against TB, even amidst a deadly pandemic such as the COVID-19.

References

Ali, I. (2021). Rituals of containment: Many pandemics, body politics, and social dramas during COVID-19 in Pakistan. *Frontiers in Sociology*, 6, 648149.

Bainbridge, M. (2020). Disease is an equal opportunity offender: COVID-19 is no exception. *The Hill*. https://thehill.com/opinion/healthcare/487573-disease-is-an-equal-opportunity-offender-and-covid-19-is-no-exception.

Balisacan, A.M., & Dela Cruz, R.M. (2021). When a pandemic strikes: Balancing Health and economy toward. *Munich Personal RePEc Archive*. https://mpra.ub.uni-muenchen.de/111259/1/MPRA_paper_111259.pdf.

Calderon, J.S., Perry, K.E., Thi, S.S., & Stevens, L.L. (2022). Innovating tuberculosis prevention to achieve universal health coverage in the Philippines. *The Lancet Regional Health - Western Pacific*, 100609. https://doi.org/10.1016/j.lanwpc.2022.100609.

Calnan, M., Moran, A., & Jassim AlMossawi, H. (2022). Maintaining essential tuberculosis services during the COVID-19 pandemic, Philippines. *Bulletin of the World Health Organization*, 100(02), 127–134. https://doi.org/10.2471/blt.21.286807.

Caren, G.J., Iskandar, D., Pitaloka, D.A.E., Abdullah, R., & Suwantika, A.A. (2022). COVID-19 pandemic disruption on the management of tuberculosis treatment in Indonesia. *Journal of Multidisciplinary Healthcare*, 15, 175–183. https://doi.org/10.2147/JMDH.S341130.

Cedeño, T.D.D., Rocha, I.C.N., Miranda, A.V., Lim, L.T.S., Buban, J.M., & Cleofas, J.V. (2023). Achieving herd immunity against COVID-19 in the Philippines. *Public Health Challenges*, 2, e61. https://doi.org/10.1002/puh2.61.

Centers for Disease Control and Prevention. (2021). Coronavirus disease 2019 (COVID-19). https://www.cdc.gov/coronavirus/2019-ncov/index.html.

Chiang, C.Y., Islam, T., Xu, C., Chinnayah, T., Garfin, A.M.C., Rahevar, K., & Raviglione, M. (2020). The impact of COVID-19 and the restoration of tuberculosis services in the Western Pacific Region. *The European Respiratory Journal*, 56(4). https://doi.org/10.1183/13993003.03054-2020.

Crismundo, K. (2022). PH inflation rises to 8% in November. *Philippine News Agency*. https://www.pna.gov.ph/articles/1190156.

Department of Budget and Management. (2021). Status of allotment releases (as of November 30, 2021). https://www.dbm.gov.ph/images/pdffiles/2019-People.

Department of Health. (2020a). Decline in reported TB cases an effect of the pandemic - DOH. https://doh.gov.ph/press-release/DECLINE-IN-REPORTED-TB-CASES-AN-EFFECT-OF-THE-PANDEMIC-DOH.

Department of Health. (2020b). *National tuberculosis control program: Manual of procedures*, 6th edition. https://doh.gov.ph/sites/default/files/publications/NTP_MOP_6th_Edition.pdf.

Department of Health. (2021). National TB control program adaptive plan: Redefining the national TB control program in the Philippines in the time of COVID-19 pandemic. https://doh.gov.ph/sites/default/files/publications/NTP%20Adaptive%20Plan.pdf.

Department of Health. (2023). National tuberculosis control program. https://ntp.doh.gov.ph/.

Dychiao, R.G.K., Capistrano, M.P.R., Flores, G.P., & Yap, C.D.D. (2022). Barriers to tuberculosis care in the Philippines. *The Lancet Respiratory Medicine*, 10(6), e55.

Eike, D., Hogrebe, M., Kifle, D., Tregilgas, M., Uppal, A., & Calmy, A. (2022). How the COVID-19 pandemic alters the landscapes of the HIV and tuberculosis epidemics in South Africa: A case study and future directions. *Epidemiologia*, 3, 297–313.

Florentino, J.L., Arao, R.M., Garfin, A.M., Gaviola, D.M., Tan, C.R., Yadav, R.P., Hiatt, T., Morishita, F., Siroka, A., Yamanaka, T., & Nishikiori, N. (2022). Expansion of social protection is necessary towards zero catastrophic costs due to TB: The first national TB patient cost survey in the Philippines. *PLOS ONE*, 17(2). https://doi.org/10.1371/journal.pone.0264689.

Hargreaves, J., Boccia, D., Evans, C., Adato, M., Petticrew, M., & Porter, J. (2011). The social determinants of tuberculosis: From evidence to action. *American Journal of Public Health*, 101(4), 654–662.

Hotez, P.J., Tiwari, H., Bandyopadhyay, A.S., & Fasce, R. (2021). Tuberculosis in the time of COVID-19: Challenges and opportunities. *Journal of Infection*, 103(1), 1–3. https://doi.org/10.2471%2FBLT.21.286807.

Jain, S., Rocha, I.C.N., Maheshwari, C., dos Santos Costa, A.C., Tsagkaris, C., Aborode, A.T., Essar, M.Y., & Ahmad, S., (2021). Chikungunya and COVID-19 in Brazil: The danger of an overlapping crisis. *Journal of Medical Virology*, 93(7), 4090.

Khatri, G., Hasan, M.M., Shaikh, S., Mir, S.L., Sahito, A.M., Rocha, I.C.N., & Elmahi, O.K.O. (2022). The simultaneous crises of dengue and COVID-19 in

Pakistan: A double hazard for the country's debilitated healthcare system. *Tropical Medicine and Health*, 50(1), 1–5.

Kuddus, M.A., Tynan, E., & McBryde, E. (2020). Urbanization: A problem for the rich and the poor? *Public Health Reviews*, 41(1). https://doi.org/10.1186/s40985-019-0116-0.

Lakner, C., Yonzan, N., Mahler, D., Aguilar, D., & Wu, H. (2021). Updated estimates of the impact of COVID-19 on global poverty: Looking back at 2020 and the outlook for 2021. *World Bank*. https://blogs.worldbank.org/opendata/updated-estimates-impact-covid-19-global-poverty-looking-back-2020-and-outlook-2021.

McQuaid, C.F., Henrion, M.Y.R., Burke, R.M., MacPherson, P., Nzawa-Soko, R., & Horton, K.C. (2022). Inequalities in the impact of COVID-19-associated disruptions on tuberculosis diagnosis by age and sex in 45 high TB burden countries. *BMC Medicine*, 20(1), 432. https://doi.org/10.1186/s12916-022-02624-6.

Miranda, A.V., Wiyono, L., Rocha, I.C.N., Cedeño, T.D.D., & Lucero-Prisno III, D.E. (2021). Strengthening virology research in the Association of Southeast Asian Nations: Preparing for future pandemics. *American Journal of Tropical Medicine and Hygiene*, 105(5), 1141.

Official Gazette of the Philippines. (1996). Proclamation No. 840, s. 1996. https://www.officialgazette.gov.ph/1996/07/30/proclamation-no-840-s-1996/.

Oliver, T.R. (2006). The politics of public health policy. *Annual Review of Public Health*, 27, 195–233. https://doi.org/10.1146/annurev.publhealth.25.101802.123126.

Querri, A., Ohkado, A., Yoshimatsu, S., Coprada, L., Lopez, E., Medina, A., Garfin, A., Bermejo, J., Tang, F., & Shimouchi, A. (2017). Enhancing tuberculosis patient detection and care through community volunteers in the urban poor, the Philippines. *Public Health Action*, 7(4), 268–274. https://doi.org/10.5588/pha.17.0036.

Rocha, I.C.N., Hasan, M.M., Goyal, S., Patel, T., Jain, S., Ghosh, A., & Cedeño, T.D.D. (2021). COVID-19 and mucormycosis syndemic: Double health threat to a collapsing healthcare system in India. *Tropical Medicine & International Health*, 26(9), 1016–1018.

Saunders, M.J., & Evans, C.A. (2020). COVID-19, tuberculosis and poverty: Preventing a perfect storm. *The European Respiratory Journal*, 56(1), 2001348. https://doi.org/10.1183/13993003.01348-2020.

Tanchuco, J.Q. (2020). In the shadows of the COVID-19 pandemic. *Acta Medica Philippina*, 54(5). https://doi.org/10.47895/amp.v54i5.2278.

TB/COVID-19 Global Study Group. (2022). Tuberculosis and COVID-19 co-infection: Description of the global cohort. *The European Respiratory Journal*, 59(3), 2102538. https://doi.org/10.1183/13993003.02538-2021.

United Nations. (2020). COVID PULSE PH: Urban poverty in the time of the pandemic. United Nations Development Programme. https://www.undp.org/philippines/publications/covid-pulse-ph-urban-poverty-time-pandemic-0.

Wi, J.A. (2021). Letter from the Philippines. *Respirology*, 26(6), 622–623. https://doi.org/10.1111/resp.14051.

Wiyono, L., Rocha, I.C.N., Cedeño, T.D.D., Miranda, A.V., & Lucero-Prisno III, D.E. (2021). Dengue and COVID-19 infections in the ASEAN region: A concurrent outbreak of viral diseases. *Epidemiology and Health*, 43, 1–5.

World Health Organization. (2020). Impact of COVID-19 on people's livelihoods, their health and our food systems. https://www.who.int/news/item/13-10-2020-impact-of-covid-19-on-people's-livelihoods-their-health-and-our-food-systems.

World Health Organization. (2021a). Tuberculosis and COVID-19. https://www.who.int/teams/global-tuberculosis-programme/covid-19.

World Health Organization. (2021b). Tuberculosis in the Philippines. https://www.who.int/countries/phl/en/.

World Health Organization. (2022a). Global tuberculosis report 2022. https://www.who.int/teams/global-tuberculosis-programme/tb-reports.

World Health Organization. (2022b). Tuberculosis deaths and disease increase during the COVID-19 pandemic. https://www.who.int/news/item/27-10-2022-tuberculosis-deaths-and-disease-increase-during-the-covid-19-pandemic.

World Health Organization. (2022c). Western Pacific regional framework to end TB: 2021–2030: Brief summary. https://www.who.int/westernpacific/publications-detail/WPR-2022-DDC-001.

World Health Organization. (2023). Tuberculosis. https://www.who.int/news-room/fact-sheets/detail/tuberculosis.

Zimmerman, A.J., Klinton, J.S., Oga-Omenka, C., Heitkamp, P., Nyirenda, C.N., Furin, J. & Pai, M. (2021). Tuberculosis in times of COVID-19. *Journal of Epidemiological Community Health*, 76(3), 310–316. https://doi.org/10.1136/jech-2021-217529.

5 "Active in the Community" and "Underlying Health Conditions"

Exploring Constructions of Blame, Responsibility, and Othering associated with Australia's COVID-19 Syndemic

Kate Senior and Richard Chenhall

The fact is that one in two Australians has at least one chronic condition and more than one in five of us are over sixty, so it is a nifty trick to get us all to believe that these people are all somehow 'other.' They are not, they *are* us, and we are all of inestimable value.

(Berger, 2021, italics in original)

The COVID-19 pandemic in Australia, as in many other countries, exposed the inequalities in the healthcare system, particularly the gaps between urban, regional, and remote settings, gaps between high and low socio-economic groups, gaps between Indigenous and non-Indigenous populations, and gaps between abled and disabled people. It is in these groups, not the Australian population, where COVID-19 had the potential to become a syndemic, demonstrating the characteristics of syndemics of being localized to regions or populations (Mendenhall, 2020; Singer et al., 2022). In Australia, these groups are characterized by high levels of co-morbidities often combined with negative social, structural, and behavioral factors influencing health and well-being.

In his analysis of the Australian outbreak, Duckett (2022, p. 1) reports that there were "over 140 deaths per 100,000 population in the poorest socio-economic quintile compared to 40 in the wealthiest quintile." This disparity became more acute in the older populations. Vaccination status also remained uneven throughout the pandemic (Duckett, 2022), with the most affluent suburbs of the north shore of Sydney reaching a 90% vaccination rate by mid-October 2021, while the mining town of Cessnock near Newcastle had only reached 58%. Furthermore, although the state of New South Wales reached its vaccination target of 80% double dose by mid-October 2021, double vaccination status was highly variable across the state, as vaccines were diverted from regional areas to the cities when they became available

DOI: 10.4324/9781003365358-6

(McPhee, 2021). Finally, access to treatment for symptoms associated with Long COVID has remained highly restricted. In 2023, dedicated Long COVID clinics are available only in the major metropolitan centers, with extremely long waiting lists. An Australian Government State by State guide to resources explains: "local services may be available. Check the website for your local health department to find services" (Australian Government, 2022). In all cases, except Sydney, New South Wales; Canberra, Australian Capital Territory; Melbourne, Victoria; and more recently Adelaide, South Australia, which have specialist clinics, people with Long COVID are directed back to their general practitioner.

By October 2021, lockdown restrictions were eased, children returned to school and people in the two most populous states in Australia faced a new normality of learning to "live with COVID-19." However, as Berger (2021) pointed out, the policy was not "living safely with COVID-19." Residents were warned, however, that the price of freedom would be spikes of the disease and resultant hospitalizations and deaths from COVID-19. These long-anticipated freedoms for many should be seen in the context of the threat that they represented to others. For example, people in aged care facilities were most adversely affected by a surge in cases during January 2023 (Belot, 2023). As Australia approached the winter months in 2023, the number of COVID-19 cases began to rise again. By April 2023, there were still an average of 3,641 cases per day, but deaths had dropped from a peak of 55 per day to 3 per day (Australian Government, 2023). The most recent weekly data for New South Wales (11–18 May 2023) Health indicated 14,699 cases, 1,322 people in hospital, and 61 deaths. In addition, there have been several school closures and extensive outbreaks through juvenile and adult detention centers (NSW Health, 2023). Despite this, COVID-19 is now rarely a topic of media attention. The World Health Organization (WHO) has issued a statement indicating that COVID-19 is no longer an emergency of international concern and should instead be considered an "established and ongoing health issue." Yet, COVID-19 continues to be a significant cause for concern for the most vulnerable people in the Australian population.

In this chapter, we examine the public construction and messaging about COVID-19 risk and responsibility in Australia, specifically messaging that justifies the deaths of people with chronic diseases, the old, fragile, disabled, and socially vulnerable as an acceptable loss for the price of freedom. We explore how this messaging, perhaps inadvertently, has reinforced the impact of COVID-19 as a syndemic (Singer et al., 2017), as repeated exposure to messages about people dying with "underlying health conditions" has created additional fear and distress among already at-risk populations. Stress, engendered by victim blaming and fear, compounded with effects of social isolation, stigma, poverty, and uncertainty have profound negative effects on both physical and mental health (Brunner & Marmot, 1999; Burbank, 2011). As Berger (2021) points out, Australians were quick to see people at risk of COVID-19 as being 'the other,' thus effectively distancing them from their own concerns.

COVID-19 Arrives in Australia

As COVID-19 entered Australia, it was a disease associated with globalization and affluence. Although the first cases of COVID-19 entered via air travel, one phenomenon, the relatively affordable cruise ship holiday, was uniquely associated with the rapid transmission and spread of the disease. In March 2020, a week after the global pandemic had been declared by the WHO, the *Ruby Princess* cruise ship was allowed to dock and discharge 2,700 passengers in Sydney without testing them. Those passengers then traveled to their homes across Australia and internationally (Mao, 2020) beginning an outbreak of the disease, which ultimately killed 28 people.

Waves of the disease that followed were directly associated with working conditions. Of the first spikes in the disease in May 2020, two industries stood out: a meat-processing factory and a series of aged care homes. As this work is often seen as undesirable for Australian nationals, both sectors rely on a casual workforce with high numbers of migrant workers, often on temporary long-stay visas, who may have limited capacity to understand or implement workplace practices that would protect their own health (Boseley, 2020a,b). Additional commonalities across these workplaces that increase communicable disease risk include low socioeconomic status and language barriers, heavy workloads, high-stress environments, stigma associated with work (Marshall, 2018), discrimination/racism, enclosed and close workplaces, and high staff turnover. Furthermore, when economic desperation is combined with no provision for sick leave, the decision to stay at work when feeling unwell (and particularly with very mild symptoms) becomes much easier to understand.

The interaction of these factors was clear in *The Guardian* newspaper's report of an outbreak at Cedar Meats, an abattoir and meat packing factory in Melbourne, Victoria, which was implicated in the beginning of the first wave of the disease in the state. Workers in the processing facility worked long shifts of ten to 12 hours a day, in close proximity, and for little pay. The low wages meant that workers also often shared houses. Workers at the plant reported a range of symptoms but were sent away from testing facilities because they did not display the correct symptoms. The COVID-19 outbreak was not diagnosed until a worker tested positive after attending a hospital for a workplace injury. The company allowed workers to continue working for several days after testing positive, on advice from the Department of Health and Human Services (Boseley, 2020a). As reported in *The Guardian*, workers from non-English-speaking backgrounds reported feeling powerless to question management, stating: "I don't speak English very well...I just stay silent and work...we just come to the factory and go home. Everything they tell us to do, we don't say no" (Boseley, 2020b). Workers also reported that they were afraid of losing their jobs if they got sick and had to stay home (Boseley, 2020a). These factors became the focus of a Worksafe Victoria investigation for which the company was cleared of any breaches of the Occupational Health and Safety Act (SBS Australia, 2020). As reported by

The Age newspaper, the failures were related to advice provided by the Department of Health and Human Services (Cunningham, 2020).

This outbreak occurred at a stage when COVID-19 was still an emergent disease and clarity about the prescribed courses of action was lacking at state and national levels. However, this outbreak and many others resulted from a combination of structural factors associated with a politically, socially, and economically marginalized workforce. COVID-19 in Australia, as elsewhere across the world, exposed the gaps in health between high- and low-socioeconomic groups. Access to vaccines, tests, ability to isolate within the home, and paid COVID-19 leave are key structural determinants of COVID-19. Despite this, media coverage on the pandemic tended to link blame with the characteristics of the individuals infected. In the case of the Cedar Meats outbreak, workers and certain characteristics of workers were highlighted by the media, rather than the actions of the company or the failure of the Department of Health and Human Services to offer prompt and effective guidance. The *Sydney Morning Herald* reported that "the majority of Cedar meats workers who tested positive for COVID-19 worked in the packing area and were of Indian, Pakistani and Bangladeshi backgrounds" (Barker et al., 2020). In the next section, we examine how public health messaging and the media constructed blame and consequently increased risk in already vulnerable populations.

Public Health Messaging and the Media

In retrospect, it seems quite extraordinary that something that became a daily feature of our lives – the WHO public health briefing – occurred for the first time in history on February 5, 2020 (Smith et al., 2020). In Australia, these briefings were accompanied by daily updates by State Premiers, which contained information about the number of cases, number of deaths, hot spots for infection, as well as public health information about COVID-19 safe practices. As Islam et al. (2020) points out, this messaging simultaneously provided important and positive messages about safety precautions, including the use of personal protective equipment and hand washing, but also raised fear among the population. These official sources of information were accompanied by unofficial information circulated through social media, resulting in what Islam et al. (2020, p. 1621) describes as an infodemic, "an overabundance of information – some accurate and some not – that makes it hard for people to find trustworthy sources and reliable guidance when they need it."

A detrimental outcome of information overload was the creation of stigma for people who were diseased or who were considered potentially at risk of contracting COVID-19 and spreading it due to their circumstances. In Australia, this was highlighted in the early stages of the disease by detailed descriptions of the individuals and circumstances of the people who inadvertently spread the disease, from students attending parties to migrant workers employed in the casual workforce associated with aged care, and interstate removalists spreading COVID-19 from one state to another. Smethurst's (2022) writing in the Melbourne Newspaper, *The Age*, provides an example of this kind of messaging:

> Last year's deadly second wave in Melbourne was initially blamed on security guards who shared a cigarette lighter while huddled outside a quarantine hotel on Swanston Street. In doing some the men were said to have committed 'unacceptable breaches' along with car-pooling to work which contributed to the second wave.

COVID-19 deaths were always presented in terms of the person's age and their vaccination status with the attempt being to make associations between natural risk (the elderly) and chosen risk (vaccination status). In aged care settings, COVID-19 deaths were explained as "being below or within the expected range" in the sense that older people's deaths were not in any way extraordinary. The Australian Government Department of Health (2022) stated that "Over the course of the pandemic all-cause mortality in residential aged care was below expected numbers in 2020 and within the expected range in 2021."

In reporting COVID-19 deaths of young people, or double vaccinated people, a new phrase crept into the daily vernacular; the deaths of these people could be explained because they had "underlying health conditions" (Berger, 2021). People living with chronic diseases and disabilities were highly vulnerable to COVID-19. In addition to biological risks, as described elsewhere in this volume, reduced access to essential health services, reduced social connections, and reliance on care workers whose vaccination status was not mandated until November 2021 (NDIS, 2021) well after vaccination became mandatory for aged care workers (National Disability Practitioners, 2021), and difficulty understanding and complying with complex and rapidly changing public health information (Shakespeare et al., 2021), all contributed to higher risk for COVID-19 morbidity and mortality. These factors were exacerbated by the very slow rollout of the vaccine (Duckett, 2022). Bik-Multanowska and colleagues (2022, p. 2), in their study of Australian parents with chronic disease, found that these factors combined to cause serious mental distress:

> Parents with a chronic health condition may be disproportionately affected and have a heightened risk for worse mental health outcomes due to layering of risks of being a parent during the pandemic and having a chronic health condition, each associated with its own stressors and risks for developing negative mental health outcomes.

However, in every press conference and every media release about COVID-19 fatalities, people with chronic diseases and disabilities received the message that their lives were not as valuable through the reiteration of the justification of deaths being due to "underlying health conditions." As such, by 2021, disability organizations in Australia condemned the use of the words "underlying health conditions" with Stephen Duckett commenting in his support of the statement released by Disability People's Australia.

> it is more or less dismissing the importance of that death and excusing the death because they had an underlying condition. It is about (The Government) trying to avoid accountability for the failure of managing the pandemic or the failures of managing vaccine rollout by saying that this death, although it occurred, isn't a really important death.
>
> (Hall, 2021)

In addition to local public health and media portrayals as some deaths being less important than others, across the world, guidelines were being developed to maximize benefit in medical rationing and transparent decision-making based on maximum benefit (Moosa & Luyckx, 2021). As Italy became overwhelmed by the number of cases, they were forced to allocate intensive care and ventilation only to those patients who had the best chance of survival, usually young, healthy people (Emanuel et al., 2020). By April, the same scenario played out in India as cases surged (GRID COVID-19 Study group, 2020). In the UK, Chen and McNamara (2020, p. 515) documented a rise in "do not resuscitate orders for people with disabilities" and commented that "it is likely that persons with a disability experienced heightened rates of anxiety owing to the narrative that they would be prevented from accessing treatment due to scarce medical resources."

Considering this, concerns mounted that people with chronic diseases or disability would not be afforded the same level of care or would be subjected to discrimination regarding their access to medical treatment. The peak bodies for people with disabilities commissioned the production of a Statement of Concern. A key concern was that "people with a disability should not be arbitrarily denied health care and medical treatment based on impairment" (PWD Australia, 2020, p. 3). In addition to the compounding health effects of reduced access to care and essential support, COVID-19 and the government response to it resulted in significant distress for people living with chronic diseases and/or disabilities as they internalized messages about their life being of lesser value and fear that they might be denied lifesaving treatment.

As Smith and colleagues (2023, p. 14) comment, "Exposure to communications (e.g., vignettes, media) that frames a group in a particular way fosters danger appraisal which leads to public stigma." Stigma, in turn, contributes to stress, which further contributes to both susceptibility of disease and the potential of serious outcomes (Smith et al., 2023). The stigmatization and potential ostracization of people with COVID-19 or at risk of COVID-19 is mediated by power. Smith and colleagues described danger appraisal as a key response to COVID-19 messaging and found that "community members who identified as white, cisgender and heterosexual consistently reported high levels of danger appraisal than those who identified with racial/ethnic, gender and or sexual orientation minority groups" (Smith, 2020, p. 17). In other words, people who are already othered by the dominant society are further marginalized by that societies' assessment of the risk the group poses to their own health and well-being.

Yet the rhetoric in public health messaging and the media remained one of individual responsibility and blame. People who unknowingly spread the disease are described as being "active in the community" without any inter-rogation of the time between being notified of exposure, test results, and the pressure to continue working. And those who died without being in the morally justified categories of the fragile elderly or the unvaccinated were justified based on existing risks due to "underlying health conditions." This choice in rhetoric accomplished two things. First, it created a sense of dis-tancing, of othering, to rationalize that the needs of the few (those at risk and benefiting most from lockdowns, social distancing, and mask mandates) should not hinder the freedoms and economic prosperity of the many. Sec-ond, as commentators have pointed out, the strategy deflected blame away from inadequate government responses to the pandemic (Smethurst, 2022).

Indigenous Australians and COVID-19: The Case of Wilcannia

Existing social inequities, failure of government response, and a rhetoric of blame compounded to create a syndemic of COVID-19 in Australia's most marginalized communities. Worldwide, Indigenous communities were dis-proportionately affected by COVID-19, with significantly higher proportions of cases in populations and higher death rates (Khanlou et al., 2022) due to the interplay of existing diseases and the social determinants of health and structural racism within health services and systems (Shim & Starks, 2021).

Indigenous Australians were at high risk of COVID-19 due to high exist-ing levels of chronic disease in the community (Finlay & Wenitong, 2020). As Yashadhana and colleagues (2020) explain that 15.6% of Indigenous Australians have three or more chronic conditions, compared to 7.6% of non-Indigenous Australians. These rates are highest in remote communi-ties, where chronic disease is exacerbated by a range of social determinants, such as poor access to health services, access to water and sanitation, lack of food security, and overcrowded housing. Similarly, Fitts and colleagues (2020) point out, many houses lacked the "health hardware" in terms of ac-cess to sinks, soap, and running water to practice COVID-19 safe hygiene. For example, the 2015 Census revealed that 40% of households in central Northern Territory and 20% in the North did not have access to functioning facilities for food preparation. Up to 40% of people in Central Australia did not have access to functioning facilities for washing people (Foster & Hall, 2021). Furthermore, overcrowded houses provide little opportunity for so-cial distancing and intergenerational families in one house also contributed to high levels of risk for older people. Being confined to a house also meant it was difficult for people to escape domestic violence situations and stresses engendered by drug and alcohol misuse. In addition, as Finlay and Wenitong (2020) argue, despite the vulnerability of the Indigenous population, very little public health material was specifically developed for them.

Despite theoretically high risk due to factors such as pre-existing comorbidities and higher levels of smoking and overcrowded housing, as a population group, Indigenous Australians did not experience disproportionately higher levels of COVID-19. Remote communities in Australia were initially protected by their isolation. Other communities in remote areas of Australia moved quickly to close off their townships from outsiders. Strong responses from Indigenous community-controlled health services managed COVID-19 exposure and risk within these contained communities (Crooks et al., 2020). Health leaders and Aboriginal community-controlled services lobbied for the dissemination of appropriate health information, increased testing and contract tracing, and strategies for housing the homeless, training safely and protecting their elders (see Eades et al., 2020). Nevertheless, the pandemic had important effects on the provision of health services in these communities where there is a heavy reliance on fly-in fly-out agency nurses and locum doctors (Fitts et al., 2020), which were not operating during COVID-19 lockdowns. The long-term impacts of this rupture in the continuity of care may yet to be realized. Furthermore, vaccine hesitancy was widespread in Indigenous communities, particularly remote communities, due to the inconsistencies of the national vaccine roll-out and the failure of health promotion to counter anti-vaccination messages (Reilly et al., 2021).

The Case of Wilcannia

Despite the efforts by Aboriginal community-controlled services, local COVID-19 syndemics did emerge in select communities where the ability to protect their most vulnerable was compromised. The developing syndemic in the small rural town of Wilcannia revealed the institutional racism embedded in policymaking towards Indigenous people, which put economic priorities associated with tourism and transport above the needs of the town. Wilcannia recorded the highest rates of transmission of the disease in New South Wales, with one-third of the town's population of 720 affected (Allam, 2021).

The situation in Wilcannia was, however, something that should have been expected and planned for, given its location on the Barrier Highway which connects New South Wales to South Australia and experiences high levels of poverty. The vulnerability of the community had been communicated in detail by the Maari Ma Aboriginal Health Organization in 2020 (Green, 2021). Efforts by the community to lockdown, so they were not exposed to the virus by visiting tourists, were not supported as the highway remained an important transport corridor. Wilcannia residents resorted to making their own signs warning "it is too dangerous to stop in Wilcannia" (Wahlquist, 2021). Yet, the danger was not for the tourists but for the resident population living in circumstances that made them vulnerable. Ironically, tourist posts on grey nomad websites provided the same message of risk for years, although tourists saw the danger stemming from the resident population of Indigenous people. The media reported with incredulity that people in Wilcannia did not have the capacity to physically distance themselves and that mobile homes were being relocated to the area to counter the effects of overcrowded homes (Gooley, 2021). Khanlou and colleagues (2022) put that the experience of racism is a systemic risk factor with strong influences on both physical and mental health (Paradies, 2007).

The effects of COVID-19 were further exacerbated by police and army personnel undertaking door-to-door compliance checks of the community, to ensure that people were isolated in their homes. People who either had COVID-19 or were at high risk of COVID-19 were removed from their homes in police vans to hospital or isolation units (Green, 2021). As Green (2021, p. 1), reporting in *The Conversation*, observed:

> Aboriginal people with mental illness or disorders, who require regular treatment and medication being picked up in police vans [rather than ambulances] and taken to hospital because they "may have COVID-19." The people of Wilcannia told me this was because police vans are "easier" to clean.

Wilcannia also has a history of over-policing and surveillance, reflective of the poor relationships between Indigenous people and the police throughout Australia (Cunneen, 2020). For example, in 1995 the town had a population of 1,000 people (800 Indigenous) and 11 police, which Cunneen and Libesman (1995, p. 9) describe as "a police population ratio nearly six times that of the State as a whole." In addition, the Barkindji people of the region have memories of forced removals of family members from what were unsuitable living conditions to the Missions (sometimes hundreds of kilometers away) by the Aborigines Protection Board (Hardy, 1976). The stress engendered by the increased surveillance and removal of people from their homes during the COVID-19 pandemic cannot be underestimated in the context of this history.

For Indigenous people in Wilcannia and elsewhere in Australia, specific COVID-19 syndemics emerged related to pre-existing health conditions, reduced continuity of care, stress, and mental health issues caused by the uncertainty and confusion caused by the pandemic and pandemic-related responses, the inability to move away from dangerous situations such as crowded living situations, and heightened surveillance by police. All these factors are underpinned by institutionalized racism, exposed in areas of greatest tension.

Conclusion

Medical anthropologists cautiously suggested not to consider the COVID-19 pandemic a global syndemic (Mendenhall, 2020; Singer et al., 2022), because the clustering of political and social factors which may negatively influence disease comorbidities and their outcomes vary across the globe. These factors were also variable within countries, as the situation in Australia highlighted. The most vulnerable people were those who were marginalized and positioned as being the 'other.'

COVID-19 made the inequalities in health across Australia visible and manifest in everyday decision-making. From vaccination rates to death rates, the impacts were greatest in the most socio-economically marginal groups; people from ethnic minorities, older people, people with disabilities, and Indigenous people, particularly those living in remote communities. As everywhere, COVID-19 compounded the effects of pre-existing health issues by reducing access to services and creating new problems caused by anxiety and social isolation, financial instability, and stigma.

The COVID-19 syndemic experienced by people with disabilities and chronic diseases and people in aged care settings needs also to be considered including the mental health effects of chronic stress and the stigma of living a life that was continually reinforced as being less valuable than other members of society (People with Disabilities Australia, 2020, 2021). For Indigenous Australians, the COVID-19 syndemic is underpinned by a particular kind of stress that is caused by the intergenerational effects of racism, combined with the continuing health and well-being effects of the social determinants of health, such as overcrowded housing.

The experience of the COVID-19 syndemics among marginalized population groups brings the impact of the interplay of the social determinants of health and diseases or health conditions into sharp focus. For some people in Australia, these effects were compounded by structural racism, stigma, and othering that had been simmering beneath the surface, but arose during periods of heightened tension, flamed by both media stories and government attempts to shift blame.

References

Allam, L. (2021). Willcania Covid Crisis: Government.

Australian Government Department of Health. (2022). Getting help for long Covid. https://www.health.gov.au/sites/default/files/documents/2022/11/getting-help-for-long-covid_0.pdf.

Australian Government Department of Health and Aged Care (2023). Covid-19 Reporting, https://www.health.gov.au/topics/covid-19/reporting

Belot, H. (2023). Deaths from covid in Australia's aged care pass 5000 after monthly fatalities double in January. *The Guardian*. https://www.theguardian.com/australia-news/2023/feb/03/deaths-from-covid-in-australian-aged-care-pass-5000-after-monthly-fatalities-double-in-january.

Barker, R., Fowler, M., & Dow, A. (2020). "We all eat together" Cedar Meat workers tells of fear and uncertainty. *The Sydney Morning Herald*, 6th May, 2020. https://www.smh.com.au/business/workplace/we-all-eat-together-cedar-meats-worker-tells-of-fear-and-uncertainty-20200506-p54qhq.html.

Berger, D. (2021). Opinion: underlying health conditions? That's almost all of us. *Sydney Morning Herald*, September 7. https://www.smh.com.au/national/underlying-health-conditions-that-s-almost-all-of-us-20210904-p58otg.html.

Bik-Multanowska, K., Mikocka-Walus, A., Fernando, J., & Westrupp, E. (2022). Mental distress of parents with chronic diseases during the COVID-19 pandemic in Australia: a prospective cohort study. *Journal of Psychosomatic Research*, 152. https://doi.org/10.1016/j.jpsychores.2021.110688.

Brunner, E., & Marmot, M. (1999). Social organisation, stress and health. In *Social Determinants of Health*, eds. E. Brunner, & M. Marmot. Oxford: Oxford University Press, pp. 17–23.

Boseley, M. (2020a). Cedar Meats knew of two coronavirus cases for several days before telling meatworks staff they could stay home. *The Guardian*, 8th May, 2020. https://www.theguardian.com/world/2020/may/08/cedar-meats-knew-of-two-covid-19-cases-for-several-days-before-telling-staff-they-could-stay-home#:~:text=3%20.

Boseley, M. (2020b). Worksafe investigates coronavirus cluster at Cedar Meats as workers speak out. *The Guardian*, 13th May, 2020. https://www.theguardian.com/australia-news/2020/may/13/worksafe-investigates-coronavirus-cluster-at-cedar-meats-as-workers-speak-out.

Burbank, V. (2011). *An Ethnography of Stress, the Social Determinants of Health in Aboriginal Australia*. New York: Palgrave Macmillan.

Chen, B., & McNamara, D.M. (2020). Disability discrimination, medical rationing and COVID-19. *Asian Bioethics Review*, 12, 511–518.

Crooks, K., Casey, D., & Ward J.S. (2020). First Nations people leading the way in COVID-19 pandemic planning, response and management. *Medical Journal of Australia*, 213(4), 151–152.

Cunneen, C. (2020). *Conflict, Politics and Crime: Aboriginal Communities and the Police*. Abingdon: Routledge.

Cunneen, C., & Libesman, T. (1995). *Indigenous People and the Law in Australia*. Sydney: Butterworths Legal Studies Series.

Cunningham, M. (2020). COVID-positive Cedar Meats worker was turned away from testing twice: inquiry. *The Age*, 18th November, 2020. https://www.theage.com.au/national/victoria/parliamentary-inquiry-into-contact-tracing-to-hear-from-chief-scientist-cedar-meats-20201118-p56fjv.html.

Duckett, S. (2022). Public health management of the COVID-19 pandemic in Australia: the role of the Morrison Government. *International Journal of Environmental Research and Public Health*, 19. https://doi.org/10.3390/ijerph191610400.

Eades, S., Eades, D., McCaullay, L., Nelson, P., Phelan, P. & Stanley, F. (2023). Australias Fisrt Nations'response to the Covid-19 pandemic, *The Lancet*, 396 (10246), 237–238.

Emanuel, E.J., Persad, G., Upshur, R., Thome, B., Parker, M., Glickman, A., Zhang, B.A., Boyle, C., Smith, M., & Phillips, J.P. (2020). Fair allocation of scare medical resources in the time of COVID-19. *New England Journal of Medicine*, 382, 2049–2055.

Fitts, M.S., Russell, D., Mathew, S., Liddle, Z., Mulholland, E., Comerford, C., & Wakerman, J. (2020). Remote health service vulnerabilities and responses to the COVID-19 pandemic. *Australian Journal of Rural Health*, 28, 613–617. https://doi.org/10.1111/ajr.12672.

Finlay, S., & Wenitong, M. (2020). Aboriginal community-controlled health organisations are taking a leading role in Covid-19 communication. *Australia and New Zealand Journal of Public Health*, 44(4), 251–251. https://doi.org/10.1111/1753-6405.13010.

Foster, T., & Hall, N.L. (2021). Housing conditions and health in Indigenous Australian communities: current status and recent trends. *International Journal of Environmental Health Research*, 31(3), 325–343.

Green, S. (2021). COVID in Wilcannia: a national disgrace we all saw coming. *The Conversation*. https://researchoutput.csu.edu.au/ws/portalfiles/portal/197605401/169118625_published_article.pdf.

Gooley, C, 2021, 'Humanitatian crisis' in Wilcannia as NSW considers extra quarantine, *The Sydney Morning Herald*, September 1, 2021.

GRID COVID-19 Study Group. (2020). Combating the COVID-19 pandemic in a resource-constrained setting: insights from initial response in India. *BMJ Global Health*, 5, e003416.

Hall, A. (2021). Disability advocates criticise use of 'underlying health conditions' in Covid-19 death reporting. *SBS News*. https://www.sbs.com.au/news/article/disability-advocates-criticise-use-of-underlying-health-conditions-in-covid-19-death-reporting/3nyyt97zk.

Hardy, B. (1976). *Lament for the Barkindji, the Vanished Tribes of the Darling River Region*. Adelaide: Rigby.

Islam, M.S., Sarkar, T., Khan, S.H., Mostofa Kamal, A.H., Hasan, S.M.M., Kabir, A., Yeasmin, D., Islam, M.A., Amin Chowdhury, K.I., Anwar, K.S., Chughtai, A.A., & Seale, H. (2020). COVID-19-related infodemic and its impact on public health: a global social media analysis. *American Journal of Tropical Medicine and Hygiene*, 103(4), 1621–1629. https://doi.org/10.4269/ajtmh.20-0812.

Khanlou, N., Vazquez, L.M., Pashang, S., Connolly, J.A., Ahmad, F., & Ssawe, A. (2022). 2020 syndemic: convergence of COVID-19, gender-based violence and racism pandemics. *Journal of Racial and Ethnic Health Disparities*, 9, 2077–2089. https://doi.org/10.1007/s40615-021-01146-w.

Marshall, A, 2018, Abattoir jobs aplenty but regional workers are spare, *Farm Weekly* May 22, 2018.

Mao, F. (2020). Coronavirus: how did Australia's Ruby Princess cruise debacle happen? *BBC News*, 24th March, 2020. https://www.bbc.com/news/world-australia-51999845.

McPhee, S. (2021). Shock and disappointment: regions left confused after Pfizer dose diverted. *The Sydney Morning Herald*. https://www.smh.com.au/national/nsw/shock-and-disappointment-regions-left-confused-after-pfizer-doses-diverted-20210731-p58enk.html.

Mendenhall, E. (2020). The Covid-19 syndemic is not global: context matters. *The Lancet*, 396(10264), 1731.

Moosa, M.R., & Luyckx, V.A. (2021). The realities of rationing in health care. *Nature Reviews. Nephrology*, 17(7), 435–436. https://doi.org/10.1038/s41581-021-00404-8.

National Disability Practitioners. (2021). COVID vaccination not to be mandated for disability support workers. https://www.ndp.org.au/in-the-news/latest-news/covid-vaccination-not-to-be-mandated-for-disability-support-workers.

NDIS Quality and Safeguards Commission. (2021). Public health orders. https://www.ndiscommission.gov.au/resources/covid-19-resources-and-information/worker-vaccination.

NSW Government Health. (2023). Locally acquired COVID-19 cases - up to 4pm 6 July 2023. https://www.health.nsw.gov.au/Infectious/covid-19/Pages/stats-local.aspx.

Paradies, Y. (2007). Racism. In *Social Determinants of Indigenous Health*, eds. B. Carson, T. Dunbar, R.D. Chenhall, & R. Bailie. Crows Nest: Allen and Unwin, pp. 65–86.

People with a Disability Australia. (2020). Covid 19, human rights, disability and ethical decision making statement of concern. https://dpoa.org.au/wp-content/uploads/2020/04/Statement-of-Concern-COVID-19-Human-rights-disability-and-ethical-decision-making_Final.pdf.

People with Disability Australia. (2021). Disability advocates condemn use of 'underlying health conditions' as COVID death explainer. https://pwd.org.au/disability-advocates-condemn-use-of-underlying-health-conditions-as-covid-death-explainer/.

Reilly, L, Adams, M and Rees, S. J, 2021, The intensifying thrat of COVID-19 among First Nations people of Australia: making up for lost time, JAMA Health Forum, 2 (12).

SBS Australia. (2020). Cedar Meats abattoir at the centre, of Victoria's largest first wave coronavirus outbreak cleared in probe. *SBS News*, 15th December, 2020. https://www.sbs.com.au/news/article/cedar-meats-abattoir-at-centre-of-victorias-largest-first-wave-coronavirus-outbreak-cleared-in-probe/yrozpho09.

Shakespeare, T.O., Ndagire, F., & Seketi, Q.E. (2021). Triple Jeopardy: disabled people and the Covid 19 pandemic. *The Lancet*, 397, 1331–1333.

Shim, R.S., & Starks, S.M. (2021). COVID-19, structural racism and mental health inequities: policy implications of an emerging syndemic. *Psychiatric Services*, 72(10), 1193–1196. https://doi.org/10.1176/appi.ps.202000725.

Singer, M., Bulled, N., & Leatherman T. (2022). Are there global syndemics? *Medical Anthropology*, 41(1), 4–18. https://doi.org/10.1080/01459740.2021.2007907.

Singer, M., Bulled, N., Ostrach, B., & Mendenhall, E. (2017). Syndemics and the biosocial conception of health. *The Lancet*, 389, 941–950.

Smethurst, A. (2022). Blaming individuals for spreading covid lets governments off the hook. *The Age*, 29th July, 2021. https://www.theage.com.au/politics/victoria/blaming-individuals-for-spreading-covid-lets-government-off-the-hook-20210729-p58e4w.html.

Smith, J. A & Judd, J, 2020, Vulnerability and the power of privilege in a pandemic. *Health Promotion Journal of Australia*, 31 (2), 158–160.

Smith, R. A., Zhu, X., Martin, M. A., Myrick, J. G., Lennon, R. P., Small, M. L., Van Scoy, L. J., & Data4Action Research Group. (2023). Longitudinal study of an emerging COVID-19 stigma: Media exposure, danger appraisal, and stress. *Stigma and Health,* 8(1), 12–20. https://doi.org/10.1037/sah0000359

Yashadhana, A., Pollard-Wharton, N., Zwi, A.B., & Biles, B. (2020). Indigenous Australians at increased risk of COVID-19 due to existing health and socioeconomic inequities. *The Lancet Regional Health. Western Pacific*, 1, 100007. https://doi.org/10.1016/j.lanwpc.2020.100007.

Wahlquist, C. (2021). 'Scared and angry' warnings ignored before Delta ripped through Wilcannia. *The Guardian*, 10th September, 2021. https://www.theguardian.com/australia-news/2021/sep/11/scared-and-angry-warnings-ignored-before-delta-ripped-through-wilcannia.

6 Understanding the COVID-19 Syndemic in South Africa

Concrete Responses and a Call to Action

Peter van Heusden, Kezia Lewins, Louis Reynolds and Laurel Baldwin-Ragaven

When SARS-CoV-2 reached South Africa in March 2020, its effects reverberated throughout a complex landscape of infectious and non-communicable disease (NCD) burdens, an overstretched public health system, and a political context of entrenched structural violence characterized by inequality and centuries of racialization. The vast majority of South Africans already faced syndemic vulnerability (Singer et al., 2017) before the virus arrived in the country. The pandemic thus became the perfect *syndemic tsunami*, leading to heightened coronavirus transmission rates, exacerbating pre-existing disease states, intensifying adverse social conditions, and burdening an already dysfunctional health system. This resulted in increased morbidity and mortality from COVID-19.

How the COVID-19 pandemic played out within the most unequal society in the world is both tragic and instructive. Barely 25 years into a fledgling democracy, when the pandemic began, South Africa suffered from the consequences of decades of Human Immunodeficiency Virus/Acquired Immunodeficiency Syndrome (HIV/AIDS) mismanagement, which wiped out at least one generation, mass unemployment particularly among the youth, food insecurity, and the effects of climate change. Additionally, essential infrastructure including water, electricity, and housing was collapsing or had never been provided; there was rampant corruption in government and corporate sectors; and, both private and public health systems were victims of distorted servicing priorities and motivations (Competition Commission of South Africa, 2019; Office of Health Standards Compliance, 2018). Thus, even prior to the global COVID-19 pandemic, South Africa was home to a vulnerable population that had been ravaged by multiple "synergistic, interacting epidemics" (Singer et al., 2017).

It is no wonder then that the arrival of SARS-CoV-2 wreaked havoc on South Africa. By February 11 2023, South Africa had over 4 million laboratory-confirmed COVID-19 cases (National Institute for Communicable Diseases, 2023a), with around 104,600 hospital-based deaths recorded up to 2022 (National Institute for Communicable Diseases, 2022). Further, between May 2020 and January 2023, the Medical Research Council estimated

DOI: 10.4324/9781003365358-7

341,123 excess deaths, equivalent to another 573 deaths per 100,000 population over what had been anticipated (Bradshaw et al., 2022).

In this chapter, we describe how the South African state failed in its constitutional mandate to provide universal access to the social determinants of health and to quality healthcare, the resulting interaction of biological and social drivers contributing to a pre-COVID-19 syndemic in South Africa, and how this syndemic and its associated patterns of "organized abandonment" exacerbated the effects of the COVID-19 pandemic. While, as far as we know, the term "organized abandonment" – a way to understand "how the state and capitalist interests devise means to subordinate and render particular groups of people vulnerable to precarity, injury and premature death" (Bhandar, 2018) – has not previously been applied in the South African context, it seems fitting here as it deepens the understanding of syndemic impacts.

We further explore how the country's fraught history determined and continues to determine life chances, and how legacies of colonialism and apartheid still influence peoples' opportunities. We expand on how the antecedent disease burden together with health system failures set the stage for devastating COVID-19 outcomes. Through case summaries, we illustrate the colliding synergies of viral transmission, multimorbidity, and chronic failures to address unmet basic needs. We illuminate the experiences of people with comorbidities whose differential access to healthcare facilities dependent on race and socio-economic status demonstrate how missed opportunities and engineered neglect resulted in unequal and diverse COVID-19 experiences across society's fault lines (Baldwin-Ragaven, 2020). By understanding these contextually specific syndemic pathways, we are able to signpost critical responses and suggest appropriate multi-dimensional interventions.

Historical Background to the Bio-politics of Health in South Africa

The history of South Africa is one of settler-colonialism and is deeply racialized. Notwithstanding the explicit rejection of fixed biologically determined "races" at the advent of the democratic era in the early 1990s, official South African data such as those collected and reported on by Statistics South Africa (StatsSA), the country's national statistical agency, remain stratified by late apartheid-era "population group" categories. In many ways, the post-apartheid government's decision to retain the racialized characterization of multiple outcomes including economics, health, educational status, social conditions, and life chances measurements speaks to the failure of the country to fulfill its constitutional imperatives of redress. The post-apartheid democratic dispensation has largely failed to fundamentally alter most people's lives (Leibbrandt et al., 2012; Noble & Wright, 2013).

While not subscribing to these categorizations other than as social and political constructs, we offer an explanatory note on South African racialized terminology: "Black African" refers to the majority in the country who speak various African languages; "Indian/Asian" to descendants of people from South and South-East Asia who were either brought by the British as indentured laborers or came as traders; "Coloured" to descendants of the indigenous South African Khoi and San people, former slaves from Dutch colonial countries and "mixed-race" descendants of all groups; and "White" to persons of European descent. The use of these labels is both commonplace and highly contentious. We reproduce them here because of their presence throughout the literature we draw on.

The health challenges South Africa faces are historical, political, socio-economic, and environmental (Coovadia et al., 2009a). In the 1980s, the scourge of HIV/AIDS emerged almost unnoticed as the political struggle against apartheid gained momentum and took center stage. This, despite the brutal last-ditch efforts of the (former) Nationalist government to stamp out resistance through states of emergency, mass detentions of anti-apartheid activists, death squads, and targeted assassinations (Laurence, 1990). By the mid-1980s, however, it was clear that apartheid was unsustainable, even as the apartheid regime's repression continued to frustrate attempts at community-level democratic organizing (Marais, 2008, p. 51). The dawn of democracy was close and with it the prospects of a new constitution based on human rights, freedoms, and an integrated national health service that would deliver healthcare according to people's needs rather than based on skin color or means.

After challenging negotiations, the previously banned African National Congress (ANC) was voted into power in the first democratic and free elections in April 1994. Of significance, the ANC Health Plan promised to establish a "single comprehensive, equitable and integrated National Health system" (African National Congress, 1994a) a move cautiously welcomed by the medical establishment (Ncayiyana, 1994, p. 55).

The new government faced enormous historic and spatial impediments from the outset. The country was burdened by massive inequalities after centuries of colonization, racial and gender discrimination, and a highly exploitative migrant labor system that destroyed family and community life (Baldwin-Ragaven et al., 1999). Decades of apartheid firmly entrenched racial, ethnic, and tribal divisions by setting up disparate quasi-independent "homelands" for separate linguistic groups, often in barren tracts of land far from any sustainable economic hubs. In urban areas, Black people had been forcibly removed from desirable properties and relocated to socially and economically marginalized areas on the periphery of cities and towns without basic infrastructure and service provision; and, over time, the rapid and informal expansion of such areas, known as townships or "locations" exacerbated infrastructure deficits (Mbambo & Agbola, 2020). Cynically, "self-government" was offered to these rural "homelands" and urban "Black Local Authorities," ensuring the creation of captive populations subjected to underfunded, poorly functioning, and illegitimate authorities (Turok, 1994).

The burden of disease inherited by democratic South Africa was enormous. The poor and marginalized overwhelmingly carried this, due to the huge wealth disparities and inequitable access to the social determinants of health (Bradshaw et al., 2003). Meanwhile, the existing health system continued to be racially segregated, fragmented between the private and public sectors, and inequitably distributed between urban suburbs, peri-urban slums, informal settlements, and rural areas. The former Bantustans inherited from apartheid each had its own, separately administered, and unequal, health system (de Beer, 1984).

In February 1997, the new human rights-based South African Constitution came into effect, with intentions of redressing inequities and restoring dignity and social justice. When compared to other national constitutions globally, it is almost unique in enshrining socio-economic rights as justiciable rights (Heyns & Brand, 1998). The Bill of Rights in the Constitution encompasses entitlements to healthcare services and education, together with a broad range of other positive claims that address the key social determinants of health. However, these came to be rhetorical promises as social justice took a back seat while a neoliberal macroeconomic policy came to take center stage in the wake of a negotiated settlement, and the formerly broad-based and active civil society were politically demobilized.

It was against this backdrop, nearly 25 years after the democratic vote, when the COVID-19 pandemic arrived in South Africa, that the country had been unable to overcome its colonial and apartheid past. Income inequality was racially skewed and had increased rather than decreased since 1994, to a level that made South Africa the most economically unequal country in the world (International Monetary Fund, 2020; World Bank, 2014). The "face" of such grinding poverty in South Africa remained most often female, Black, rural, and those raising young children (Bittar, 2020; Statistics South Africa, 2018). As flagged in 2017, by the one-time contender for president and ANC stalwart, Dr. Nkosazana Dlamini Zuma, "The face of poverty is feminine especially in South Africa because women suffer triple oppression. We are oppressed because we are poor, Black and female. The triple and persistent challenges of poverty, inequality and unemployment affect women more than they do men" (quoted in Shaban, 2017). This was reiterated five years later by the current president of South Africa Cyril Ramaphosa who emphasized, "The face of poverty in our country is the face of an African woman" (Makhaye, 2022).

Statistics bear out this fact. Black African women are most likely to be unemployed, followed by Black African men, Coloured women, and Coloured men (Statistics South Africa, 2021a). Broad systemic shifts in the South African labor market towards casualized labor and precarious employment (Barchiesi, 2008) negatively affect Black people the most. Such deeply rooted processes of economic exploitation and unfair racialized and gendered discrimination, along with engineered neglect and corruption, have become commonplace in the post-democratic period. These conditions are the hallmark of ongoing structural violence, which Oppong et al. (2015, p. 189) describe as "an arrangement of social institutions in a manner that prevents the realization of human potential, including freedom of choice, high quality of life, and basic survival." Two poignant quotes, one from before and the other after the advent of democracy, convey the continuity of the real struggles for a dignified life in South Africa:

> Township life alone makes it a miracle for anyone to live up to adulthood.
>
> (Biko, 1987)

And:

> The stones in the road sit like kids on the pavement
>   and ask you all the time for a rand
> The wind comes and goes like a man that doesn't worry about his kids...
> The people are stompies [cigarette ends] stuffed into matchboxes.
>
> (Trantraal, 2017)

The extension of healthcare services to the entire population, designed to mitigate the effects of poverty and discrimination, have fallen short of the mark. Despite the post-1994 incorporation of the previously racialized and fragmented public health services into a single national health service under the National Health Department, the South African health system remains vastly inequitable. Although there is a national network of provincially administered tertiary, regional, and district hospitals; community health centers; and primary care clinics established to provide comprehensive public health services, the health system is under-resourced, demoralized, and plagued by high levels of corruption (Cullinan, 2006; Rispel et al., 2016).

Notwithstanding several world-class hospitals in some major cities, the public sector is critically dysfunctional and service delivery remains unequally distributed between urban and rural areas. While receiving less than half the national spending on health, the public health system must provide for 83% of the population, who depend on it for care and who carry the overwhelming share of the disease burden because of poverty. In contrast, the mercenary private healthcare sector (The Competition Commission, 2019; Solanki et al., 2020) accounts for more than half the country's total health expenditure. Of the total health expenditure, 45% comes through health insurance schemes that cover only 17% of the population, while 14% comes from out-of-pocket payments in the private sector by those without health insurance (Ataguba & Akazili, 2010).

Furthermore, the health system remains highly racialized, with Black African (and to a lesser extent Coloured) adults less likely to live within five kilometers of a health facility, less likely to have had a recent health consultation, and more likely to use the overburdened public health system than their White counterparts (McLaren et al., 2014). While there have been attempts to broaden access and provide universal healthcare through a National Health

Insurance (NHI), the NHI Bill languishes in the legislative process without implementation (Parliament of South Africa, 2022). This perfect storm led to an impossible situation in public health terms when SARS-CoV-2 arrived – a true crisis landing on the crises of health bio-politics (Reynolds, 2020).

Co-existing Syndemic Disease Burdens in South Africa

These fundamentally unequal, disparate, and fragmented societal and health system that dominates the post-apartheid health landscape, provide the context for South Africa's *quadruple burden of disease* (Bradshaw et al., 2003). Furthermore, the experience of pre-existing co-occurring infectious and non-communicable diseases (NCDs) cumulatively contribute to current and existing cycles of social, economic, and political disadvantage and marginalization. While we discuss these at individual and community levels, we are cognizant of the intergenerational nature of such circles of biological and social vulnerability.

Aligning with poverty (Statistics South Africa, 2020a), Black African and Coloured population groups bear the brunt of South Africa's quadruple burden of disease: HIV/AIDS and tuberculosis (TB); poor maternal and perinatal health outcomes coupled with malnutrition; violence and injuries; and, an increasing prevalence of NCDs, especially those associated with the nutritional transition, diabetes and hypertension, including chronic kidney disease (CKD) (Pillay-van Wyk et al., 2016). Furthermore, because of the health system inequities discussed, the same people who suffer the quadruple burden remain undiagnosed or untreated and fail to be effectively managed even when connected to a health facility (Husain et al., 2017; Ramkisson et al., 2017). While age has emerged overwhelmingly as the most significant risk factor for severe COVID-19 infection as well as death from the disease globally (US CDC, 2023), the COVID-19 pandemic in South Africa showed a skewed demographic profile of adverse outcomes in younger patients (Phaswana-Mafuya et al., 2021) that likely reflects the quadruple burden.

HIV/AIDS, TB, and Co-infections

The South African HIV/AIDS epidemic burgeoned throughout the 1980s and 1990s, during the critical period of the democratic transition. The government under then-President Thabo Mbeki (1999–2008) refused to accept that HIV caused AIDS and obstructed attempts to institute antiretroviral treatment programs including for the prevention of mother-to-child transmission (Chigwedere et al., 2008). Chigwedere and colleagues (2008, p. 410) estimated that between 2000 and 2005, this refusal resulted in the unnecessary loss of at least 330,000 lives or 2.2 million person-years. The prevalence of HIV/AIDS in the adult population in 2005 was approximately 18.8%, with about 5.5 million South Africans HIV-infected (UNAIDS, 2006).

At the peak of the HIV/AIDS pandemic in 2014/2015, South Africa was reported to have "the highest estimated incidence and prevalence of TB, the second highest number of diagnosed multidrug-resistant (MDR) TB cases, and the largest number of HIV-associated TB cases" (Churchyard et al., 2014, p. 244). Mudzengi and colleagues (2017) found the economic burden and time lost for patients with co-occurring diseases to be "catastrophic" and particularly noted the lack of social and income protection as well as the absence of health service integration. The failure of the state to adequately and appropriately respond to the AIDS crisis wiped out an entire generation of economically active adults and resulted in more than 2 million children younger than 17 years losing one or both parents over this period (Breckenridge et al., 2019, p. 502).

The contested and hard-won rollout of the now largest antiretroviral treatment (ART) program in the world began in 2004 (South African History Online, 2019). In the years since access to these life-saving drugs has steadily blunted the impact of HIV/AIDS on mortality in South Africa. Nonetheless, according to the most recent national survey (Simbayi et al., 2019), HIV infection prevalence remains high, affecting at least 14% of the total population and 16% of Black African people. The highest infection rates (33%) are in women aged 35–39 years, with poverty, gender-based violence, and the low socio-economic status of women driving disparities in infection rates (Mabaso et al., 2019). An estimated 74% of people living with HIV are on ART, with 67% of those achieving viral load suppression. South Africa thus still falls far short of the United Nations Programme on HIV/AIDS (UNAIDS) 95–95–95 targets (UNAIDS, 2022).

One in five people living globally with HIV resides in South Africa (Statistics South Africa, 2021b; UNAIDS, 2021), and 60% have TB as a co-occurring infection (Kalonji & Mahomed, 2019). South Africa's first national tuberculosis prevalence study, conducted between 2017 and 2019 (Department of Health, 2021, p. 17), resulted in an estimated prevalence of 852 cases of pulmonary TB per 100,000 population, substantially higher than previous estimates. However, these too are likely to be undercounted. More than half of patients with confirmed TB infection by GeneXpert had chest X-ray abnormalities but displayed no TB symptoms, suggesting subclinical TB commonly occurs and is responsible for increasing drug resistance (Berhanu et al., 2023; Kendall et al., 2021). Furthermore, the risk of TB infection in South Africa is correlated with a higher body mass index (BMI), alcohol consumption, and belonging to Black African population groups (Maja & Maposa, 2022).

While the co-occurrence of HIV and TB has previously been described as a syndemic (Kwan & Ernst, 2011), in South Africa these diseases occur in the context of persistent malnutrition (Ojo et al., 2022; Singer, 2011), which impacts immune function both directly and indirectly via diseases such as diabetes, along with a social context of persistent inequality, high levels of interpersonal violence and stress (Mendenhall, 2014; Mendenhall et al., 2022). Increasingly, these synergistic interactions of the social and the biological are being joined by an epidemic of non-communicable diseases, which we describe below.

Non-communicable Diseases (NCDs)

With an increasingly urban and poor population, South Africa is undergoing a nutritional transition involving increased consumption of processed foods high in sodium, fat, and sugar (Nnyepi et al., 2015). While overweight and obesity (OWOB) are most prevalent in high-income groups internationally (Goetjes et al., 2021), the South African nutritional transition is driving an increased incidence of OWOB in lower-income groups, paralleling a trend seen in other low- and middle-income countries (Templin et al., 2019).

The second National Burden of Disease Study (NBDS-2), covering the years 1997–2012, showed a marked increase in deaths from diabetes with the disease climbing from the tenth to the sixth leading cause of death (Pillay-van Wyk et al., 2016). Drawing on the South African National Health and Nutrition Examination Survey (SANHANES-1), Stokes and colleagues (2017, p. 1) showed that approximately 10% of the South African population has diabetes (comparable with the United States) with the prevalence of this disease markedly higher (25%) among the Indian population. South Africa lacks a comprehensive diabetes screening program, largely due to budgetary constraints (Voigt, 2021). This contributes to the SANHANES-1's alarming finding that diabetes went undetected, and thus untreated and unmanaged, in 54% of Black African and 38% of Coloured people, compared to only 7% of white and 14% of Indian people (Stokes et al., 2017, p. 8).

Apart from a diagnosis of full-blown diabetes, Pillay-van Wyk and colleagues (2022, p. 601) describe a "public health crisis" of high fasting plasma glucose (FPG), or pre-diabetes. In their study, 30% of the country's population was found to be pre-diabetic (HbA1c between 5.7 and 6.5%), with over-representation in Black African (31%) and Coloured groups (36%). This condition is associated with an increased risk of cardiovascular disease (CVD), chronic kidney disease (CKD), and TB even in non-diabetic individuals. Deaths associated with elevated FPG increased by 32% between 2000 and 2012 (Pillay-van Wyk et al., 2022, p. 597–601).

While much of the medical literature is focused on single diseases, connections must be drawn between hypertension, diabetes, CKD, obesity, and diet – with disease awareness and self-management. In a 2017 study of Cape Town teachers (age 46 ± 8.5 years), CKD was present in 6% and correlated with diabetes and hypertension (Adeniyi et al., 2017). Diabetes is strongly associated with increased BMI (Stokes et al., 2017), while increased vegetable consumption negatively correlates with the risk of weight gain (Nour et al., 2018). However, Black Africans are less likely to consume the WHO-recommended 400g a day of fresh fruit and vegetables, largely for reasons of availability and affordability (Cois et al., 2022; Wilkinson et al., 2003). Global food insecurity, food deserts, and inadequate nutrition have become a reality as the political economy of food production impacts the poor most substantially.

Finally, many of those living with hypertension are unaware that they suffer from the condition. Being Black African, living in informal urban housing (Berry et al., 2017) and poverty (Peer et al., 2021) are all associated with undiagnosed and untreated hypertension. Kapwata et al. (2018) found that poor CVD case management was associated with "a lack of accessible healthcare," within "impoverished municipalities" and among the poorest households, often leading to "increased CVD-related morbidity and mortality" (Kapwata & Manda, 2018, p. 205). The management of chronic diseases, including diabetes and hypertension, requires frequent healthcare visits. In one survey, attending to one's chronic health condition amounted to a catastrophic expense for about a quarter of public healthcare users (Mutyambizi et al., 2019). These social, economic, and political contexts all intersect and manifest as ill health in individuals of specific segments of the population, who are then simultaneously further deprived through inadequate resource and intervention provision at all levels. Adverse economic events such as job loss or stoppage of a social grant are associated with an increase in systolic blood pressure (Gangaidzo et al., 2022), further demonstrating how macro-level political and economic decisions directly impact the physiological and psycho-social aspects of both individual and population health.

The NCD situation in South Africa illustrates not only the implications of a single disease but the knock-on and interacting physiological effects of multiple diseases embedded within the South African social context that both contribute to and are affected by these diseases. As a precursor to COVID-19, these synergistic relationships between these pre-existing conditions provide the context upon which SARS-CoV-2 would land, thus creating the perfect syndemic storm.

Alcohol Use and Violence

Alcohol use, especially heavy episodic drinking (HED), is a major contributor to the overall burden of disease. In South Africa, HED is associated with and exacerbates NCDs as well as TB, HIV/AIDS, road injuries, interpersonal violence (IPV), and cardiovascular disease (Matzopoulos et al., 2022). IPV has an additional impact on health as it is associated with and is a risk factor for CVD; furthermore, there is a mutually reinforcing relationship between IPV and drug, alcohol, and tobacco use (Thurston et al., 2022; Waldrop & Cohen, 2014). Heavy alcohol consumption (Probst et al., 2018), and HED (Trangenstein et al., 2018), are concentrated among the poor of South African society. The dynamic and complex relationship between socio-economic conditions, risky behaviors associated with HIV/AIDS transmission, and interpersonal violence has been previously described as a syndemic (Hatcher et al., 2022). Moreover, alcohol consumption often takes place in crowded, poorly ventilated settings, which are associated with TB transmission and suppression of immune response, further exacerbating cycles of vulnerability.

Notwithstanding the biopsychosocial interconnections that exist between multiple diseases, the historical origins – and the intervening political and socio-economic patterning – also need acknowledgment. In particular, the insidious use of alcohol as a weapon of racialized and capitalist social control is illustrative. In colonial and apartheid South Africa, the "dop" (tot) system[1] as a form of remuneration has had an intergenerational legacy on HED, IPV, rural poverty, and a fetal alcohol syndrome rate at least 14 times higher than the global average (SABC News, 2018). The role of alcohol in fueling accidents and trauma pre-COVID (Corrigall & Matzopoulos, 2012; Mathews et al., 2009; Matzopoulos et al., 2014) was not lost on the political decision to include a ban on alcohol sales as part of the lockdown strategy to reduce virus transmission and divert non-COVID-19 cases from accessing the healthcare system (Barron et al., 2022). Notably, rates of trauma-related accidents and injuries were reduced considerably under this ban.

Maternal and Child Health

A full exploration of maternal and child health is not possible here. As such, we draw attention to a few key issues. Despite improvements after the introduction of ARTs, South Africa still did not meet its Millennium Development Goals (MDGs) for maternal and child health. The reasons why women die during pregnancy and childbirth are complex and reflect health system factors such as poor clinical assessment, delay in referral, not following standard protocols, and not responding to abnormalities in monitoring patients (Moodley & Pattinson, 2014), as well as generalized inaccessible healthcare, and socio-economic deprivation. As discussed earlier, these contribute to a layered constellation of multiple burdens on the syndemically vulnerable, leading to high rates of maternal death from HIV, TB, pneumonia as well as hypertension and obstetric hemorrhage. Mothers and children are also victims of the "double burden" of malnutrition, which manifests as underweight children with stunted growth and overweight mothers (with the risk factors discussed earlier), results of poverty and inadequate access to healthy nutrition (Kimani-Murage, 2013; Modjadji & Madiba, 2019; Sanders et al., 2019).

Despite being the most food-secure country on the African continent (The Economist, 2022), food insecurity is still a pressing national issue. Approximately half or "30 million people lack regular access to enough safe and nutritious food – whether that's due to unavailability or being unable to afford it" (FoodForward SA, 2022). According to the Household Affordability Index 55.5% of the population were in the uppermost poverty level, surviving on 1335 ZAR or less per month (approximately 75 USD), as of February 2022 (Pietermaritzburg Economic Justice & Dignity Group, 2022). Furthermore, this income was less than a third of the average household food basket, a defined set of basic food items, and thus explains why stunting in under five-year-olds remains at 25% for girls and 30% for boys (Pietermaritzburg Economic Justice & Dignity Group, 2022).

The extent of social and economic vulnerability in South Africa is further highlighted in that prior to the COVID-19 pandemic, over a third or approximately 18 million South Africans received some form of state support, relief, or grant (Statistics South Africa, 2020b). The vast majority of these subsidies were either child support or old age grants (12 and 3.6 million, respectively), representing approximately two-thirds of each demographic receiving government assistance (van der Merwe, 2022). Research from the SANHANES on food insecurity in households with children and adolescents indicated that in 2012, neither decreased child dependence (the presence of youth who could theoretically contribute to household income after school leaving) nor the fact that a household received government grants, pensions, or remittances, mitigated against household hunger (Mkhize et al., 2022). Thus, being dependent on the state for survival at either end of the life course does not substantially reduce social vulnerability.

The South African Syndemic before COVID-19

The weakness of the public health system renders much of the disease burden suffered by the poor majority in South Africa invisible, while the spatial planning inherited from apartheid – and exacerbated in subsequent years – concentrates the poor within high-density housing at some distance from most employment opportunities, reachable using crowded and often dangerous forms of transport. These bio-social relationships are depicted in Figure 6.1. It is onto this canvas of relentless precarity that the COVID-19 pandemic landed in South Africa.

The Emergence of COVID-19 and the Healthcare Response in South Africa

On 5 March 2020, the National Institute for Communicable Diseases (NICD) in South Africa reported the first confirmed case of COVID-19 in the country (National Institute for Communicable Diseases, 2020) in a traveler who recently returned from a holiday in Italy. At that time, most early introductions of SARS-CoV-2 to South Africa were from Europe, where the virus was rapidly spreading at the time (Tegally et al., 2021). The virus' introduction into wealthier South African suburbs rapidly spread, leading to the first of several deadly waves of infection (occurring in June–July 2020).

The initial spread of COVID-19 in South Africa was associated with intense scrutiny of a small number of overwhelmingly White and relatively wealthy (Naidoo, 2020) individuals infected with the disease. However, the rapidity of infection soon overwhelmed local health authorities' systems of tracing, tracking, and reporting (Giandhari et al., 2021). The earlier individualized focus was replaced by daily updates of infection rates and, after 28 March 2020, announcements of the number of deaths (Pillay-van Wyk et al., 2020). The test statistics were generated from a network of private

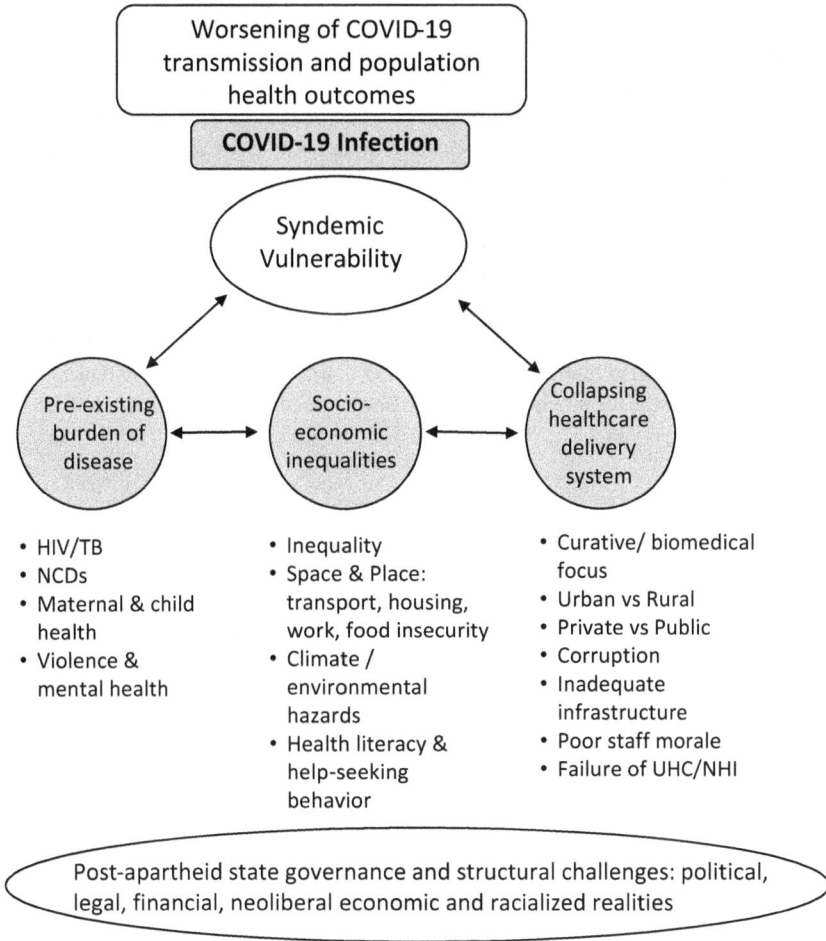

Figure 6.1 Syndemic pathways leading to worsening COVID-19 transmission and population health outcomes in South Africa.

and public laboratories conducting PCR, with an approximately even split of tests, illustrative of the continued impact of the separate but unequal, health system in South Africa.

In response to the rapid spread of SARS-CoV-2 and to ease the impact of the disease on the healthcare system, the South African government declared a state of emergency and imposed an initial month of "lockdown" from 26 March 2020. All but essential workers were required to stay at home. Much of 2020 and, to a lesser extent, 2021 was spent under gradually easing restrictions on work, travel, schooling, and social activities (South African Government, 2021).

The lockdown and the pandemic itself have had devastating economic consequences. At the start of 2022, the expanded unemployment rate was at an all-time high of 45.5%. The loss of 2.2 million jobs during the COVID-19 lockdown and restrictions only added to the toll of chronic mass unemployment (Köhler et al., 2021). Yet, South Africa is also home to five USD billionaires, and 10% of the population owns four-fifths of the wealth (Schotte et al., 2017).

While for many, at least at first, the lockdown was the face of the pandemic, those tasked with the pandemic response faced other emergencies. The country's health response was mired by shortages of, for example, personal protective equipment (PPE) and oxygen, as well as by hospital fires, corruption scandals, and the intimidation and murder of whistleblowers. These contributed to the further decline of the healthcare sector and severe burnout among healthcare workers (Haffajee, 2021; le Roux et al., 2020; le Roux & Dramowski, 2020; Singh, 2020). Global and local competition, stockouts and price gouging meant that testing supplies, reagents, and PPE were not available, and the rationing of testing, particularly within the public sector, became commonplace. Those with the financial means and/or health insurance made use of private testing labs, where faster polymerase chain reaction (PCR) turnaround times contrasted with week-or-more long delays within the increasingly overwhelmed public testing system (Lewins et al., 2022). Meanwhile, state initiatives such as community screening via the deployment of community healthcare workers to geographically remote as well as infection hot spot areas were quickly phased out as the program faced problems of limited laboratory capacity, resistance to "community-based screening" and the apparent futility of trying to implement "social distancing" in a context of housing shortage and limited social support (David & Mash, 2020; Nachega et al., 2021; Porter et al., 2020). Thus, while perceived to be the holy grail of pandemic containment, daily statistics were severely limited, and skewed by historical resource maldistribution. This led to large gaps in terms of understanding who was already sick or likely to be at risk of falling ill, and thus further skewed state-led interventions. As we discuss below, these initial aggressive testing and data-sharing failures also distorted the likelihood of becoming severely ill with COVID-19 as well as one's chance of receiving timely and adequate care, and ultimately recovering.

The overall biomedical response was *hospicentric*, designed to cater for severe cases to be admitted and treated in pre-identified, designated tertiary-level COVID-19 hospitals (all located in major cities and towns), supported by makeshift field hospitals and later in the pandemic, by the building of alternative building technology (ABT) units. Despite additional funding allocation, the COVID-19 prevention strategy had faltered by mid-2020 and was never truly resuscitated (van den Heever, 2020). In the face of climbing case numbers, hospital facilities developed their own treatment protocols in response to the novel coronavirus. Admission criteria to intensive care units (ICU) differed across, and even between, the private and public sectors, further impacting equitable access to healthcare facilities and treatment once within facilities. By 11 February 2023, of the over 4 million people who tested positive for COVID-19 in South Africa, around 550,000 were hospitalized (National Institute for Communicable Diseases, 2023a, p. 3), with varied outcomes described below.

As evident globally, the postponing of 'non-essential' health services and the reallocation of health personnel and resources to COVID-19 units has had massive consequences on healthcare and the population's overall health and well-being. In a country such as South Africa, with its pre-existing disease and syndemic burdens, taking stock of this cost is only beginning. As discussed below, the syndemically vulnerable are once again those most at risk of physiological, psychological, and social effects as the pandemic ends, with a return to some form of 'normalcy.'

The COVID-19 Syndemic in South Africa

As per Figure 6.1, the impact of the COVID-19 pandemic needs to be considered within the context of pre-existing diseases, socio-economic inequalities, and the collapsing health sector. Above, we illustrated how the COVID-19 pandemic, response, and outcomes are themselves reflective of and further exacerbate these conditions, as well as the position and experience of the syndemically vulnerable. As evinced globally, the South African case demonstrates the disparity in who was at risk of severe COVID-19 disease and/or death. In this regard, the studies we cite reflect international data, such as Apea et al.'s (2021) study of London hospitals that found Black and Asian patients were 30% and 49%, respectively, more likely to die within 30 days of a COVID-19 admission than White patients of similar health and age. As geographic and socio-economic differentials were ruled out in their study, they concluded structural racism was important and affected inequities and outcomes.

Notwithstanding data limitations due to systemic challenges of accurate capturing as well as non-availability in the public domain, we elaborate on limited access to healthcare for most people living in South Africa, resulting in inequities of health outcomes, observable at individual and population levels. Certain groups of people, namely the elderly, African women, and rural and township communities were systematically and structurally unable to protect themselves from the deleterious effects of SARS-CoV-2 infection, the exacerbation of NCDs, and the socio-economic deterioration of life itself during lockdown and thereafter.

Comorbidities

As discussed previously, comorbidities are common and generally inadequately diagnosed and treated among vulnerable populations in South Africa. Worse still, for known NCD patients, the COVID-19 pandemic shifted essential resources away from chronic care toward the emerging crisis. A focus on this new disease curtailed "non-essential" healthcare services threatening NCD patients' daily well-being and survival. Jassat and colleagues (2021) found that during the first year of the pandemic (March 2020 to March 2021), the more comorbidities present, the greater the risk of in-hospital mortality. Death rates from SARS-CoV-2 infection were higher among those with the following co-occurring diseases: hypertension (37.4%), diabetes (27.4%), HIV (9.1%), and TB (3.6%). Furthermore, HIV patients not on ARTs were also at greater risk of death than those on medication (Jassat et al., 2021). Such pre-existing syndemic vulnerability, characterized by a chronic inflammatory state and compromised immunity, provided a physiological pathway for severe COVID-19 illness (Jassat et al., 2021; WHO, 2021).

While the elderly and disabled in South Africa, especially those living in long-term care facilities, also experienced high mortality (Maree & Khanyile, 2020; Cowper et al, 2020), the presence of co-morbidities in younger populations diversified the 'typical' demographics of those who presented with severe COVID-19 illness. For people who survived their disease, this has implications for subsequent healthcare, as long COVID-19 layered additional ailments on top of existing ones, and in some cases triggered new NCDs and/or unmasked old ones. An upside of the extent of multimorbidity associated with COVID-19 was that such newly diagnosed NCD patients received diagnoses, health education, and were started on effective treatment regimens.

Much health literature examined the knock-on effects of COVID-19 on the provision of other healthcare services, often finding that prevention, treatment, and care programs across the health system were disrupted, particularly during lockdown and because of the reallocation of resources and personnel into COVID-19 care. This particularly affected countries in the Global South with weak health systems where TB and HIV control programs have been negatively impacted (Abdool Karim & Baxter, 2022). For example, Larki and colleagues (2021) note that a six-month disruption of ART delivery due to COVID-19 in sub-Saharan Africa could result in over 500,000 additional deaths from AIDS-related diseases, including TB. Recently, UNAIDS (2022) has also documented the long-term effects on control measures for vulnerable groups due to the pandemic. Similar disruptions in routine childhood immunizations, elective surgeries, mental health services, and cancer care have become evident in lengthy hospital waiting lists for many conditions, together with recent outbreaks of measles and cholera (National Institute for Communicable Diseases, 2023b, 2023c). As discussed earlier, the social and health system inequities within South Africa mean that the burden of this is again borne by the socio-economically vulnerable.

The impact of the pandemic itself is a double-edged sword, depending on the NCD disease/condition concerned. For example, while TB alone was not considered a significant risk factor for severe COVID-19, the pandemic had lasting and complex effects on TB management. For example, people's susceptibility to TB was affected both positively and negatively by the lockdown and social distancing. Practitioners struggled to differentiate between the clinical presentation of each disease. Co-infection was shown to cause case ambiguity and symptom suppression, and sometimes higher rates of disease severity, in-hospital mortality, long-term lung complications, and a likelihood of future susceptibility to infection. However, beneficial strategies and interventions were also shared across disease responses (Dheda et al., 2022). Furthermore, TB testing and screening in South Africa have yet to reach pre-COVID-19 levels. Patients are presenting in facilities with advanced illnesses, and TB mortality rates are still high (Jeranji, 2022). Even where COVID-19 as a disease did not directly affect individuals and communities, its indirect effects have been felt. Madhu Pai describes the simultaneous impacts of COVID-19 and TB as a "syndemic that feeds on social inequalities and poverty" (Dheda et al., 2022; Pai, 2020).

Disparities in Access to Higher Levels of Care

As mentioned, the official COVID-19 pandemic response was hospicentric. Hospitals were the only source of reliable data on mortality related to the disease. Hospital data, however, give some insight into inequities in the provision and quality of healthcare, as well as the impact of the pandemic on the broader, non-hospitalized population.

Hospital data from the first four COVID-19 waves (until February 2022) illustrate the complex ways in which the health system is intimately interconnected with and exacerbates existing social inequalities and biological risk of the syndemically vulnerable. Jassat and colleagues (2022) found that Black African patients experienced an increased rate of COVID-19 mortality. Black African people were likely to be admitted at a younger age, to be women, and were more likely to have comorbidities. They were also less likely to have received supplemental oxygen, to have been ventilated, and/or to have been treated within an ICU – regardless of in which sector they sought care (although more did seek care in the public sector). The researchers argue that the intersection of age, gender, race, and socio-economic status is reflective of people's differential "exposure, susceptibility to infection, and differences in access to care" (Jassat et al., 2022, p. 10).

Access to ICU care differed sharply between the public and private sectors, with 90% of COVID-19 patients who died in public sector hospitals dying outside the ICU, compared to 40% of those in private sector hospitals. Socio-economic factors overwhelmingly allocated Black African patients to public sector hospitals (Jassat et al., 2022). The explanations are complex and include historic structural inequalities; community vulnerability; inadequate resource and infrastructure provision across multiple levels of the COVID-19 response; corruption and redirection of budgets; patient multimorbidity; delays in presentation for healthcare and inadequate provision of healthcare. Jassat and colleagues (2022) echo Phaswana-Mafuya and colleagues (2021) who found that COVID-19 had heterogeneous effects, disproportionately affecting Black Africans, the marginalized, and low socio-economic groups. This was true especially among Black African women who had significantly higher rates of hospitalization and were hospitalized at younger ages. The significance of the pandemic is that it played out in ways that yet again reproduced existing inequalities of racialization, class-based and gender-based inequities across society and within the health sector.

Historical healthcare system inequity, particularly between the public and private sectors, underpins these discrepancies. Private specialists have traditionally located their consulting rooms in private hospitals, where they also admit their patients, excluding most of the population who lack health insurance. By 1990, privatization had led to 62% of general doctors and 66% of specialists being in private practice (Coovadia et al., 2009b, p. 826). In the wealthiest province, Gauteng, only three in ten hospitals are in the public sector. The ongoing impact of these disparities was reflected in differential access to facilities and outcomes during COVID-19.

In addition, illustrative of the spatial inequalities in the distribution of healthcare facilities, Gauteng and the Western Cape – provinces that contain 45% of the country's hospitals serving just over a third of the country's population – documented 50.7% of all COVID-19 cases, 51.9% of hospital admissions, and 47.5% of all COVID-19 deaths (National Institute for Communicable Diseases, 2023a).The implications for vulnerable populations living in peri-urban or rural areas, especially those in other provinces, are late presentation, increased risk of complications, and adverse outcomes.

Global patterns of inequity also shaped the South African response and outcomes. COVID-19 vaccination hoarding by high-income countries and restrictions to access imposed by the problematic agreement on Trade Related Aspects of Intellectual Property Rights (TRIPS) negatively affected middle-income countries' timely access to vaccines (World Trade Organisation, n.d.; Motari et al., 2021). Vaccine rates remain comparatively low across the Global South, with South Africa only reaching 51.6% of the adult population by May 2023 (SACoronavirus). Although healthcare workers first received access in February 2021 as part of a national research project, most of the population could only access COVID-19 vaccines from May 2021 as the third wave began (Health Justice Initiative, 2022; Moodley et al., 2021) which subsequently had the largest death toll. According to Runciman et al., the demand for vaccines amongst the most vulnerable was the highest, with 67% wanting a vaccine (Runciman et al., 2021). However, access, particularly in the public sector, was severely limited by logistic limitations in making online appointments, the often-inconvenient allocation to specific roll-out centers, and the lack of enablement factors such as transport to vaccination sites (Xezwi, 2021). By September 2021, Alexander (2021) found "50% of the insured population had received a vaccination compared with only 25% of the uninsured."

For those facing the disease unvaccinated, Biccard and colleagues (2021, p. 1885), reporting on the African COVID-19 Critical Care Outcomes Study across Africa, found that "mortality in critically ill patients with COVID-19 is higher in African countries than reported from studies" on other continents. They argue this was principally due to "insufficient critical care resources," patient comorbidity, and the "severity of organ dysfunction at admission" (Biccard et al., 2021, p. 1893).

The Impact of the National Lockdown

The national lockdown severely restricted movement in South Africa, impacting schooling, social interactions, and non-essential retail, including the sale of alcohol, throughout most of 2020. Due to these restrictions, many people lost their sources of income, exacerbating the need for more social assistance. In May 2020, all existing government grants were augmented for a six-month period. A new Social Relief of Distress (SRD) Grant was introduced for registered citizens, permanent residents, or UN Convention refugees receiving no other form of income or grant. This short-term relief, the equivalent of 350 ZAR per month (less than 0.75 USD/day), was intended to avert starvation. By October 2022, there were 7.5 million SRD grant recipients (Khumalo, 2022), and, at least 46% of the population was recorded as receiving some type of government grant (Human, 2022). While the battle for a Basic Income Grant goes on, it is suggested that societal need requires the SRD to be extended for at least another year, to over another 10 million recipients (Human, 2022). Despite the patchwork of COVID-19-related grants made available, almost a quarter of South African households reported skipping a meal in the previous week (van der Berg et al., 2022).

The economic impacts of the lockdown were strongly gendered, with about two-thirds of employment loss being borne by women. School and daycare center closures increased women's childcare and homeschooling responsibilities (Casale & Shepherd, 2021). Such domestic arrangements also put women at higher risk for intimate partner violence. As discussed in depth in Chapter 8, gender-based violence (GBV) in South Africa was at catastrophic proportions even prior to the COVID-19 pandemic and increased to such an extent that President Ramaphosa declared GBV South Africa's "second pandemic." Despite government initiatives to establish call centers, shelters, and women and children empowerment initiatives, Dekel and Abrahams (2021, pp. 1–10) reaffirmed that "insensitive pandemic control measures" [actually] "magnified the risk of escalation of abuse in families already experiencing IPV prior to COVID-19."

The COVID-19 pandemic in South Africa also saw a dramatic increase in maternal mortality through an exacerbation of previously identified weaknesses in maternal healthcare, including reduced ante-natal visits and problems with transport to and capacity at hospitals (Ahmed et al., 2021; Jeranji, 2021) as well as the impact of COVID-19 infection during pregnancy (Budhram et al., 2021).

The COVID-19 pandemic and the lockdown led to a marked reduction in routine childhood immunization coverage. Data from January 2021 show that measles vaccine coverage had fallen below the targets required to be effective (UNICEF, 2021). Towards the end of 2022 and into 2023 there was an outbreak of measles in the country, with the largest number of cases occurring in three of the most impoverished provinces: the North-West, Limpopo, and Eastern Cape (National Institute for Communicable Diseases, 2023c).

Conclusion

During the COVID-19 pandemic in South Africa, over 300,000 "excess deaths" were inequitably concentrated in the most vulnerable parts of society. The syndemic interplay between population disparities and the systemic sociopolitical conditions responsible for these, all of which predated the arrival of the SARS-CoV-2, provided fertile ground with devastating consequences, not only for individuals and their families but for the collective and its consciousness. Yet this was not inevitable. To quote epidemiologist Larry Brilliant, "outbreaks are inevitable, epidemics are optional" (Jain, 2014). Although there are examples of transcendent behaviors and positive outcomes, such as the heroic and often selfless performance of healthcare professionals in saving patients' lives in ICU, South Africa has emerged more structurally embattled from these intersections. Countries such as New Zealand, Australia, China, Vietnam, and Thailand on the other hand showed that COVID-19 outbreaks could be controlled, and their robust interventions illustrated a path that South Africa could have followed. Thailand is economically and in population size a reasonable match for South Africa. It managed to keep cases to a minimum until mid-2021 and, as of 2023, never had excess mortality reach more than 40% of pre-pandemic levels (Mathieu et al., 2020b). South Africa, by contrast, had excess mortality that peaked at over 160% of pre-pandemic levels (Mathieu et al., 2020a).

The many missed opportunities to embrace the Primary Healthcare (PHC) approach loom large over the South African landscape. Ironically, the roots of "primary healthcare" are in South Africa, in the work of Sidney and Emily Kark at their clinic in Pholela in Kwa-Zulu Natal in the 1940s. The Karks' experiment offered preventative, curative, and promotive medical intervention in a single center that worked with local health assistants to both provide grassroots data collection on the state of health in the district as well as build strong links between health promotion, community work, and resource provision (Kark & Kark, 1983; Phillips, 2014). Embraced by the WHO in the 1978 Alma Ata Declaration, PHC became a call for health through reconstruction of the socio-economic order at scales both global and local (WHO, 1978), a call that was in turn embraced through the ANC's 1994 Health Plan (African National Congress, 1994c) and the Reconstruction and Development Programme (RDP) (African National Congress, 1994b). Such radical visions were always under threat, however, first from the medical establishment itself with its hospicentric approaches and, secondly, through the interests vested in the maintenance of the existing social and economic order. The Pholela clinic was thus shut down, the RDP Office was dismantled, and the vision of comprehensive primary healthcare has remained rhetoric rather than practice in South Africa (Naledi et al., 2011; Visagie & Schneider, 2014).

How the COVID-19 pandemic played out in South Africa has rendered it even more syndemically vulnerable to the next infectious disease occurrence or natural disaster assault. Political and socio-economic conditions have worsened: there are crises of governance, finance, and social injustice that further permeate our collective social fabric. There have always been those advocating alternative approaches to the "organized abandonment" that state power and private wealth promoted in South Africa. In Thailand, for example, "village health volunteers" connected with a network of health facilities played a key role in identifying not only COVID-19 cases but also where to focus interventions during periods of "lockdown" and increased hunger (Noknoy et al., 2021). In Kerala State in India, a strong program of local government-led health promotion enabled coordination between Accredited Social Health Activists (ASHAs), women's self-help groups, and other community actors to quickly identify and respond to the pandemic (Chandra & Sinha, 2022; Dutta & Fischer, 2021; Israelsen & Malji, 2021). In South Africa, a previous pandemic, that of HIV/AIDS, saw widespread mobilization and the emergence of a new generation of "community health-care workers" (Heywood, 2009; Schneider et al., 2008) and patient self-advocacy formations. As COVID-19 emerged, NGOs such as the People's Health Movement in South Africa turned to community health workers, organizing training workshops to enable rapid health promotion in the face of this emerging threat.

In parallel, the widespread sense of crisis provoked both by the growing pandemic and the lockdown that followed led to the formation of Community Action Networks (CANs) in major cities. These volunteer-based CANs mobilized resources to identify vulnerable households and share tasks such as education and food distribution (Odendaal, 2021; van Ryneveld et al., 2020). Taking a complementary approach, health departments in Gauteng and the Western Cape provinces (Moolla et al., 2020) turned to telehealth approaches to connect patients with services. Lewins and colleagues (2022) reported on the operation of one such Gauteng-based "family-patient liaison" unit, where they sought to connect with the households of COVID-19 patients, facilitate access to resources and address psycho-social problems associated with COVID-19 patients' ongoing needs for care.

While admirable, much more than boutique "emergency responses" is needed to address the ongoing syndemic vulnerabilities of most of South Africa's population. Community healthcare workers remain poorly integrated into the broader healthcare system, the healthcare system remains fragmented between private and public sectors, and the broader perpetuation of the legacies of colonialism and apartheid continues to bedevil a primary healthcare approach in the South African context. Calls made during the height of the pandemic for a "bottom-up," people-centric, and "whole of society" approach to the pandemic went largely ignored (Munshi et al, 2020).

"Health," says the WHO (1978), is "more than simply the absence of disease but is rather a state of complete physical, mental, and social well-being." Illness, syndemic theory holds, is more than a simple medical question. While with the emergence of widespread immunity through vaccination, infection, and, unfortunately, the deaths of millions, COVID-19 has now largely joined influenza as an endemic disease, likely to cause hundreds or thousands rather than hundreds of thousands of deaths in South Africa each year. The COVID-19 pandemic that devastated South Africa from 2020 to 2022 should act as a clarion call for the need for a radical reconstruction of society and the urgent need to address syndemic vulnerabilities through a community-oriented public healthcare approach.

Note

1 The dop system is over 300-years old, having been institutionalized in colonial South Africa, particularly in the Western Cape agricultural sector between farm owners and laborers. London's research (1999) found that a fifth of farm workers were still being paid a portion of their wages in alcohol, and just under half had previously received alcohol as a salary in exchange for employment.

References

Abdool Karim, Q., & Baxter, C. (2022). COVID-19: Impact on the HIV and tuberculosis response, service delivery, and research in South Africa. *Current HIV/AIDS Reports*, 19(1), 46–53. https://doi.org/10.1007/s11904-021-00588-5.

Adeniyi, A.B., Laurence, C.E., Volmink, J.A., & Davids, M.R. (2017). Prevalence of chronic kidney disease and association with cardiovascular risk factors among teachers in Cape Town, South Africa. *Clinical Kidney Journal*, 10(3), 363–369. https://doi.org/10.1093/ckj/sfw138.

African National Congress. (1994a). *Policy Documents 1994: A National Health Plan for South Africa – ANC*. African National Congress. https://www.anc1912. org.za/policy-documents-1994-a-national-health-plan-for-south-africa/.

African National Congress. (1994b). *The Reconstruction and Development Programme*. Umanyano Publishers.

African National Congress. (1994c, May 30). A national health plan for South Africa. *African National Congress Policy Documents*. https://www.anc1912.org.za/ policy-documents-1994-a-national-health-plan-for-south-africa/.

Ahmed, T., Rahman, A.E., Amole, T.G., Galadanci, H., Matjila, M., Soma-Pillay, P., Gillespie, B.M., El Arifeen, S., & Anumba, D.O.C. (2021). The effect of COVID-19 on maternal newborn and child health (MNCH) services in Bangladesh, Nigeria and South Africa: Call for a contextualised pandemic response in LMICs. *International Journal for Equity in Health*, 20(1), 77. https://doi.org/10.1186/ s12939-021-01414-5.

Alexander, K. (2021, December 3). Vaccine mandates are not a panacea. News24. https://www.news24.com/news24/opinions/fridaybriefing/kate-alexander-vaccine-mandates-are-not-a-panacea-20211202.

Apea, V.J., Wan, Y.I., Dhairyawan, R., Puthucheary, Z.A., Pearse, R.M., Orkin, C.M., & Prowle, J.R. (2021). Ethnicity and outcomes in patients hospitalised with COVID-19 infection in East London: An observational cohort study. *BMJ Open*, 11(1), e042140. https://doi.org/10.1136/bmjopen-2020-042140.

Ataguba, J.E.-O., & Akazili, J. (2010). Health care financing in South Africa: Moving towards universal coverage. *Continuing Medical Education*, 28(2), 74–78. http://www.cmej.org.za/index.php/cmej/article/viewFile/1782/1466.

Baldwin-Ragaven, L. (2020). Social dimensions of COVID-19 in South Africa: A neglected element of the treatment plan. *Wits Journal of Clinical Medicine*, 2(SI), 33–38. https://doi.org/10.18772/26180197.2020.v2nSIa6.

Baldwin-Ragaven, L., London, L., & Gruchy, J.D. (1999). *An Ambulance of the Wrong Colour: Health Professionals, Human Rights and Ethics in South Africa*. Juta and Company Ltd.

Barchiesi, F. (2008). Wage labor, precarious employment, and social inclusion in the making of South Africa's postapartheid transition. *African Studies Review*, 51(2), 119–142.

Barron, K., Parry, C.D.H., Bradshaw, D., Dorrington, R., Groenewald, P., Laubscher, R., & Matzopoulos, R. (2022). Alcohol, violence and injury-induced mortality: Evidence from a modern-day prohibition. *The Review of Economics and Statistics*, 1–45. https://doi.org/10.1162/rest_a_01228.

Berhanu, R.H., Lebina, L., Nonyane, B.A.S., Milovanovic, M., Kinghorn, A., Connell, L., Nyathi, S., Young, K., Hausler, H., Naidoo, P., Brey, Z., Shearer, K., Genade, L., & Martinson, N.A. (2023). Yield of facility-based targeted universal testing for tuberculosis (TUTT) with Xpert and mycobacterial culture in high-risk groups attending primary care facilities in South Africa. *Clinical Infectious Diseases: An Official Publication of the Infectious Diseases Society of America*, ciac965. https://doi.org/10.1093/cid/ciac965.

Berry, K.M., Parker, W., Mchiza, Z.J., Sewpaul, R., Labadarios, D., Rosen, S., & Stokes, A. (2017). Quantifying unmet need for hypertension care in South Africa through a care cascade: Evidence from the SANHANES, 2011-2012. *BMJ Global Health*, 2(3), e000348. https://doi.org/10.1136/bmjgh-2017-000348.

Bhandar, B. (2018, September 21). Organised state abandonment: The meaning of Grenfell. *Critical Legal Thinking*. https://criticallegalthinking.com/2018/09/21/organised-state-abandonment-the-meaning-of-grenfell/.

Biccard, B.M., Gopalan, P.D., Miller, M., Michell, W.L., Thomson, D., Ademuyiwa, A., Aniteye, E., Calligaro, G., Chaibou, M.S., Dhufera, H.T., Elfagieh, M., Elfiky, M., Elhadi, M., Fawzy, M., Fredericks, D., Gebre, M., Bayih, A.G., Hardy, A., Joubert, I., … Govender, V. (2021). Patient care and clinical outcomes for patients with COVID-19 infection admitted to African high-care or intensive care units (ACCCOS): A multicentre, prospective, observational cohort study. *The Lancet*, 397(10288), 1885–1894. https://doi.org/10.1016/S0140-6736(21)00441-4.

Biko, S. (1987). *I Write What I Like: A Selection of His Writings*. Heinemann.

Bittar, A. (2020, August 14). *Poverty on the Rise in South Africa*. The Borgen Project. https://borgenproject.org/poverty-in-south-africa/.

Bradshaw, B., Laubscher, R., Dorrington, R., Groenewald, P & Moultrie, T. (2022, November 23). *Report on Weekly Deaths in South Africa [Text]*. South

African Medical Research Council. https://www.samrc.ac.za/reports/report-weekly-deaths-south-africa.

Bradshaw, D., Groenewald, P., Laubscher, R., Nannan, N., Nojilana, B., Norman, R., Pieterse, D., Schneider, M., Bourne, D.E., Timaeus, I.M., Dorrington, R., & Johnson, L. (2003). Initial burden of disease estimates for South Africa, 2000. *South African Medical Journal*, 93(9), Article 9.

Breckenridge, T.A., Black-Hughes, C., Rautenbach, J., & McKinley, M. (2019). HIV/AIDS orphans in South Africa: NGO interventions supporting transitions to alternative care. *International Social Work*, 62(2), 502–517. https://doi.org/10.1177/0020872817732377.

Budhram, S., Vannevel, V., Botha, T., Chauke, L., Bhoora, S., Balie, G.M., Odell, N., Lombaard, H., Wise, A., Georgiou, C., Ngxola, N., Wynne, E., Mbewu, U., Mabenge, M., Phinzi, S., Gubu-Ntaba, N., Goldman, G., Tunkyi, K., Prithipal, S., ... Yates, L.M. (2021). Maternal characteristics and pregnancy outcomes of hospitalized pregnant women with SARS-CoV-2 infection in South Africa: An International Network of Obstetric Survey Systems-based cohort study. *International Journal of Gynaecology and Obstetrics*, 155(3), 455–465. https://doi.org/10.1002/ijgo.13917.

Casale, D., & Shepherd, D. (2021). The gendered effects of the COVID-19 crisis and ongoing lockdown in South Africa. *Evidence from NIDS-CRAM Waves 1–5*. https://cramsurvey.org/wp-content/uploads/2021/07/3.-Casale-D.-_-Shepherd-D.-2021-The-gendered-effects-of-the-Covid-19-crisis-and-ongoing-lockdown-in-South-Africa-Evidence-from-NIDS-CRAM-Waves-1-%E2%80%93-5.pdf.

Chandra, R., & Sinha, S. (2022). India fighting COVID-19: Experiences and lessons learned from the successful Kerala and Bhilwara models. *Disaster Medicine and Public Health Preparedness*, 16(6), 2314–2318. https://doi.org/10.1017/dmp.2021.115.

Chigwedere, P., Seage, G.R., Gruskin, S., Lee, T.-H., & Essex, M. (2008). Estimating the lost benefits of antiretroviral drug use in South Africa. *Journal of Acquired Immune Deficiency Syndromes (1999)*, 49(4), 410–415. https://doi.org/10.1097/qai.0b013e31818a6cd5.

Churchyard, G.J., Mametja, L.D., Mvusi, L., Ndjeka, N., Hesseling, A.C., Reid, A., Babatunde, S., & Pillay, Y. (2014). Tuberculosis control in South Africa: Successes, challenges and recommendations. *South African Medical Journal = Suid-Afrikaanse Tydskrif Vir Geneeskunde*, 104(3 Suppl 1), 244–248. https://doi.org/10.7196/samj.7689.

Cois, A., Abdelatief, N., Steyn, N., Turawa, E.B., Awotiwon, O.F., Roomaney, R.A., Neethling, I., Joubert, J.D., Pacella, R., Bradshaw, D., & Pillay van-Wyk, V. (2022). Estimating the burden of disease attributable to a diet low in fruit and vegetables in South Africa for 2000, 2006 and 2012. *South African Medical Journal = Suid-Afrikaanse Tydskrif Vir Geneeskunde*, 112(8b), 617–626. https://doi.org/10.7196/SAMJ.2022.v112i8b.16486.

Competition Commission of South Africa. (2019). *Healthcare Market Inquiry – The Competition Commission*. https://www.compcom.co.za/wp-content/uploads/2020/01/Final-Findings-and-recommendations-report-Health-Market-Inquiry.pdf.

Coovadia, H., Jewkes, R., Barron, P., Sanders, D., & McIntyre, D. (2009a). The health and health system of South Africa: Historical roots of current public health challenges. *Lancet (London, England)*, 374(9692), 817–834. https://doi.org/10.1016/S0140-6736(09)60951-X.

Coovadia, H., Jewkes, R., Barron, P., Sanders, D., & McIntyre, D. (2009b). The health and health system of South Africa: Historical roots of current public health challenges. *The Lancet*, 374(9692), 817–834. https://doi.org/10.1016/S0140-6736(09)60951-X.

Corrigall, J., & Matzopoulos, R. (2012). Violence, alcohol misuse and mental health: Gaps in the health system's response. *South African Health Review*, 2012/2013(1), 103–114. https://doi.org/10.10520/EJC133695.

Cowper, B., Jassat, W., Pretorius, P., Geffen, L., Legodu, C., Singh, S., & Blumberg, L. (2020). COVID-19 in long-term care facilities in South Africa: No time for complacency. *SAMJ: South African Medical Journal*, 110(9). https://doi.org/10.7196/samj.2020.v110i10.15214.

Cullinan, K. (2006, January 29). Health services in South Africa: A basic introduction. *Health-e News Service*. https://health-e.org.za/2006/01/29/health-services-in-south-africa-a-basic-introduction/.

David, N., & Mash, R. (2020). Community-based screening and testing for coronavirus in Cape Town, South Africa: Short report. *African Journal of Primary Health Care & Family Medicine*, 12(1), 2499. https://doi.org/10.4102/phcfm.v12i1.2499.

de Beer, C. (1984). *The South African Disease: Apartheid, Health, and Health Services*. Southern African Research Service.

Dekel, B., & Abrahams, N. (2021). 'I will rather be killed by corona than by him…': Experiences of abused women seeking shelter during South Africa's COVID-19 lockdown. *PLOS ONE*, 16(10), e0259275. https://doi.org/10.1371/journal.pone.0259275.

Department of Health. (2021). *The First National TB Prevalence Survey—South Africa 2018*. https://www.knowledgehub.org.za/elibrary/first-national-tb-prevalence-survey-south-africa-2018.

Dheda, K., Perumal, T., Moultrie, H., Perumal, R., Esmail, A., Scott, A.J., Udwadia, Z., Chang, K.C., Peter, J., Pooran, A., von Delft, A., von Delft, D., Martinson, N., Loveday, M., Charalambous, S., Kachingwe, E., Jassat, W., Cohen, C., Tempia, S., … Pai, M. (2022). The intersecting pandemics of tuberculosis and COVID-19: Population-level and patient-level impact, clinical presentation, and corrective interventions. *The Lancet Respiratory Medicine*, 10(6), 603–622. https://doi.org/10.1016/S2213-2600(22)00092-3.

Dutta, A., & Fischer, H.W. (2021). The local governance of COVID-19: Disease prevention and social security in rural India. *World Development*, 138, 105234. https://doi.org/10.1016/j.worlddev.2020.105234.

FoodForward SA. (2022, September 16). Repurpose the surplus & help us end hunger. *FoodForward SA*. https://foodforwardsa.org/2022/09/16/repurpose-the-surplus-help-us-end-hunger/.

Gangaidzo, T., von Fintel, M., Schutte, A.E., & Burger, R. (2022). Stressful life events, neighbourhood characteristics, and systolic blood pressure in South Africa. *Journal of Human Hypertension*, 1–7. https://doi.org/10.1038/s41371-022-00695-9.

Giandhari, J., Pillay, S., Wilkinson, E., Tegally, H., Sinayskiy, I., Schuld, M., Lourenço, J., Chimukangara, B., Lessells, R., Moosa, Y., Gazy, I., Fish, M., Singh, L., Khanyile, K.S., Fonseca, V., Giovanetti, M., Alcantara, L.C.J., Petruccione, F., & Oliveira, T. de. (2021). Early transmission of SARS-CoV-2 in South Africa: An epidemiological and phylogenetic report. *International Journal of Infectious Diseases*, 103, 234–241. https://doi.org/10.1016/j.ijid.2020.11.128.

Goetjes, E., Pavlova, M., Hongoro, C., & Groot, W. (2021). Socioeconomic inequalities and obesity in South Africa—A decomposition analysis. *International Journal of Environmental Research and Public Health*, 18(17), 9181. https://doi.org/10.3390/ijerph18179181.

Haffajee, F. (2021, June 7). Reflection: Corruption in a pandemic: R15bn (and counting) – I want to pay my taxes to gift of the givers. *Daily Maverick*. https://www.dailymaverick.co.za/article/2021-06-07-corruption-in-a-pandemic-r15bn-and-counting-i-want-to-pay-my-taxes-to-gift-of-the-givers/.

Hatcher, A.M., Gibbs, A., McBride, R.-S., Rebombo, D., Khumalo, M., & Christofides, N.J. (2022). Gendered syndemic of intimate partner violence, alcohol misuse, and HIV risk among peri-urban, heterosexual men in South Africa. *Social Science & Medicine*, 295, 112637. https://doi.org/10.1016/j.socscimed.2019.112637.

Health Justice Initiative. (2022, July). *Vaccine Timeline*. Health Justice Initiative (HJI). https://healthjusticeinitiative.org.za/vaccine-equity/vaccine-timeline/.

Heyns, C., & Brand, D. (1998). Introduction to socio-economic rights in the South African Constitution. *Law, Democracy & Development*, 2(2), Article 2. https://doi.org/10.4314/ldd.v2i2.

Heywood, M. (2009). South Africa's treatment action campaign: Combining law and social mobilization to realize the right to health. *Journal of Human Rights Practice*, 1(1), 14–36. https://doi.org/10.1093/jhuman/hun006.

Human, B.L. (2022, February 23). Finance Minister announces 2022 social grant increases. *GroundUp News*. https://www.groundup.org.za/article/finance-minister-announces-2022-social-grant-increases/.

Husain, N.E., Noor, S.K., Elmadhoun, W.M., Almobarak, A.O., Awadalla, H., Woodward, C.L., Mital, D., & Ahmed, M.H. (2017). Diabetes, metabolic syndrome and dyslipidemia in people living with HIV in Africa: Re-emerging challenges not to be forgotten. *HIV/AIDS - Research and Palliative Care*, 9, 193–202. https://doi.org/10.2147/HIV.S137974.

International Monetary Fund. (2020, January 30). *Six Charts Explain South Africa's Inequality*. IMF. https://www.imf.org/en/News/Articles/2020/01/29/na012820six-charts-on-south-africas-persistent-and-multi-faceted-inequality.

Israelsen, S., & Malji, A. (2021). COVID-19 in India: A comparative analysis of the Kerala and Gujarat development models' initial responses. *Progress in Development Studies*, 21(4), 397–418.

Jain, K. (2014, December 10). Epidemics are optional. *Harvard Gazette*. https://news.harvard.edu/gazette/story/2014/12/epidemics-are-optional/.

Jassat, W., Cohen, C., Tempia, S., Masha, M., Goldstein, S., Kufa, T., Murangandi, P., Savulescu, D., Walaza, S., Bam, J.-L., Davies, M.-A., Prozesky, H.W., Naude, J., Mnguni, A.T., Lawrence, C.A., Mathema, H.T., Zamparini, J., Black, J., Mehta, R., ... Zwane, N. (2021). Risk factors for COVID-19-related in-hospital mortality in a high HIV and tuberculosis prevalence setting in South Africa: A cohort study. *The Lancet HIV*, 8(9), e554–e567. https://doi.org/10.1016/S2352-3018(21)00151-X.

Jassat, W., Ozougwu, L., Munshi, S., Mudara, C., Vika, C., Arendse, T., Masha, M., Welch, R., Govender, N., Ebonwu, J., Groome, M., Joseph, A., Madhi, S.A., Cohen, C., & Blumberg, L. (2022). The intersection of age, sex, race and socio-economic status in COVID-19 hospital admissions and deaths in South Africa (with corrigendum). *South African Journal of Science*, 118(5/6), Article 5/6. https://doi.org/10.17159/sajs.2022/13323.

Jeranji, T. (2021, March 5). 30% increase in maternal deaths during COVID-19 lockdown reported. *Spotlight.* https://www.spotlightnsp.co.za/2021/03/05/30-increase-in-maternal-deaths-during-covid-19-lockdown-reported/.

Jeranji, T. (2022, September 15). As testing volumes improve, government outlines TB recovery plan. *Spotlight.* https://www.spotlightnsp.co.za/2022/09/15/as-testing-volumes-improve-government-outlines-tb-recovery-plan/.

Kalonji, D., & Mahomed, O.H. (2019). Health system challenges affecting HIV and tuberculosis integration at primary healthcare clinics in Durban, South Africa. *African Journal of Primary Health Care & Family Medicine*, 11(1), Article 1.

Kapwata, T., & Manda, S. (2018). Geographic assessment of access to health care in patients with cardiovascular disease in South Africa. *BMC Health Services Research*, 18(1), 197. https://doi.org/10.1186/s12913-018-3006-0.

Kark, S.L., & Kark, E. (1983). An alternative strategy in community health care: Community-oriented primary health care. *Israel Journal of Medical Sciences*, 19(8), 707–713.

Kendall, E.A., Shrestha, S., & Dowdy, D.W. (2021). The epidemiological importance of subclinical tuberculosis. a critical reappraisal. *American Journal of Respiratory and Critical Care Medicine*, 203(2), 168–174. https://doi.org/10.1164/rccm.202006-2394PP.

Khumalo, J. (2022, October 10). Govt expecting 3 million more to receive R350 social relief distress grant. *News24.* https://www.news24.com/news24/politics/government/govt-expecting-3-million-more-to-receive-r350-social-relief-distress-grant-20221010.

Kimani-Murage, E.W. (2013). Exploring the paradox: Double burden of malnutrition in rural South Africa. *Global Health Action*, 6(1), 19249. https://doi.org/10.3402/gha.v6i0.19249.

Köhler, T., Bhorat, H., Hill, R., & Stanwix, B. (2021, May 31). *COVID-19 and the Labour Market: Estimating the Employment Effects of South Africa's National Lockdown.* Africa Portal; Development Policy Research Unit (DPRU). https://www.africaportal.org/publications/covid-19-and-labour-market-estimating-employment-effects-south-africas-national-lockdown/.

Kwan, C.K., & Ernst, J.D. (2011). HIV and tuberculosis: A deadly human syndemic. *Clinical Microbiology Reviews*, 24(2), 351–376. https://doi.org/10.1128/CMR.00042-10.

Larki, M., Sharifi, F., Manouchehri, E., & Latifnejad Roudsari, R. (2021). Responding to the essential sexual and reproductive health needs for women during the COVID-19 pandemic: A literature review. *The Malaysian Journal of Medical Sciences: MJMS*, 28(6), 8–19. https://doi.org/10.21315/mjms2021.28.6.2.

Laurence, P. (1990). *Death Squads: Apartheid's Secret Weapon.* Penguin Books.

le Roux, C., & Dramowski, A. (2020). Personal protective equipment (PPE) in a pandemic: Approaches to PPE preservation for South African healthcare facilities. *SAMJ: South African Medical Journal*, 110(6), 1–3. https://doi.org/10.7196/SAMJ.2020.v110i6.14831.

le Roux, C., Stinson, K., Dawood, F., Jansen van Vuuren, N., & Dramowski, A. (2020). *South African Medical Students' Perspectives on COVID-19 and Clinical Training.* https://repository.up.ac.za/handle/2263/82072.

Leibbrandt, M., Finn, A., & Woolard, I. (2012). Describing and decomposing post-apartheid income inequality in South Africa. *Development Southern Africa*, 29(1), 19–34. https://doi.org/10.1080/0376835X.2012.645639.

Lewins, K., Seabi, T.M., Seotsanyana, L., Maphelela, K., Nyirenda, T., & Benvie, C. (2022). Reflections on first wave COVID-19 practice: Insights from family–patient liaisons. *South African Review of Sociology*, 51(3–4), 165–187. https://doi.org/10.1080/21528586.2022.2035252.

Lewins, K., van Heusden, P., & Baldwin-Ragaven, L. (2022). Testing times: COVID-19 testing and healthcare workers in South Africa. In C. Vindrola-Padros, & G.A. Johnson (Eds.), *Caring on the Frontline during COVID-19: Contributions from Rapid Qualitative Research* (pp. 199–227). Springer. https://doi.org/10.1007/978-981-16-6486-1_10.

London, L. (1999). The 'dop' system, alcohol abuse and social control amongst farm workers in South Africa: A public health challenge. *Social Science & Medicine*, 48(10), 1407–1414. https://doi.org/10.1016/S0277-9536(98)00445-6.

Mabaso, M., Makola, L., Naidoo, I., Mlangeni, L.L., Jooste, S., & Simbayi, L. (2019). HIV prevalence in South Africa through gender and racial lenses: Results from the 2012 population-based national household survey. *International Journal for Equity in Health*, 18(1), 167. https://doi.org/10.1186/s12939-019-1055-6.

Maja, T.F., & Maposa, D. (2022). An investigation of risk factors associated with tuberculosis transmission in South Africa using logistic regression model. *Infectious Disease Reports*, 14(4), 609–620. https://doi.org/10.3390/idr14040066.

Makhaye, C. (2022, August 9). 'Even in this day, the face of poverty is African women', says Ramaphosa. *Daily Maverick*. https://www.dailymaverick.co.za/article/2022-08-09-even-in-this-day-the-face-of-poverty-is-african-women-says-ramaphosa/.

Marais, H. (2008). *South Africa: Limits to Change: The Political Economy of Transition*. University of Cape Town Press.

Maree, G., & Khanyile, S. (2020). *The Impact of COVID-19 on Long Term Care Facilities*. https://hdl.handle.net/10539/29766.

Mathews, S., Abrahams, N., Jewkes, R., Martin, L.J., & Lombard, C. (2009). Alcohol use and its role in female homicides in the Western Cape, South Africa. *Journal of Studies on Alcohol and Drugs*, 70(3), 321–327. https://doi.org/10.15288/jsad.2009.70.321.

Mathieu, E., Ritchie, H., Rodés-Guirao, L., Appel, C., Giattino, C., Hasell, J., Macdonald, B., Dattani, S., Beltekian, D., Ortiz-Ospina, E., & Roser, M. (2020a). Excess mortality during COVID-19 pandemic (Our World in Data). *Our World in Data*. https://ourworldindata.org/excess-mortality-covid.

Mathieu, E., Ritchie, H., Rodés-Guirao, L., Appel, C., Giattino, C., Hasell, J., Macdonald, B., Dattani, S., Beltekian, D., Ortiz-Ospina, E., & Roser, M. (2020b). Thailand: Coronavirus pandemic country profile (our world in data). *Our World in Data*. https://ourworldindata.org/coronavirus/country/thailand.

Matzopoulos, R., Cois, A., Probst, C., Parry, C.D.H., Vellios, N., Sorsdahl, K., Joubert, J.D., Pillay-van Wyk, V., Bradshaw, D., & Pacella, R. (2022). Estimating the changing burden of disease attributable to alcohol use in South Africa for 2000, 2006 and 2012. *South African Medical Journal = Suid-Afrikaanse Tydskrif Vir Geneeskunde*, 112(8b), 662–675. https://doi.org/10.7196/SAMJ.2022.v112i8b.16487.

Matzopoulos, R.G., Truen, S., Bowman, B., & Corrigall, J. (2014). The cost of harmful alcohol use in South Africa. *South African Medical Journal*, 104(2), Article 2.

Mbambo, S.B., & Agbola, S.B. (2020). The impact of the COVID-19 pandemic in townships and lessons for urban spatial restructuring in South Africa. *African Journal of Governance & Development*, 9(1.1), Article 1.1.

McLaren, Z.M., Ardington, C., & Leibbrandt, M. (2014). Distance decay and persistent health care disparities in South Africa. *BMC Health Services Research*, 14(1), 541. https://doi.org/10.1186/s12913-014-0541-1.

Mendenhall, E. (2014). Syndemic suffering in Soweto: Violence and inequality at the nexus of health transition in South Africa. *Annals of Anthropological Practice*, 38(2), 300–316. https://doi.org/10.1111/napa.12058.

Mendenhall, E., Kim, A.W., Panasci, A., Cele, L., Mpondo, F., Bosire, E.N., Norris, S.A., & Tsai, A.C. (2022). A mixed-methods, population-based study of a syndemic in Soweto, South Africa. *Nature Human Behaviour*, 6(1), Article 1. https://doi.org/10.1038/s41562-021-01242-1.

Mkhize, S., Libhaber, E., Sewpaul, R., Reddy, P., & Baldwin-Ragaven, L. (2022). Child and adolescent food insecurity in South Africa: A household-level analysis of hunger. *PLOS ONE*, 17(12), e0278191. https://doi.org/10.1371/journal.pone.0278191.

Modjadji, P., & Madiba, S. (2019). The double burden of malnutrition in a rural health and demographic surveillance system site in South Africa: A study of primary schoolchildren and their mothers. *BMC Public Health*, 19(1), 1087. https://doi.org/10.1186/s12889-019-7412-y.

Moodley, J., & Pattinson, R.C. (2014). Sixth Comprehensive Report on Confidential Enquiries into Maternal Deaths in South Africa: A case study. *BJOG: An International Journal of Obstetrics and Gynaecology*, 121(S4), 53–60. https://doi.org/10.1111/1471-0528.12869.

Moodley, K., Blockman, M., Pienaar, D., Hawkridge, A.J., Meintjes, J., Davies, M.-A., & London, L. (2021). Hard choices: Ethical challenges in phase 1 of COVID-19 vaccine roll-out in South Africa. *South African Medical Journal*, 111(6), Article 6.

Moolla, M.S., Broadhurst, A., Parker, M.A., Parker, A., & Mowlana, A. (2020). Implementing a video call visit system in a coronavirus disease 2019 unit. *African Journal of Primary Health Care & Family Medicine*, 12(1), Article 1. https://doi.org/10.4102/phcfm.v12i1.2637

Motari, M., Nikiema, J.-B., Kasilo, O.M.J., Kniazkov, S., Loua, A., Sougou, A., & Tumusiime, P. (2021). The role of intellectual property rights on access to medicines in the WHO African region: 25 years after the TRIPS agreement. *BMC Public Health*, 21(1), 490. https://doi.org/10.1186/s12889-021-10374-y.

Mudzengi, D., Sweeney, S., Hippner, P., Kufa, T., Fielding, K., Grant, A.D., Churchyard, G., & Vassall, A. (2017). The patient costs of care for those with TB and HIV: A cross-sectional study from South Africa. *Health Policy and Planning*, 32(suppl_4), iv48–iv56. https://doi.org/10.1093/heapol/czw183.

Munshi, P.B., Cairncross, L. Reynolds, T. Naledi, S. Cox, M. Stevens, I. Schoeman, N. Vidima, J. van Duuren, L., & Louskieter, S. (2020, July 13). *COVID-19: What a People-Centred Response to Covid-19 Would Look Like*. Daily Maverick. https://www.dailymaverick.co.za/article/2020-07-14-what-a-people-centred-response-to-covid-19-would-look-like/.

Mutyambizi, C., Pavlova, M., Hongoro, C., Booysen, F., & Groot, W. (2019). Incidence, socio-economic inequalities and determinants of catastrophic health expenditure and impoverishment for diabetes care in South Africa: A study at two public hospitals in Tshwane. *International Journal for Equity in Health*, 18(1), 73. https://doi.org/10.1186/s12939-019-0977-3.

Nachega, J.B., Grimwood, A., Mahomed, H., Fatti, G., Preiser, W., Kallay, O., Mbala, P.K., Muyembe, J.-J.T., Rwagasore, E., Nsanzimana, S., Ngamije, D., Condo, J.,

Sidat, M., Noormahomed, E.V., Reid, M., Lukeni, B., Suleman, F., Mteta, A., & Zumla, A. (2021). From easing lockdowns to scaling up community-based coronavirus disease 2019 screening, testing, and contact tracing in Africa—Shared approaches, innovations, and challenges to minimize morbidity and mortality. *Clinical Infectious Diseases*, 72(2), 327–331. https://doi.org/10.1093/cid/ciaa695.

Naidoo, Y. (2020, March 15). SA citizens diagnosed with Covid-19 after Italian ski trip in 'high spirits'. *Sunday Times*. https://www.timeslive.co.za/sunday-times/news/2020-03-15-sa-citizens-diagnosed-with-covid-19-after-italian-ski-trip-in-high-spirits/.

Naledi, T., Barron, P., & Schneider, H. (2011). Primary health care in SA since 1994 and implications of the new vision for PHC re-engineering. *South African Health Review*, 2011(1), 17–28. https://doi.org/10.10520/EJC119087.

National Institute for Communicable Diseases. (2020, March 5). First case of COVID-19 coronavirus reported in South Africa. *NICD*. https://www.nicd.ac.za/first-case-of-covid-19-coronavirus-reported-in-sa/https/nicd.ac.za/first-case-of-covid-19-coronavirus-reported-in-sa/.

National Institute for Communicable Diseases. (2022, December 17). *COVID-19 Hospital Surveillance Update: Week 50, 2022.* https://www.nicd.ac.za/wp-content/uploads/2022/12/NICD-COVID-19-Hospital-Surveillance-update-Week-50-2022.pdf.

National Institute for Communicable Diseases. (2023a, February 11). *COVID-19 Weekly Epidemiology Brief: Week ending 11 February 2023 (Week 6 of 2023).* https://www.nicd.ac.za/wp-content/uploads/2023/02/COVID-19-Weekly-Epidemiology-Brief-week-6-2023-.pdf.

National Institute for Communicable Diseases. (2023b, March 30). *Cholera Outbreak in South Africa (30 March 2023).* NICD. https://www.nicd.ac.za/cholera-outbreak-in-south-africa-30-march-2023/.

National Institute for Communicable Diseases. (2023c, March 31). *South African Measles Outbreak Update 2023 (31 March).* NICD. https://www.nicd.ac.za/south-african-measles-outbreak-update-2023-31-march/.

Ncayiyana, D. (1994). Coming to grips with the future of health care—The ANC National Health Plan. *South African Medical Journal*, 84, 55–56.

Nnyepi, M.S., Gwisai, N., Lekgoa, M., & Seru, T. (2015). Evidence of nutrition transition in Southern Africa. *Proceedings of the Nutrition Society*, 74(4), 478–486. https://doi.org/10.1017/S0029665115000051.

Noble, M., & Wright, G. (2013). Using indicators of multiple deprivation to demonstrate the spatial legacy of apartheid in South Africa. *Social Indicators Research*, 112(1), 187–201. https://doi.org/10.1007/s11205-012-0047-3.

Noknoy, S., Kassai, R., Sharma, N., Nicodemus, L., Canhota, C., & Goodyear-Smith, F. (2021). Integrating public health and primary care: The response of six Asia–Pacific countries to the COVID-19 pandemic. *British Journal of General Practice*, 71(708), 326–329. https://doi.org/10.3399/bjgp21X716417.

Nour, M., Lutze, S.A., Grech, A., & Allman-Farinelli, M. (2018). The relationship between vegetable intake and weight outcomes: A systematic review of cohort studies. *Nutrients*, 10(11), 1626. https://doi.org/10.3390/nu10111626.

Odendaal, N. (2021). Recombining place: COVID-19 and community action networks in South Africa. *International Journal of E-Planning Research (IJEPR)*, 10(2), 124–131. https://doi.org/10.4018/IJEPR.20210401.oa11.

Office of Health Standards Compliance. (2018, June 11). Statement on the OHSC annual inspection report for the public-sector health establishments inspected during the 2016/17 financial year. *Office of Health Standards Compliance.* https://ohsc.org.za/ohsc-annual-inspection-report-for-the-public-sector-health-establishments-inspected-during-the-2016-17-financial-year/.

Ojo, T., Ruan, C., Hameed, T., Malburg, C., Thunga, S., Smith, J., Vieira, D., Snyder, A., Tampubolon, S.J., Gyamfi, J., Ryan, N., Lim, S., Santacatterina, M., & Peprah, E. (2022). HIV, tuberculosis, and food insecurity in Africa—A syndemics-based scoping review. *International Journal of Environmental Research and Public Health,* 19(3), Article 3. https://doi.org/10.3390/ijerph19031101.

Oppong, J.R., Mayer, J., & Oren, E. (2015). The global health threat of African urban slums: The example of urban tuberculosis. *African Geographical Review,* 34(2), 182–195. https://doi.org/10.1080/19376812.2014.910815.

Pai, M. (2020, September 26). Tuberculosis and Covid-19: Fighting a deadly syndemic. *Forbes.* https://www.forbes.com/sites/madhukarpai/2020/09/26/tuberculosis-and-covid-19-fighting-a-deadly-syndemic/.

Parliament of South Africa. (2022, August 22). *National Health Insurance (NHI) Bill.* https://www.parliament.gov.za/project-event-details/54.

Peer, N., Uthman, O.A., & Kengne, A.-P. (2021). Rising prevalence, and improved but suboptimal management, of hypertension in South Africa: A comparison of two national surveys. *Global Epidemiology,* 3, 100063. https://doi.org/10.1016/j.gloepi.2021.100063.

Phaswana-Mafuya, N., Shisana, O., Jassat, W., Baral, S.D., Makofane, K., Phalane, E., Zuma, K., Zanga, N., & Chadyiwa, M. (2021). Understanding the differential impacts of COVID-19 among hospitalised patients in South Africa for equitable response. *SAMJ: South African Medical Journal,* 111(11), 1084–1091. https://doi.org/10.7196/samj.2021.v111i11.15812.

Phillips, H. (2014). The return of the pholela experiment: Medical history and primary health care in post-apartheid South Africa. *American Journal of Public Health,* 104(10), 1872–1876. https://doi.org/10.2105/AJPH.2014.302136.

Pietermaritzburg Economic Justice & Dignity Group. (2022). *Household Affordability Index—December 2022.* https://pmbejd.org.za/wp-content/uploads/2023/01/December-2022-Household-Affordability-Index-PMBEJD_28122022.pdf.

Pillay-van Wyk, V., Bradshaw, D., Groenewald, P., Seocharan, I., Manda, S., Roomaney, R.A., Awotiwon, O., Nkwenika, T., Gray, G., Buthelezi, S.S., & Mkhize, Z.L. (2020). COVID-19 deaths in South Africa: 99 days since South Africa's first death. *SAMJ: South African Medical Journal,* 110(11), 1093–1099. https://doi.org/10.7196/samj.2020.v110i11.15249.

Pillay-van Wyk, V., Cois, A., Kengne, A.P., Roomaney, R.A., Levitt, N., Turawa, E.B., Abdelatief, N., Neethling, I., Awotiwon, O.F., Nojilana, B., Joubert, J.D., Pacella, R., & Bradshaw, D. (2022). Estimating the changing burden of disease attributable to high fasting plasma glucose in South Africa for 2000, 2006 and 2012. *South African Medical Journal,* 594–606. https://doi.org/10.7196/SAMJ.2022.v112i8b.16659.

Pillay-van Wyk, V., Msemburi, W., Laubscher, R., Dorrington, R.E., Groenewald, P., Glass, T., Nojilana, B., Joubert, J.D., Matzopoulos, R., Prinsloo, M., Nannan, N., Gwebushe, N., Vos, T., Somdyala, N., Sithole, N., Neethling, I., Nicol, E., Rossouw, A., & Bradshaw, D. (2016). Mortality trends and differentials in South Africa from

1997 to 2012: Second national burden of disease study. *The Lancet Global Health*, 4(9), e642–e653. https://doi.org/10.1016/S2214-109X(16)30113-9.

Porter, J.D., Mash, R., & Preiser, W. (2020). Turnaround times - The Achilles' heel of community screening and testing in Cape Town, South Africa: A short report. *African Journal of Primary Health Care & Family Medicine*, 12(1), e1–e3. https://doi.org/10.4102/phcfm.v12i1.2624.

Probst, C., Parry, C.D.H., Wittchen, H.-U., & Rehm, J. (2018). The socioeconomic profile of alcohol-attributable mortality in South Africa: A modelling study. *BMC Medicine*, 16(1), 97. https://doi.org/10.1186/s12916-018-1080-0.

Ramkisson, S., Pillay, B.J., & Sibanda, W. (2017). Social support and coping in adults with type 2 diabetes. *African Journal of Primary Health Care and Family Medicine*, 9(1), 1–8. https://doi.org/10.4102/phcfm.v9i1.1405.

Reynolds., L. (2020). The coronavirus crisis and the struggle for health. *Amandla*, 69. https://aidc.org.za/the-coronavirus-crisis-and-the-struggle-for-health/.

Rispel, L.C., de Jager, P., & Fonn, S. (2016). Exploring corruption in the South African health sector. *Health Policy and Planning*, 31(2), 239–249. https://doi.org/10.1093/heapol/czv047.

Runciman, C., Roberts, B., Alexander, K., Bohler-Muller, N., & Bekker, M. (2021). UJ-HSRC COVID-19 Democracy Survey, Willingness to take a Covid-19 vaccine: A research briefing. Johannesburg: University of Johannesburg. https://www.uj.ac.za/wp-content/uploads/2022/02/2022-02-02-r5-vaccine-acceptance-and-hesitancy.pdf.

SABC News. (2018, August 2). High human cost of dop system spurs social responsibility. *SABC News - Breaking News, Special Reports, World, Business, Sport Coverage of All South African Current Events. Africa's News Leader.* https://www.sabcnews.com/sabcnews/sa-has-highest-number-of-children-living-with-foetal-alcohol-syndrome/.

SACoronavirus. (2023, May 8). Latest vaccine statistics. https://sacoronavirus.co.za/latest-vaccine-statistics/.

Sanders, D., Hendricks, M., Kroll, F., Puoane, T., Ramokolo, V., Swart, R., & Tsolekile, L. (2019). The triple burden of malnutrition in childhood: Causes, policy implementation and recommendations. In Shung-King, M., Lake, L., Sanders, D., & Hendricks, M. (Eds). *South African Child Gauge 2019* (pp. 145–160). Cape Town: Children's Institute, University of Cape Town.

Schneider, H., Hlophe, H., & van Rensburg, D. (2008). Community health workers and the response to HIV/AIDS in South Africa: Tensions and prospects. *Health Policy and Planning*, 23(3), 179–187. https://doi.org/10.1093/heapol/czn006.

Schotte, S., Zizzamia, R., & Leibbrandt, M. (2017). *Social Stratification, Life Chances and Vulnerability to Poverty in South Africa* [Working Paper]. http://localhost:8080/handle/11090/883.

Shaban, A.R.A. (2017, July 8). 'The face of poverty is feminine especially in South Africa' – Dlamini Zuma. *Africanews*. https://www.africanews.com/2017/07/08/the-face-of-poverty-is-feminine-especially-in-south-africa-dlamini-zuma/.

Simbayi, L., Zuma, K., Zungu, N., Moyo, S., Marinda, E., Jooste, S., Mabaso, M., Ramlagan, S., North, A., van Zyl, J., Mohlabane, N., Dietrich, C., Naidoo, I., & SABSSM V Team. (2019). *South African National HIV Prevalence, Incidence, Behaviour and Communication Survey, 2017*. HSRC Press. https://www.hsrcpress.ac.za/books/south-african-national-hiv-prevalence-incidence-behaviour-and-communication-survey-2017.

Singer, M. (2011). Toward a critical biosocial model of ecohealth in Southern Africa: The Hiv/Aids and nutrition insecurity syndemic. *Annals of Anthropological Practice*, 35(1), 8–27. https://doi.org/10.1111/j.2153-9588.2011.01064.x.

Singer, M., Bulled, N., Ostrach, B., & Mendenhall, E. (2017). Syndemics and the biosocial conception of health. *The Lancet*, 389(10072), 941–950. https://doi.org/10.1016/S0140-6736(17)30003-X.

Singh, K. (2020, December 21). Inside 17 public hospitals: Health workers forced to wear torn PPE, blitz inspections reveal. *News24*. https://www.news24.com/news24/southafrica/news/inside-17-public-hospitals-health-workers-forced-to-wear-torn-ppes-report-finds-20201221.

Solanki, G.C., Cornell, J.E., Besada, D., Morar, R.L., & Wilkinson, T. (2020). The competition commission health market inquiry report: An overview and key imperatives. *South African Medical Journal*, 110(2), 88. https://doi.org/10.7196/SAMJ.2020.v110i2.14455.

South African Government. (2021, November). *About Alert System*. https://www.gov.za/covid-19/about/about-alert-system.

South African History Online. (2019, August 27). *Prevention/Treatment*. https://www.sahistory.org.za/article/preventiontreatment.

Statistics South Africa. (2018). *Men, Women and Children—Findings of the Living Conditions Survey 2014 / 2015*. Statistics South Africa. https://www.statssa.gov.za/publications/Report-03-10-02%20/Report-03-10-02%202015.pdf.

Statistics South Africa. (2020a, February 4). *How Unequal Is South Africa?* Statistics South Africa. https://www.statssa.gov.za/?p=12930.

Statistics South Africa. (2020b). *General Household Survey 2019*. Statistics South Africa.

Statistics South Africa. (2021a, August 24). *South African Labour Market Is More Favourable to Men Than Women*. https://www.statssa.gov.za/?p=14606.

Statistics South Africa. (2021b). South Africa's people. https://www.gov.za/about-sa/south-africas-people.

Stokes, A., Berry, K.M., Mchiza, Z., Parker, W., Labadarios, D., Chola, L., Hongoro, C., Zuma, K., Brennan, A.T., Rockers, P.C., & Rosen, S. (2017). Prevalence and unmet need for diabetes care across the care continuum in a national sample of South African adults: Evidence from the SANHANES-1, 2011-2012. *PLOS ONE*, 12(10), e0184264. https://doi.org/10.1371/journal.pone.0184264.

Tegally, H., Wilkinson, E., Lessells, R.J., Giandhari, J., Pillay, S., Msomi, N., Mlisana, K., Bhiman, J.N., von Gottberg, A., Walaza, S., Fonseca, V., Allam, M., Ismail, A., Glass, A.J., Engelbrecht, S., Van Zyl, G., Preiser, W., Williamson, C., Petruccione, F., ... de Oliveira, T. (2021). Sixteen novel lineages of SARS-CoV-2 in South Africa. *Nature Medicine*, 27(3), Article 3. https://doi.org/10.1038/s41591-021-01255-3.

Templin, T., Hashiguchi, T.C.O., Thomson, B., Dieleman, J., & Bendavid, E. (2019). The overweight and obesity transition from the wealthy to the poor in low- and middle-income countries: A survey of household data from 103 countries. *PLOS Medicine*, 16(11), e1002968. https://doi.org/10.1371/journal.pmed.1002968.

The Competition Commission. (2019, September). *Healthcare Market Inquiry*. https://www.compcom.co.za/healthcare-inquiry/.

The Economist. (2022, September 29). *Global Food Security Index (GFSI)*. Global Food Security Index (GFSI). https://impact.economist.com/sustainability/project/food-security-index.

Thurston, R.C., Chang, Y., Matthews, K.A., Harlow, S., El Khoudary, S.R., Janssen, I., & Derby, C. (2022). Interpersonal trauma and risk of incident cardiovascular disease events among women. *Journal of the American Heart Association*, 11(7), e024724. https://doi.org/10.1161/JAHA.121.024724.

Trantraal., N. (2017). Delft. https://www.asymptotejournal.com/poetry/nathan-trantraal-chokers-en-survivors/.

Trangenstein, P.J., Morojele, N.K., Lombard, C., Jernigan, D.H., & Parry, C.D.H. (2018). Heavy drinking and contextual risk factors among adults in South Africa: Findings from the International Alcohol Control study. *Substance Abuse Treatment, Prevention, and Policy*, 13(1), 43. https://doi.org/10.1186/s13011-018-0182-1.

Turok, I. (1994). Urban planning in the transition from apartheid: Part 1: The legacy of social control. *The Town Planning Review*, 65(3), 243–259.

UNAIDS. (2006). *2006 Report on the Global AIDS Epidemic*. https://data.unaids.org/pub/report/2006/2006_gr_en.pdf.

UNAIDS. (2021). Global HIV & AIDS statistics—Fact sheet. https://www.unaids.org/en/resources/fact-sheet.

UNAIDS. (2022). *South Africa: UNAIDS Country Fact Sheet*. https://www.unaids.org/en/regionscountries/countries/southafrica.

UNICEF. (2021, Winter). *Uneven Routine Immunization Coverage Threatens the Health of South Africa's Youngest Children*. https://www.unicef.org/southafrica/press-releases/uneven-routine-immunization-coverage-threatens-health-south-africas-youngest.

US CDC. (2023, April 25). *Risk for COVID-19 Infection, Hospitalization, and Death by Age Group*. Centers for Disease Control and Prevention. https://www.cdc.gov/coronavirus/2019-ncov/covid-data/investigations-discovery/hospitalization-death-by-age.html.

van den Heever, A. (2020, June 29). South Africa sets aside more money for COVID-19 but lacks a spending strategy. *The Conversation*. http://theconversation.com/south-africa-sets-aside-more-money-for-covid-19-but-lacks-a-spending-strategy-141619.

van der Berg, S., Patel, L., & Bridgman, G. (2022). Food insecurity in South Africa: Evidence from NIDS-CRAM wave 5. *Development Southern Africa*, 39(5), 722–737. https://doi.org/10.1080/0376835X.2022.2062299.

van der Merwe, M. (2022, March 6). SA pensioners in dire financial state, report shows. *Business*. https://www.news24.com/fin24/sa-pensioners-in-dire-financial-state-report-shows-20200306-2.

van Ryneveld, M., Whyle, E., & Brady, L. (2020). What is COVID-19 teaching us about community health systems? A reflection from a rapid community-led mutual aid response in Cape Town, South Africa. *International Journal of Health Policy and Management*, 11(1), 5–8. https://doi.org/10.34172/ijhpm.2020.167.

Visagie, S., & Schneider, M. (2014). Implementation of the principles of primary health care in a rural area of South Africa: Original research. *African Journal of Primary Health Care and Family Medicine*, 6(1), 1–10. https://doi.org/10.4102/phcfm.v6i1.562.

Voigt, E. (2021, October 15). In-depth: Does SA have a diabetes testing problem? *Spotlight*. https://www.spotlightnsp.co.za/2021/10/15/in-depth-does-sa-have-a-diabetes-testing-problem/.

Waldrop, A.E., & Cohen, B.E. (2014). Trauma exposure predicts alcohol, nicotine, and drug problems beyond the contribution of PTSD and depression in patients with cardiovascular disease: Data from the heart and soul study. *The American Journal on Addictions*, 23(1), 53–61. https://doi.org/10.1111/j.1521-0391.2013.12053.x.

Wilkinson, R., Marmot, M., & WHO R.O. for Europe (2003). *Social Determinants of Health: The Solid Facts*. World Health Organization. Regional Office for Europe. https://apps.who.int/iris/handle/10665/326568.

World Bank. (2014). *Gini Index—South Africa*. https://data.worldbank.org/indicator/SI.POV.GINI?end=2014&locations=ZA&start=1993&view=chart.

World Health Organisation. (1978). *Declaration of Alma-Ata*. https://www.who.int/teams/social-determinants-of-health/declaration-of-alma-ata.

World Health Organization. (2021, December 6). *COVID-19 and the Social Determinants of Health and Health Equity: Evidence Brief*. https://www.who.int/publications-detail-redirect/9789240038387.

World Trade Organisation. (n.d.). *Overview of TRIPS Agreement*. Retrieved 25 April 2023, from https://www.wto.org/english/tratop_e/trips_e/intel2_e.htm.

Xezwi, K.A., & Xezwi, B. (2021, September 30). Maverick Citizen OP-ED: We can do it! Mass vaccination can be achieved through empowered community leadership. *Daily Maverick*. https://www.dailymaverick.co.za/article/2021-09-30-we-can-do-it-mass-vaccination-can-be-achieved-through-empowered-community-leadership/.

7 COVID-19 Syndemics in Three Distinct South African Communities and the Impact on Shared Loss and Grieving

Lorena Nunez Carrasco, Gracsious Maviza, Vuyokazi Myoli, and Storm Theunissen

COVID-19 is one of the most widespread pandemics of the past century (Eisma & Tamminga, 2020). In an effort to contain the pandemic locally, the South African government initially introduced policies on physical distancing, face masks, and restrictions on social events. As cases continued to rise globally, the government of President Cyril Ramaphosa declared a state of catastrophe and imposed an alert level 5 national lockdown from March 26 until April 30, 2020. Everyone in the country was forced to adhere to regulations, which were reinforced by military deployment. Only essential services remained operating. Public transportation was limited. Inter-provincial travel was prohibited. The hard lockdown aimed at buying time and preparing the health system to respond to an imminent disaster.

The alert level 5 was downgraded to an alert level 4 throughout the month of May 2020. Under alert level 4, nighttime curfews were imposed, schools remained closed, no leisure travel was allowed, and all alcohol sales were banned. While preventing the spread of the disease in the population, these lockdowns put the survival of the poorest and women at risk. Unemployment reached a record high of 34%. The high level of unemployment and precarity were fertile ground for an increase in violence. This was demonstrated by the events of July 2021 when there was an eruption of unrest in the provinces of Gauteng and KwaZulu-Natal, two key economic centers of the country, in which 354 lives were recorded lost, and thousands of businesses were looted and closed. According to the South African Owners Association, the unrest is estimated to have cost the country about 50 billion Rands ($3.3 billion) in lost production and put at least 150,000 jobs at risk. Domestic violence, already a major problem, also worsened.

Of significant concern was the potential impact of COVID-19 on the vulnerable immune-compromised population and on the healthcare system burdened by the existing epidemics of HIV and tuberculosis (TB). South Africa has the largest number of people living with HIV in the world and has the greatest number of people receiving anti-retroviral therapy (see Chapter 6 in this volume). TB rates are also very high, largely due to the historical heritage of the precarious working conditions in the gold, platinum, and diamond

DOI: 10.4324/9781003365358-8

mines and the HIV epidemic. In the wake of the COVID-19 pandemic, these and other chronic diseases have been neglected.

According to official figures from the South African Medical Research Council, excess deaths in 2022 suggested that more than 133,000 people in the country died from COVID-19. This figure has been contested by the scientific community arguing that the excess deaths during the pandemic are 2.5 times higher than the official number reported by the government (Heywood, 2021). Unlike countries in the Global North, these deaths have occurred mostly among young people. Not only have a significant number of deaths not been recognized in the official counts, but there are also invisible effects of the pandemic. To a large extent, while the economic impact of the pandemic and subsequent lockdown is evident and devastating, the underlying and underestimated impact of the pandemic on physical and mental health has been regarded as inconsequential (Nguse & Wassenaar, 2021). Furthermore, restrictions on funerary and burial practices, so important for South African populations, directly impacted the grieving process and mental health. Mental health issues continue to be unrecognized, resources are limited, and the resources provided by the government for the management of these issues remain of low quality.

COVID-19 deeply impacted South African societies across the racial and class divide. Lockdown measures were justified in a discourse that emphasized the need to protect the population. In practice, they protected the middle and affluent classes leaving the poor and socially marginalized helpless. Direct financial subsidies were granted to manage the COVID-19 pandemic as a form of distributive, marginal justice aimed at the poorest segments of the population. However, foreign-born migrants were not included as beneficiaries of these subsidies despite constituting approximately 6% of the country's population and serving as a significant proportion of the essential workforce (Mukumbang et al., 2020).

In its interactions with existing inequalities, marginalities, and vulnerabilities of different communities in South Africa, COVID-19 became syndemic. It amplified specific contextual biosocial factors that created adverse and precarious conditions and health outcomes for different communities (Horton, 2020; Schmidt-Sane et al., 2021; Singer & Rylko-Bauer, 2021). In this chapter, we present ethnographic accounts of three distinct communities in South Africa – the AmaXhosa in the Eastern Cape, white Afrikaans speakers, and Zimbabwean migrants – to reveal how COVID-19 syndemics have played out in specific ways across diverse communities. Past work on COVID-19 syndemics has contrasted populations in different countries. In this chapter, we affirm the local nature of syndemics by comparing COVID-19 syndemics in three populations in the same country, with differing demographics, disease histories, and social conditions that collectively result in, at times, different syndemic outcomes. Syndemics in this context not only provide a frame to examine the distinct presentation of biosocial factors and their interactions in each community, but also reveals the lasting deleterious social impacts of disease epidemics.

AmaXhosa: A Syndemic of Economic Marginalization

Rural and other marginalized communities have been subjected to the most gruesome adverse effects of the COVID-19 pandemic and the related government response. Social, economic, and political inequalities were amplified by the pandemic and by the health response, as Bambra and colleagues (2020, p. 967) contend:

> Historically, people have experienced pandemics differently and unequally with higher rates of infection and mortality among the most disadvantaged communities – particularly in more socially unequal countries. Emerging evidence from a variety of countries suggests that these inequalities are being mirrored today in the COVID-19 pandemic. Both then and now, these inequalities have emerged through the syndemic nature of COVID-19 – as it interacts with and exacerbates existing social inequalities in chronic disease and the social determinants of health.

For marginalized and rural communities, such as the AmaXhosa community residing in and around King William's Town[1] in South Africa's Eastern Cape Province, the COVID-19 pandemic had a synergistic effect. Limited and informal employment opportunities, long-standing endemics of HIV and TB, alcohol use and gender-based violence, and underfunded healthcare systems, became exacerbated by the emergence of the COVID-19 pandemic (Chenneville et al., 2020).

In the poverty-stricken rural setting of King William's Town, government efforts to contain the COVID-19 pandemic—the national lockdown—resulted in unanticipated and devastating effects. In this context, large households frequently share very small and under-resourced spaces, making social distancing, and the isolation/quarantining of cases impossible. Furthermore, the lockdowns occurred during the winter months, when temperatures reach an average high of 13°C/55°F, and most people prefer to spend time inside with doors and windows sealed. Consequently, during the period of national lockdown, an increase in TB cases was observed along with a rapid spread of COVID-19. The transmission routes of COVID-19 and TB are similar – close contact with an infected person via secretions from the respiratory tract (Alene, et al., 2020; Chapter 4 of this volume). A study from Cape Town, South Africa, suggests that COVID-19 patients with TB have a 2.7 times higher risk of mortality compared to COVID-19 patients without TB (Western Cape Department of Health, 2021). The combination of TB and COVID-19 is considered a "cursed duet," with TB patients at significantly higher risk of COVID-19 infection and poor disease outcomes (TB/COVID-19 Global Study Group, 2022). With TB endemic in the region and physical distancing impossible for many, rates of TB grew in King William's Town in the wake of COVID-19.

In addition, already high rates of HIV and chronic health conditions such as diabetes further increased the likelihood of COVID-19 infection and mortality. COVID-19 and diabetes have a bi-directional relationship: people with diabetes are more susceptible to COVID-19 infection given chronic low-grade inflammation and have higher rates of hospital admissions, severe pneumonia, and higher mortality; conversely, COVID-19 is capable of damaging the pancreas which worsens diabetes blood sugar management and even induces the onset of diabetes (Lima-Martínez et al., 2021; Chapter 3 in this volume).

Although evidence to date does not suggest that people living with HIV have a higher susceptibility to COVID-19 infection, a large population-based study from the Western Cape Province, South Africa, reported higher risk of death (Western Cape Department of Health, 2021). The study cohort contained a high number of people living with HIV who were not virologically suppressed or were living with uncontrolled diabetes, potentially explaining the divergent results compared with Europe and the US. Disparities in social conditions and comorbidities are presumed to have a greater influence on disease outcomes than biological interactions with HIV (Brown et al., 2021). Such social conditions include limited access to routine healthcare services, given the over-burdened underfunded and crisis-ridden public hospitals and health clinics, resulting in the disrupted management of chronic disease conditions.

In King William's Town, people living with HIV were unable to access clinics to obtain their routine medications, worsening their HIV disease progression and heightening their risk for poor COVID-19 outcomes. This situation is evident in the account of Zuko, who struggled to access routine treatment services. Zuko, from Mtyholo village just outside of King William's Town, shares:

> Besingakwazi nokuya eklinikhi, okanye esibhedlele ngoba kuthiwa ezondawo zezona ndawo kuthiwa kusulelwana khona. Kengoku bekunzima uphuma apha endlini sithi siyahambha siya eklinikhi ngoba nalapho akuvumelekanga ukuba sishiye izindlu zethu. Sineeswekile ke thina namathambo, ngelaxesha zange sikwazi nokuya siyokufumana itreatment le siyidingayo.
>
> We couldn't even go to the clinic or hospital because it was said that that's where the most transmission [of COVID-19] happens. Now it became difficult to even leave the house to attend clinic visits because we were not even allowed to leave our homes. We have [suffered from] diabetes and bone issues and during that time we could not access the treatment [medication] we needed.

In addition to limiting access to necessary healthcare resources, South Africa's national lockdown and other restrictive policies including the ban on the sale of alcohol, contributed unexpectedly to increasing public health risk. In King William's Town, the government ban on alcohol sales increased the brewing of alcohol at home, known locally as "home brews." South Africans began sharing home-brewing tips on social media. Home-made alcohol included ginger beer and pineapple brews. As these concoctions are unstandardized and unregulated, the alcohol content and safety are unknown. In May 2020, nine people died in different villages in the Eastern Cape, including three in King William's Town, after drinking home brew mixed with potent additives like methylated spirits (Pyatt, 2020).

In King William's Town, home brews not only resulted in the deaths of community members, but they were also linked to perceived increases in intimate partner violence. Thandokazi, a 22-year-old full-time college student, attributed alcoholism and intimate partner violence to COVID-19. She argues that COVID-19 and the national lockdown resulted in a series of causal consequences: job losses, the consumption of alcohol by people who ordinarily did not drink, and violent behavior towards intimate partners. She tells the story of her neighbor, a man who lost his job during the COVID-19 lockdown and resorted to alcohol to reduce his resulting anxiety.

> Yazi sisi, imbhi into endiybone ngexesha le Covid, ngoba abantu ebend-ingazange ndababona besela before [long pause] ndithi zange ndibabone besele before COVID, kodwa kuthe kowuvalwa, abantu balahlekelwa yimisebenzi savalelwa ezindlini…ndaqala apho ukubona ukuba umntu nanini na angatshintsha. Umeza wam wazombethela apha ekhaya um-fazi wakhe ngenxa yokuba echithe umtshovalale wakhe. Ndaqala apho ke mna ukuyibona ukuba esisifo neziphumo sazo ziyingozi.
>
> You know sister, what I witnessed during the COVID era was horrible, because people I had never seen drinking before [long pause] I'm saying I had never seen them drunk before COVID, but when the country was closed (lockdown) and people lost their jobs, we were caged in our homes…that was the first time I realized that a person can change anytime. My neighbor beat his wife up here at my home with reasons that she threw away his home brewed alcohol. That is when I realized that this sickness (COVID-19) and its repercussions are dangerous.

The situation was made even worse as women could not escape the violence and victim services were inaccessible. Nduna and Tshona (2021, p. 347) indicate that

> informal sources of help for victims of abuse were limited due to closed economic activities, and community-based helping services for domestic violence were not permitted to open. Some victims of domestic violence struggled with public transportation to access informal help, visit the police, social workers and other sources of help.

In the absence of social support structures to address job loss, emergency transportation, and victim services, people were left abandoned and suffering. Government policies only offered protection from COVID-19.

Elite communities in South Africa found ways of living comfortably in the midst of a pandemic through the normalization of the "new" work-from-home industrial culture and newfound ways of maintaining social connection virtually; all made possible by the luxury and use of technology (Mbambo & Agbola, 2020). By contrast, the employment of the national lockdown for the greater social good proved to have unintended consequences in marginalized and rural communities (Bank & Sharpley, 2020), like King William's Town. In the absence of large homes for physical distancing, access to healthcare services, and financial resources to support loss of income, poor and marginalized communities suffered a synergy of biological and social conditions that heighten risk of disease morbidity and mortality (Bank & Sharpley, 2020).

Afrikaner: A Syndemic of Loss and Grief

The Afrikaner ethnic group in South Africa descended from Dutch settlers and other Western Europeans who settled at the southern tip of South Africa in the 17th and 18th centuries.[2] The Afrikaner community speak the Afrikaans language, which developed as a vernacular of Dutch, German, and French. Based on the 2011 South African National Census, Afrikaners (number of white South Africans who speak Afrikaans as a first language) only make up 5.2% of the total South African population.

The Afrikaner community,[3] especially the older generation, are known for being tough and resilient. As the common Afrikaans saying goes, "Die sterkste mens is die een wat die meeste seer dra, en stil verlang sonder dat iemand daarvan bewus is." [The strongest person is the one who hurts the most, and silently longs without anyone being aware of it.] They barely regard mental health. Nicolette, a member in the Afrikaner community, explains:

> We don't ever really discuss mental health in our culture. It's not a thing. You don't tell people you are struggling. It's like money, it's something you just keep to yourself. It also makes you sound weak, and we are not weak people, huh…it's actually funny if you think about it. But we are now beginning to realize that there are problems, and we are struggling to mentally deal with them. We have to face the fact that mental health is a thing, and it does affect us, and we should talk about it.

This view has made it difficult for the community to manage the COVID-19 pandemic, its policies, losses, and resulting mental health issues. The members in this community suffered job and financial losses, the loss of loved ones, and the loss of community, and because of these losses and their inability to provide for their families they lost their sense of pride and self-esteem. Such losses have resulted in a unique syndemic of mental health, situated in a legacy of Apartheid that has limited both the availability and utility of mental health services.

Mental health in South Africa has been treated as an inconsequential issue in the South African health sector (Nguse & Wassenaar, 2021). Mental health continues to be unrecognized as well as under-resourced. Although the South African government has made legislative policies to prioritize mental health, it has failed in its implementation. According to Willem, a member of the Afrikaner community, politicians treat their mental illness related to COVID-19 grief as inconsequential, brushing it off with statements such as "Kom al klaar daaroor. Dit is deel van die lewe." [Get over it already. It is a part of life.] This has been particularly problematic in the Afrikaner community, where issues related to mental health are rarely discussed and individuals are unlikely to admit to needing help. Furthermore, the already limited healthcare resources in South Africa were spent on the biomedical aspect of the COVID-19 pandemic and disregarded the mental impact (Nguse & Wassenaar 2021, p. 309). The COVID-19 pandemic has "amplified the existing mental health gap and constrained access to mental health care services" (Nguse & Wassenaar, 2021, p. 305). Willem explains this convergence of economic and cultural issues:

> Hoe moet ons ons geestes gesondheidskwessies hanteer as ons geen hulpbronne het om dit te hanteer nie? En die hulpbronne wat beskikbaar is, is duur vir die gemiddelde Suid-Afrikaner. Hoekom sal ons te midde van 'n pandemie vir iets so duur betaal as ons ons werk verloor het en nie eers kan bekostig om kos te koop nie. Geestesgesondheid is die laaste ding op die lys waarna gesorg moet word.
>
> How must we cope with our mental health issues if we don't have any resources to deal with them? And the resources that are available are expensive to the average South African. Why would we pay for something that expensive in the middle of a pandemic when we have lost our jobs and can't afford to even buy food. Mental health is the last thing on the list that needs to be taken care of.

During the first four months of the nationwide lockdown more than 3 million South Africans lost their jobs (Ingle et al., 2020). These job losses occurred during a time in South Africa when there were already alarming rates of unemployment. The Afrikaner community were no exception to this. Loss of employment due to shutdowns and illness, and the consequent inability to financially support self and family forced mass borrowing, increased debt, and forced a reliance on community and social services such as food parcels from local churches. In addition, Apartheid legacies and personal pride prevented middle-class Afrikaners from utilizing free or low-cost public hospital services, delaying medical care for COVID-19 infections and disease co-morbidities, and contributing to a rise in mental health issues.

Theuns, a 65-year-old male who was a car mechanic in Cape Town, suffered many losses due to the pandemic and his mental well-being was deeply affected. Theuns lost both his job and his brother. In losing his job, he struggled with his self-esteem and pride; he no longer felt "man" enough to provide for his family. The loss of employment in the Afrikaner community affected access to resources, such as food and medical treatment, elevating symptoms of anxiety and depression (Posel et al., 2021). Theuns describes his experience:

> Ek het my broer verloor, my werk verloor en my reg om saam met my familie bymekaar te kom verloor. Dit het my lewe baie moeilik gemaak en ek het gesukkel om alles te hanteer. Toe ek my werk verloor moes ek geld by familie leen en dit het my trots aangetas ek het nutteloos gevoel. Ek moes ook kospakkies by die kerk kry om seker te maak my vrou en kinders het kos om te eet. Dit het my gebreek, ek het nie soos ń man gevoel nie, ek voel nog steeds nie soos een nie.
>
> I lost my brother, lost my job, and lost my right to gather with my family. It made my life very difficult, and I struggled to cope with everything. When I lost my job, I had to borrow money from family and it affected my pride, I felt useless. I also had to get food parcels from the church to make sure my wife and children had food to eat. It broke me, I didn't feel like a man, I still don't feel like one.

Grief is an emotional response people have towards experiences of loss (Weinstock et al., 2021). Being unable to process the loss of loved ones, jobs, identities, social status, self-esteem, affects the grieving process which heightens risk for mental illness. Studies conducted in other countries have demonstrated that nation-wide lockdown is associated with depressive symptoms, anxiety symptoms, and sleeping disturbances (Choudhari, 2020; Gualano et al., 2020; Mukhtar, 2020). Erika describes her altered mental state, a consequence of pandemic losses:

> I really can't seem to function properly. It takes effort to do anything, even brushing my teeth is too much to handle. All I do is cry and sleep. And I'm just so angry, I'm fuming. Sleeping has been the only thing I can really do. When I sleep, I don't have to think of anything. I don't need to think about my son no longer being here and I don't need to live through the experience. I honestly feel sick. I wish I could go to sleep forever.

The only way members of the Afrikaner community (and many communities worldwide) can successfully grieve loss is to perform cultural rituals. These rituals are context-dependent: for the loss of a loved one, rituals would include proper funeral processes and gatherings; for financial or job loss, it would include reaching out for support, accepting the reality, and taking time to adjust. These rituals have either been altered or removed to accommodate COVID-19 prevention policies. Under alert level 5, no gatherings were allowed. Under alert level 4, funeral attendance was limited to 50 persons or less if people could not maintain a six-foot physical distance, no night vigils or after-funeral gatherings were allowed, face mask wearing and social distancing measures were required during services, and services were limited to a maximum of two hours (https://www.gov.za/covid-19). Some of these rituals for grieving, specifically related to employment loss, a more recent experience in the Afrikaner community in post-Apartheid South Africa, were never present to begin with.

Family members resented COVID-19 policies that prevented them from taking care of community members during their time of grief. Normally family and community members would collectively plan and arrange funeral services, cook food, hand out memorial letters, and most importantly offer personal support during a time of loss. Saying goodbye to loved ones for Afrikaners means having an embodied presence. Grief is normally experienced in a social setting with other family and community members. Support allows the bereaved to recover (Kasiram & Partab, 2002). Government COVID-19 pandemic policies restricting travel and social gatherings limited the support community members could provide to one another; the policies restricted people's ability to both provide comfort and to accept loss. In complicating the process of grieving, COVID-19 and government regulations have increased mental health burdens including anxiety and depression.

Nicolette expressed her desperate need to say goodbye to her deceased loved one. She described a proper goodbye as including the presence and physical support of family, friends, and community; as involving the gathering of loved ones to celebrate the life of that individual and acknowledging the new spiritual role of that person, and as witnessing that person being buried. It includes eating food together, singing and crying together, and sharing stories. Without this goodbye, Afrikaners have a difficult time processing their grief. Nicolette is also deeply affected by the desire to have done more for her mother during life, an idea that is strongly attached to pandemic-specific deaths. Without the usual social structures to manage this grief, some will develop clinical mental health issues.

> Ek kan nie meer nie…ek, ek wil nie meer nie. Dit is te moeilik. My hart is in stukkies en voel soos dit nooit weer heel sal wees nie. Die lig is uit my lewe uit en ek voel soos ek in die donker bly. Ek wil terug gaan na 'n tyd waar sy nog steeds daar is, waar ek kan se mammie ek is lief vir jou en jou kan nou maar rus, maar dit sal nie gebêre nie. Ek kon meer vir haar doen. Ek wou net bye sê.

> I can't anymore…I, I don't want too anymore. It is too difficult. My heart is in pieces and feels like it will never be whole again. The light is out of my life, and I feel like I live in darkness. I want to go back to a time when she is still there, where I can say mommy, I love you and you can rest now, but that won't happen. I could have done more for her. I just wanted to say goodbye.

COVID-19 has proven unpredictable, and despite public health disease control efforts including the national lockdown, physical distancing regulations, mask policies, and vaccines, it did not appear to be ending soon. This uncertainty further impacted the mental state of people suffering personal and financial losses. Willie talks about the effect of this uncertainty and his thoughts of what should be done.

> Dit is moeilik om te dink hoe ons voort gaan. Ons weet nie eers hoe lank Covid hier gaan wees nie en dit affekteer hoe ons treur. Niemand weet nie en dit is die grootste probleem. Ek dink rêrig die regering moet iets uit sort. Wat nou aan gaan is nie goed nie en maak die pandemie net erger.
>
> It is difficult to think about how we will go forward. We don't even know how long Covid will be here, and it affects how we grieve. Nobody knows and that is the biggest problem. I really think the government must sort something out. What's going on now isn't good and it's making the pandemic harder.

Willie's perceptions are shared by many members of this community. They fear not only the pandemic but the uncertainty of how the pandemic will affect their lives moving forward. For members of this community, COVID-19-related losses have made existing depression and anxiety symptoms worse for some and stimulated depression and anxiety symptoms in others. At present, there is no evidence to indicate that COVID-19 and mental health illness are interacting biologically, such as mental illness increasing risk of COVID-19 infection or worsening COVID-19 disease progression, or COVID-19 infection causing the onset of depression or anxiety. However, the psychosocial impact of COVID-19 and COVID-19 control policies has been clearly documented globally. In addition, existing chronic diseases such as diabetes, alcohol and/or drug addiction, cardiovascular disease, are likely to have been impacted by the mental distress of COVID-19, as outlined on work on stigma-related syndemics (Marcus et al., 2017; Ostrach et al., 2017). The effects of the mental illness/COVID-19 losses syndemic in the Afrikaner community are compounded by social and structural factors that include limited access to mental health care given high cost of private facilities and Apartheid legacies that deny poor Afrikaners access to public services, poor quality of mental healthcare services available, limited government-supported social and financial services, and a culture of stoicism and toughness that denies the need for mental healthcare.

Zimbabwean Migrants: A Syndemic of Political Precarity

South Africa has been a preferred destination for many migrants from other parts of Africa given its commitment to upholding the rights of asylum-seekers and its advanced economy. An estimated 2 million foreign-born migrants of working age (15–64) were living in South Africa in 2017, representing 5.3% of the South African labor force (African Centre for Migration & Society, 2020). Unofficially, the migrant population in South Africa today is estimated to be around 4.2 million (Garba, 2020). The South African Refugees Act provides the right for asylum-seekers and refugees to work and study, to access medical services and life-saving treatment and freedom of movement (Consortium for Refugees & Migrants in South Africa, 2008). However, limited capacity to manage the large volume of asylum-seekers and migrants, bureaucratic inefficiency, and corruption have created a backlog in the system (Masuku, 2020). Consequently, many migrants remain undocumented, unable to find meaningful long-term employment, relegated to the informal sector, face precarious employment conditions, are compelled to reside in underprivileged communities, and are unable to access medical services that require nationally approved identification.

In addition, there is the shared perception that migrants deprive South Africans of employment, business opportunities, and place a strain on social services and amenities. This is supported by data from the Centre for Migration and Society that indicates, all things being equal, migrants do have a higher probability of being employed and owning businesses than South Africans (African Centre for Migration & Society, 2020). This constitutes the main driver of xenophobic feelings that often turn violent (Choane et al., 2011). Although these geopolitical tensions have always been present, most have been brought to the surface by the overwhelming effects of the pandemic which has paralyzed economies and investment in basic services, adversely affecting migrants.

While the national lockdown negatively affected all people living in South Africa, migrants disproportionally experienced the negative impacts of the pandemic given their existing vulnerabilities (Mukumbang et al., 2020). The hard lockdowns and the disease control measures implemented by the South African government to curb the pandemic rendered migrants incomeless, invisible, and, in some instances, stranded (Sizani, 2020; Zanker & Moyo, 2020). Migrants from Zimbabwe[4] were unable to return home when international borders closed. Interviews with selected Zimbabwean migrants revealed that many lost their jobs and had no money for their basic upkeep. One of the respondents narrated that:

> COVID-19 really affected me [...]. I was used to a decent life with decent meals, clothing, and accommodation. But with COVID-19, we both lost our jobs, my husband and I, and eventually, our savings were finished. It was the longest two years.
>
> (M5)

Another migrant stated that they got help from their siblings in better-performing economies like the United Kingdom and America, stating, "I remember I stayed the whole of 2021 without working at all. At some point, my rentals were paid by my brother and sisters who were overseas. It was tough" (M1).

The economic vulnerability experienced by migrants directly impacted their mental well-being increasing levels of depression as some lost not only jobs and housing, but also beloved family members (Jesline et al., 2021; York, 2022). Furthermore, migrants could not send remittances to their dependents back home, increasing the impact of COVID-19 on extended families. Evidence shows that migrants living under such circumstances of vulnerability in sub-Saharan Africa have consistently poorer mental health outcomes than others (Bempong et al., 2019). One migrant was notably bitter and aggrieved, stating that he failed to take care of his mother. He harbored bitterness and anger, blaming himself that he could not fulfill his obligation to his mother, who depended on him for survival. He put it this way:

I felt defeated; I really had episodes of depression. I was not working and could not properly take care of my family here in South Africa, but at least I was with them. What really broke me was that I could not support my ailing mother. I had no money and could not travel just to be with her, at least.

(M4)

Migrants who managed to retain their jobs were vulnerable in other ways. Several studies from countries and regions around the world acknowledge that migrants dominate key sectors in the urban environment (e.g., distribution, food processing, or health care), which were deemed essential during COVID-19 lockdowns (Jesline et al., 2021; OECD, 2020). Most Zimbabweans in South Africa work in typical migrant sectors such as hospitality, retail, cleaning, and vending (Angu & Masiya, 2022). Given their dominance in essential sectors, their vulnerability to COVID-19 exposure was increased (Jesline et al., 2021; York, 2022). A Zimbabwean migrant working in the health sector in Johannesburg narrated that:

I am a nurse in a private health facility. I was forced to work daily; I had bills to pay and children to take care of. Every time I stepped out of the house felt like I was gambling with my life; it was really depressing.

(M2)

Working in spite of the risks was necessary as migrants were not considered in any of the South African government plans to mitigate the effects of the pandemic (Carrasco 2021; Mukumbang et al., 2020; Zanker & Moyo, 2020). Three economic measures were adopted to address some of the socio-economic hardship that COVID-19 control measures had caused: six months of a Social Relief of Distress grant of 350 Rands (20 USD) to all unemployed individuals; a temporary increase in the value of child and social support grants; and a Business Relief Fund of 500 million Rand (30 million USD) for businesses affected by the COVID-19 pandemic. In addition, the government provided tax subsidies for small businesses and individuals and lowered contributes to the Unemployment Insurance Fund. Migrants were unable to access any of these. To be considered for the Business Relief Fund, businesses must be 100% South African owned (Business Insider South Africa, 2020a). Foreign-born migrants (documented or undocumented) did not receive payments from their Unemployment Insurance Fund as the electronic system used to distribute the funds did not recognize foreign passport numbers (Business Insider South Africa, 2020b). Similarly, access to food parcels, government food relief programs, and the Social Relief of Distress grants required a South African national ID or special permit, which many migrants do not possess (Bornman & Oatway, 2020; Reuters, 2020).

Given lack of official documentation, a situation further worsened by the closure of the Department of Home Affairs responsible for renewing and issuing residence permits, migrants became vulnerable to harassment and extortion by law enforcement agents (Garba, 2020). During COVID-19 lockdowns there were reports that migrants were more likely to be arrested for minor offenses (Ntshidi, 2020). Fears of being arrested, detained, or deported, prevented migrants from seeking tests or care for COVID-19 symptoms, decreasing the possibilities for early detection, diagnosis, contact tracing, and treatment (Mukumbang et al., 2020). This increased the risk of clustered outbreaks among migrants (Blumberg et al., 2020) as well as poor disease outcomes or death.

Even prior to COVID-19, migrants in South Africa faced health-related vulnerabilities. Most migrants entering South Africa come from regions with endemic malaria, HIV, and TB (Faturiyele et al., 2018; Pindolia et al., 2014; Vearey, 2018), diseases known to have biological interactions with COVID-19 (Bulled & Singer, 2020). In addition, there is equally large burden of non-communicable diseases among migrants living in South Africa (Vearey et al. 2017), primarily due to poor living conditions and high levels of stress. Diseases such as diabetes, obesity, asthma, and cardiovascular disease are also recognized as having poor biological interactions with COVID-19, increasing vulnerability to infection and worsening disease outcomes (Singer & Rylko-Bauer, 2021). Migrants in South Africa face challenges accessing preventative and curative healthcare services including the lack of migration-aware and mobility-competent health system programs (Vearey et al., 2017). There is an overall poor engagement of South Africa's public healthcare system with migrants, and as such, testing and treatment responses within public health system failed to engage with migrants during the COVID-19 pandemic (Vearey, 2014).

The COVID-19 pandemic exposed several fault lines in different societies (Schmidt-Sane, et al., 2021). For the Zimbabwe migrant community in South Africa, their lives have always been characterized by cleavages of hostility in the form of xenophobia as well as vulnerability and precarity related to housing and working conditions, unequal access to healthcare and social services, and higher risk for exploitation and abuse (Crush & Tawodzera, 2017; Crush et al., 2017; Culbertson, 2009; Merry et al., 2017; Mukumbang et al., 2020). The lockdown worsened these conditions as migrants found themselves suddenly jobless, evicted from their homes, food insecure, and trapped in homes, dormitories or camps where physical distancing proved difficult (Botes & Thaldar, 2020; Ray, 2020). Migrants were ineligible for state subsidies and as such were compelled to continue to work resulting in greater exposure to COVID-19. Furthermore, border closures due to hard lockdowns and the observance of disease control measures to contain the virus rendered migrants immobile, further restricting their already weak social support structures. For Zimbabwean migrants in South Africa, COVID-19 became a syndemic of social and political precarity.

Conclusion

The South African government put in place a 'state of exception' to manage a national emergency, one that "appears as the legal form of what cannot have legal form" (Agamben, 2005, p. 1). The imposed restrictions, enforced by a military presence, resulted in significant losses throughout South Africa. For the AmaXhosa in the King William's Town, the Afrikaans, and Zimbabwean migrants in Johannesburg, the losses and uncertainty experienced due to COVID-19 have created and continue to fuel feelings of uncertainty, distress, anxiety, fear, anger, and hopelessness; conditions considered as precursors and prodromes of mental health illnesses such as anxiety and depression (Batterham et al., 2013; IOM, 2020) and secondary health concerns – neglect of self-care, respiratory infections, and substance abuse (Mukhtar, 2020). These social and biological conditions synergistically interact in unique ways in each population to worsen COVID-19 vulnerability and disease outcomes. The failure of the state to take an integrated approach to COVID-19 that acknowledges layered challenges faced by different communities renders certain populations invisible and amplifies existing inequalities (Schmidt-Sane et al., 2021).

Notes

1 A study on bereavement in the times of COVID-19 was conducted in rural King William's Town focusing on the AmaXhosa people. Semi-structured interviews were conducted in participants' homes and participant observation was achieved primarily through the rapport-establishing process as well as during the conversations with participants. These interviews were conducted primarily in isiXhosa. However, due to the complicated nature of the different dialects in the isiXhosa language, some English was also used in the interviews. All participants were isiXhosa-speaking locals.

2 Afrikaner | South African History Online, *From European to "Africaander,"* https://www.sahistory.org.za/article/afrikaner.

3 There are 16 participants in this research consisting of both male and female individuals from five white Afrikaans-speaking families. The participants are all from a middle-class socio-economic background and this affects the kinds of narratives

they provided. The participants are situated in different regions within South Africa: one family resides in Cape Town, three families reside in Johannesburg, and the last family resides in Limpopo.
4 The insights offered here are based on a qualitative study conducted among the community of Zimbabwean migrants from Tsholotsho residing in Johannesburg. The study focused on transnational migrants from families that had experienced at least one COVID-19 death between March 2020 and December 2021.

References

African Centre for Migration & Society. (2020). *Fact sheet on foreign workers in South Africa: overview based on statistics South Africa data (2012–2017).* Johannesburg: ACMS. http://www.migration.org.za/fact-sheet-on-foreign-workers-in-south-africa-overview-based-on-statistics-south-africa-data-2012-2017/.

Agamben, G. (2005). State of exception. Trans Kevin Attell. Chicago: University of Chicago Press.

Alene, K.A., Wangdi, K., & Clements, A.C.A. (2020). Impact of the COVID-19 pandemic on tuberculosis control: an overview. *Tropical Medicine and Infectious Disease,* 5(3), 123. https://doi.org/10.3390/tropicalmed5030123.

Angu, P., & Masiya, T. (2022). *South African-based African migrants' responses to COVID-19: strategies, opportunities, challenges and implications.* LANGAA RP-CIG Project MUSE muse.jhu.edu/book/102003

Bambra, C., Riordan, R., Ford, J., & Matthews, F. (2020). The COVID-19 pandemic and health inequalities. *Journal of Epidemiology and Community Health,* 74(11), 964–968. https://doi.org/10.1136/jech-2020-214401.

Bank, S., & Sharpley, N. (2020). A state of (greater) exception? Funerals, custom and the "war on COVID" in rural South Africa. *South African Review of Sociology,* 51(3–4), 143–164. https://doi.org/10.1080/21528586.2021.2015717.

Batterham, P.J., Christensen, H., & Calear, A.L. (2013). Anxiety symptoms as precursors of major depression and suicidal ideation. *Depress Anxiety,* 30, 908–916.

Bempong, N.E., Sheath, D., Seybold, J., et al. (2019). Critical reflections, challenges and solutions for migrant and refugee health: 2nd M8 Alliance expert meeting. *Public Health Reviews,* 40, 3.

Blumberg, L., Jassat, W., Mendelson, M., et al. (2020). The COVID-19 crisis in South Africa: protecting the vulnerable. *South African Medical Journal.* https://doi.org/10.7196/SAMJ.2020.v110i9.15116.

Bornman, J., & Oatway, J. (2020). South Africa: migrants excluded from government food aid. *All Africa.* https://allafrica.com/stories/202005130663.html.

Botes, W.M., & Thaldar, D.W. (2020). COVID-19 and quarantine orders: a practical approach. *South African Medical Journal,* 110, 1. https://doi.org/10.7196/samj.2020v110i6.14794.

Brown, L.B., Spinelli, M.A., & Gandhi, M. (2021). The interplay between HIV and COVID-19: summary of the data and responses to date. *Current Opinion in HIV and AIDS,* 16(1), 63–73. https://doi.org/10.1097/COH.0000000000000659.

Bulled, N., & Singer, M. (2020) In the shadow of HIV & TB: a commentary on the COVID epidemic in South Africa. *Global Public Health,* 15(8), 1231–1243. https://doi.org/10.1080/17441692.2020.1775275.

Business Insider South Africa. (2020a). UIF Covid-19 payout trouble: these are the most common problems holding back the cash. *Business Insider South Africa.* https://www.businessinsider.co.za/how-to-avoid-uif-problems-2020-5.

Business Insider South Africa. (2020b). Prime less 5% for honest small businesses – and plus 10% for chancers: Covid-19 help details. *Business Insider South Africa.* https://www.businessinsider.co.za/help-for-my-business-during-the-coronavirus-disaster-in-south-africa-2020-3.

Carrasco, L.N. (2021). Dying in COVID times, an account of the experiences of migrants in South Africa. In *Every body counts: Death, Covid-19 and migration understanding the consequences of pandemic measures on migrant families.* Methoria: The Last Rights Project.

Chenneville, T., Gabbidon, K., Hanson, P., & Holyfield, C. (2020). The impact of COVID-19 on HIV treatment and research: a call to action. *International Journal of Environmental Research and Public Health*, 17(12), 4548. https://doi.org/10.3390/ijerph17124548.

Choane, M., Shulika, L.S., & Mthombeni, M. (2011). An analysis of the causes, effects and ramifications of xenophobia in South Africa. *Insight Africa*, 3, 129–142.

Choudhari R. (2020). COVID 19 pandemic: mental health challenges of internal migrant workers of India. *Asian Journal of Psychiatry*, 54, 102254. https://doi.org/10.1016/j.ajp.2020.102254.

Consortium for Refugees and Migrants in South Africa. (2008). *Protecting refugees, asylum seekers and immigrants in South Africa.* Johannesburg. www.cormsa.org.za.

Crush, J., & Tawodzera, G. (2017). *Living with xenophobia: Zimbabwean informal enterprise in South Africa.* Southern African Migration Programme. https://scholars.wlu.ca/samp/21/.

Crush, J., Tawodzera, G., Chikanda, A., et al. (2017). *South Africa case study: the double crisis–mass migration from Zimbabwe and xenophobic violence in South Africa.* Southern African Migration Programme. https://scholars.wlu.ca/samp/4/.

Culbertson, P.E. (2009). *Xenophobia: the consequences of being a Zimbabwean in South Africa.* School of Public Affairs, Master's Thesis, The American University in Cairo.

Eisma, M.C., & Tamminga, E. (2020). Grief before and during the COVID-19 pandemic: multiple group comparisons. *Journal of Pain and Symptom Management*, 60(6), e1–e4. https://doi.org/10.1016/j.jpainsymman.2020.10.004.

Faturiyele, I., Karletsos, D., Ntene-Sealiete, K., et al. (2018). Access to HIV care and treatment for migrants between Lesotho and South Africa: a mixed methods study. *BMC Public Health*, 18, 668.

Garba, N.W.F. (2020). Covid-19 in South Africa: whither migrants? *African Arguments.* https://africanarguments.org/2020/06/17/covid-19-in-south-africa-whither-migrants/.

Gualano, M.R., Lo Moro, G., Voglino, G., et al. (2020). Effects of Covid-19 lockdown on mental health and sleep disturbances in Italy. *International Journal of Environmental Research in Public Health*, 17, 4779.

Heywood, M. (2021). 264,809 deaths later: Covid-19's terrifying toll on South Africa, almost three times the official figure. *Daily Maverick.* https://www.dailymaverick.co.za/article/2021-10-20-264809-deaths-later-covid-19s-terrifying-toll-on-south-africa-almost-three-times-the-official-figure/.

Horton, R. (2020). Offline: COVID-19 is not a pandemic. *The Lancet*, 396(10255), 874.

Ingle, K., Brophy, T., & Daniels R.C. (2020). National Income Dynamics Study–Coronavirus Rapid Mobile Survey (NIDS-CRAM) panel user manual. Technical Note Version 1. Cape Town: Southern Africa Labour and Development Research Unit.

International Organization for Migration. (2020). IOM reiterates importance of addressing mental health impacts of COVID-19 on displaced and migrant populations. https://www.iom.int/news/iom-reiterates-importance-addressing-mental-health-impacts-covid-19-displaced-and-migrant.

Jesline, J., Romate, J., Rajkumar, E., & George, A.J. (2021). The plight of migrants during COVID-19 and the impact of circular migration in India: a systematic review. *Humanities and Social Sciences Communications*, 8(1), 231. https://doi.org/10.1057/s41599-021-00915-6.

Kasiram, M.I. & Partab, R. (2002). Grieving through culture and community: A South African perspective. *Social Work*, 38(1), 39–44.

Lima-Martínez, M.M., Carrera Boada, C., Madera-Silva, M.D., et al. (2021). COVID-19 and diabetes: a bidirectional relationship [COVID-19 y diabetes mellitus: una relación bidireccional]. *Clínica e Investigación en Arteriosclerosis (English Edition)*, 33(3), 151–157. https://doi.org/10.1016/j.artere.2021.04.004.

Marcus, R., Singer, M., Lerman, S., & Ostrach, B. (2017). *Foundations of biosocial health: stigma and illness interactions*. Lanham, MD: Lexington Books.

Masuku S. (2020, May 12). How South Africa is denying refugees their rights: what needs to change. *The conversation*. https://theconversation.com/how-south-africa-is-denying-refugees-their-rights-what-needs-to-change-135692. Accessed 30 July 2020

Mbambo, S.B., & Agbola, S.B. (2020). The impact of the COVID-19 pandemic in townships and lessons for urban spatial restructuring in South Africa. *African Journal of Governance & Development*, 9(1.1), 329–351.

Mbiba, B. (2010). Burial at home? Dealing with death in the diaspora and Zimbabwe's new diaspora: displacement and the cultural politics of survival. In J. McGregor & R. Primorac (Eds.), *Zimbabwe's New Diaspora: Displacement and the Cultural Politics of Survival* (pp. 144–163). New York: Berghahn Books.

Merry, L., Pelaez, S., & Edwards, N.C. (2017). Refugees, asylum-seekers and undocumented migrants and the experience of parenthood: a synthesis of the qualitative literature. *Globalization and Health*, 13(1), 1–17.

Mukhtar, S. (2020). Psychological health during the coronavirus disease 2019 pandemic outbreak. *International Journal of Social Psychiatry*, 66, 512–516.

Mukumbang, F.C., Ambe, A.N. & Adebiyi, B.O. (2020). Unspoken inequality: how COVID-19 has exacerbated existing vulnerabilities of asylum-seekers, refugees, and undocumented migrants in South Africa. *International Journal of Equity Health*, 19, 141. https://doi.org/10.1186/s12939-020-01259-4.

Nduna, M., & Tshona, S.O. (2021). Domesticated poly-violence against women during the 2020 Covid-19 lockdown in South Africa. *Psychology Studies*, 66(3), 347–353. https://doi.org/10.1007/s12646-021-00616-9.

Nguse, S. & Wassenaar, D. (2021). Mental health and COVID-19 in South Africa. *South African Journal of Psychology*, 51(2), 304–313. https://doi.org/10.1177/00812463211001543.

Ntshidi, E. (2020). 130 people arrested in Soweto for breaching lockdown laws, other offences. *Eyewitness News*. https://ewn.co.za/2020/05/11/police-arrest-130-people-in-soweto-for-breaching-lockdown-laws.

Organisation for Economic Co-operation and Development. (2020, November 26). *COVID-19 and key workers: what role do migrants play in your region?* OECD. https://www.oecd.org/coronavirus/policy-responses/Covid-19-and-key-workers-what-role-do-migrants-play-in-your-region-42847cb9/.

Ostrach, B., Lerman, S., & Singer, M. (Eds). (2017). *Stigma syndemics: new directions in biosocial health*. Lanham, MD: Lexington Books.

Pindolia, D.K., Garcia, A.J., Huang, Z., et al. (2014). Quantifying cross-border movements and migrations for guiding the strategic planning of malaria control and elimination. *Malaria Journal*, 13(1), 1–11.

Posel, D., Oyenubi, A., & Kollamparambil, U. (2021). Job loss and mental health during the COVID-19 lockdown: evidence from South Africa. *PLoS ONE*, 16(3), e0249352. https://doi.org/10.1371/journal.pone.0249352.

Pyatt, J. (2020, May 25). Fourteen people die and ten more are fighting for their lives after drinking home brew to get around South Africa alcohol ban. https://www. dailymail.co.uk/news/article-8355213/Fourteen-people-die-ten-fighting-lives-drinking-home-brew-South-Africa.html.

Ray, S.C. (2020). Covid-19 special collection. *African Journal of Primary Health Care and Family Medicine*, 12. https://doi.org/10.4102/PHCFM.V12I1.2466.

Reuters. (2020). Migrants and those without ID face hunger in South vAfrica. *New York Post*. https://nypost.com/2020/05/20/migrants-and-those-without-id-face-hunger-in-south-africa/.

Schmidt-Sane, M., Leach, M., MacGregor, H., et al. (2021). Local Covid-19 syndemics and the need for an integrated response. *IDS Bulletin*, 52(1). https://doi.org/10.19088/1968-2021.103.

Singer, M., & Rylko-Bauer, B. (2021). The syndemics and structural violence of the COVID pandemic: anthropological insights on a crisis. *Open Anthropological Research*, 1(1), 7–32.

Sizani, M. (2020, March 27). Covid-19: police shut immigrant-owned spaza shops after Minister's xenophobic statement. *Daily Maverick*. https://www.dailymaverick.co.za/article/2020-03-27-covid-19-xenophobia-alert-police-shut-immigrant-owned-spaza-shops-after-ministers-statement/

The TB/COVID-19 Global Study Group. (2022). Tuberculosis and COVID-19 co-infection: description of the global cohort. *European Respiratory Journal*, 59(3), 2102538. https://doi.org/10.1183/13993003.02538-2021.

Vearey, J. (2014). Healthy migration: a public health and development imperative for South (ern) Africa: forum-opinion. *South African Medical Journal*, 104(10), 663–664.

Vearey, J. (2018). Moving forward: why responding to migration, mobility and HIV in south(ern) Africa is a public health priority. *Journal of International AIDS Society*, 21, e25137.

Vearey, J.O., Modisenyane, M., & Hunter-Adams, J. (2017). Towards a migration-aware health system in South Africa: a strategic opportunity to address health inequity. *South African Health Review*, 2017(1), 89–98.

Weinstock, L., Dunda, D., Harrington, H., & Nelson, H. (2021). It's complicated—adolescent grief in the time of Covid-19. *Frontiers in Psychiatry*, 12, 166. https://doi.org/10.3389/fpsyt.2021.638940.

Western Cape Department of Health in collaboration with the National Institute for Communicable Diseases, South Africa. (2021). Risk factors for coronavirus disease 2019 (COVID-19) death in a population cohort study from the Western

Cape Province, South Africa. *Clinical Infectious Diseases*, 73(7), e2005–e2015. https://doi.org/10.1093/cid/ciaa1198

York, J. (2022). How Covid-19 has made life more dangerous for migrant workers. Retrieved from Migration Data Portal: The bigger picture. https://www.migrationdataportal.org/blog/how-covid-19-has-made-life-more-dangerous-migrant-workers.

Zanker, F.L., & Moyo, K. (2020). The corona virus and migration governance in South Africa: business as usual? *Africa Spectrum*, 55(1), 100–112.

8 The Iatrogenic Syndemic of COVID-19/Diabetes Mellitus/Black Fungus in India

Evidence of the Shortcomings of Neoliberal Healthcare Policies

Nicola Bulled

In 2021, India experienced a sudden and unexpected second wave of COVID-19. Close to 30 million cases were officially reported, with a true toll estimated at closer to 500 million cases (Gamio & Glanz, 2021). The surge rapidly overwhelmed India's already tenuous health infrastructure. National oxygen supplies were quickly depleted, hospital beds filled to overcapacity, ventilators were in short supply, and COVID-19-specific treatments and supplies dwindled. Desperate patients lined up outside hospitals, unable to gain entrance let alone admittance. Poorly managed distribution of oxygen and the reliance on industrial oxygen supplies resulted in black market dealings and soaring prices. Providers were forced to take desperate measures, including prescribing steroids and zinc to alleviate symptoms, even in patients they were unable to closely monitor.

Patients and their families without the benefit of a health professional consultation cobbled together treatment strategies to alleviate suffering and prevent death (The Lancet, 2021). Anecdotal evidence suggests that treatment plans offered by doctors for one individual were used to address the symptoms of others, including reports of shared drug treatments. General advice offered on social media was implemented without awareness of potential side effects or cautionary use warnings. Such treatments included the use of oxygen concentrators and easily accessible and cheap antibiotics (Sulis et al., 2021), steroids, and vitamins. In mid-May reports surfaced of the Karnataka Youth Congress (a political party) distributing the steroid Dexahim as part of a COVID-19 home isolation kit (India Today, 2021a).

As the surge of COVID-19 pushed India's healthcare system to a point of almost complete collapse, a second epidemic began to emerge. Clustered outbreaks occurred of a rare disease, mucormycosis commonly referred to as "black fungus," caused by environmental molds found in soil and decaying organic matter (Jeong et al., 2019). The prevalence of mucormycosis in the year 2019–2020 ranged from 0.005 to 1.7 per million people worldwide, with the incidence in India about 80 times greater than in industrialized nations (Prakash & Chakrabarti, 2019; Skiada et al., 2020). At least 14,872 cases of mucormycosis had been reported in India as of May 28, 2021

DOI: 10.4324/9781003365358-9

(Raut & Huy, 2021) with 200 deaths (Biswas, 2021a, 2021b). Two states declared an epidemic and the central government declared it a prominent disease in India (CNN, 2021).

The disease involves the fungal hyphae invading the respiratory tract and destroying tissues in the sinuses and surrounding structures resulting in dark disfiguring patches on the face, blindness, cranial nerve palsies, and brain invasion (Kontoyiannis & Lewis, 2015). Treatment requires prompt initiation of aggressive and costly surgical intervention and antifungal agents (Cornely et al., 2019). Compounding the crises in India were reported shortages of amphotericin B, the main antifungal used to treat mucormycosis, which gave rise to a black market for drugs that were already too expensive for most people to afford (India Today, 2021d; National Geographic, 2021). Even under ideal conditions, with prompt surgical debridement and adequate antifungal therapy mortality from black fungus is high, with estimates ranging from 50% to 85% (Palejwala et al., 2016; Roden et al., 2005).

As exposure to the mold is common, black fungus is not contagious and generally the fungi are not harmful in healthy individuals, Indian doctors became curious about the rise in cases. They realized that the majority of people with mucormycosis were COVID-19 patients, recently recovered ones, immunosuppressed individuals, or individuals with underlying conditions, particularly diabetes mellitus (Gandra et al., 2021; Ghazi et al., 2021; Rocha et al., 2021; Singh et al., 2021). More than 80% of patients with COVID-19-associated mucormycosis had elevated blood glucose levels at presentation (Singh et al., 2021). The clusters of COVID-19/black fungus/ diabetes mellitus in India suggested disease interactions that extended beyond biologies to social conditions that enhanced deleterious outcomes of co-morbidities.

In this chapter, I explore the syndemic of COVID-19/black fungus/diabetes mellitus, and specifically the role of the indiscriminate use of steroids to treat COVID-19 patients in response to an overwhelmed health system. It explores how the social inequities in India created the ideal context for syndemic outbreaks, with marginalized groups at greatest risk given poor living conditions (i.e., densely populated slums with limited ability to physically distance and inadequate access to clean water) increasing exposure to black fungus and COVID-19, existing health conditions including undiagnosed diabetes, and an overreliance on poorly regulated pharmaceuticals given limited access to quality healthcare. Finally, I argue for a re-articulation of national and global public health principles away from the neoliberal public health agenda towards one that prioritizes individual behavior change, assumes agency, and consequently places both the responsibility and the burden of health on citizens. Governments must assume responsibility for ensuring healthy environments, improved living conditions, adequate access to quality foods, and affordable healthcare, which will reduce each of the epidemics of COVID-19, diabetes mellitus, and black fungus independently and as a syndemic.

The COVID-19/Diabetes Mellitus Syndemic in India

People with existing diseases are known to both be at higher risk for COVID-19 and suffer more severe outcomes (World Heart Federation, 2020). In India, 86% of COVID-19 patients had comorbidities (Thakur, 2020). In Italy, 96.2% of COVID-19 patients who died in hospitals had co-morbidities (Yadav et al., 2020). The most commonly reported comorbidities that have been shown to predict poor prognosis in COVID-19 patients include hypertension, diabetes, cardiovascular disease, and chronic lung disease (Guan et al., 2020; Kluge et al., 2020; Thakur, 2020; Wang et al., 2020; Yang et al., 2020a; Yang et al., 2020b). Patients with comorbidities such as diabetes have underlying immune system deficiencies, which may make them more susceptible to infection and COVID-19 complications (Pal & Bhadada, 2020).

An ecological study of the association of diabetes with state-level COVID-19 cases and deaths per million from February to November 2020 found a statistically significant positive correlation (Gaur et al., 2017). The syndemic nature of COVID-19 and diabetes has been described (Singer & Rylko-Bauer, 2021), with multiple pathways suggested. Biologically, people with uncontrolled diabetes have compromised innate immune systems, the first line of defense against COVID-19, allowing for the unchecked proliferation of virus within the body (Pal & Bhadada, 2020). Increasing stress levels resulting from COVID-19 infection cause the release of hyperglycemic hormones, which prompt an increase in blood glucose, further suppressing the immune system. In addition, an exaggerated pro-inflammatory or cytokine response, characteristic of diabetes (Geerlings & Hoepelman, 1999), can lead to rapid deterioration, shock, and acute respiratory distress syndrome. Furthermore, people with diabetes have reduced expression of the angiotensin-converting enzyme 2 critical to regulating blood pressure and wound healing. In short, there appear to be multiple pathways facilitating adverse interactions between COVID-19 and diabetes.

Patients with diabetes are commonly prescribed an ACE inhibitor and angiotensin receptor blocker (Pal & Bhadada, 2020). ACE2 is an epithelial cell membrane glycoprotein expressed on the lungs, kidney, intestine, and blood vessels. SARS-CoV-2 uses ACE2 as a receptor for entry into host pneumocyte lung cells (Wrapp et al., 2020). As such, any condition that upregulates ACE2 is likely to facilitate infection with COVID-19. While ACE2 expression is reduced in patients with diabetes, ACE inhibitor and angiotensin receptor blocker drugs increase the expression of ACE2 (Fang et al., 2020). Thus, standard treatment measures for diabetes might be a contributing cause for the severe and fatal COVID-19 disease seen in patients with diabetes. Pal and Bhadada (2020) have recommended alternative treatment strategies such as a calcium channel blocker that does not upregulate ACE2 levels, despite organizations worldwide recommending the continuation of standard treatment measures.

The failure of healthcare systems to adjust chronic disease management highlights the social parameters of the COVID-19/diabetes syndemic. Not only did health providers not adjust treatment regimens to respond to the threat of COVID-19, but patients routine healthcare services were disrupted because of the COVID-19 threat. COVID-19 lockdowns left many with co-morbidities unable to access services or acquire necessary treatments (Yadav et al., 2020). A survey of 155 countries conducted by the World Health Organization (2020) revealed that 53% had partially or completely impaired services for non-communicable diseases. The problem was further exacerbated by the reassignment of health staff from facilities managing non-communicable disease care to COVID-19 facilities. Disruptions of medical supplies and diagnostics also resulted from nationwide lockdowns. In India, some outpatient services were temporarily closed and hospitals completed converted into designated COVID-19 wards (Basu, 2020).

India is deemed the diabetes capital of the world, home to over 77 million people with diabetes (*Diabetes Atlas, 9th Edition*, 2019). Not only are those numbers large, noncompliance with medications by many results in poorly controlled diabetes (Guariguata et al., 2014). A survey of 13,055 blood samples in four states in India revealed that the prevalence of diabetes was higher in urban compared to rural areas, with rates highest in urban men in the 55–64 age group (Anjana et al., 2011). Rapid urbanization and an increasingly sedentary lifestyle, a consequence of the built urban environment, lacking green space, and safe opportunities for informal physical activities, as well as calorie-dense diets, contribute to the high prevalence of diabetes in India (Nanditha et al., 2016).

Further compounding these epidemic challenges are significant social, economic, and political inequities. A large proportion of urban Indian residents live in informal settlements or slums.[1] The 2011 Indian census shows that one of six urban Indians resides in a slum. Informal settlements in India are legally structured and recognized by the government as either notified versus non-notified slums. Approximately 59% of slums in India are non-notified, which limits residents from access to critical health, sanitation, and education services (Agarwal & Taneja, 2005; Nolan et al., 2017; Osrin et al., 2011; Subbaraman et al., 2012). Estimates indicate that over 35% of slum households do not have access to clean drinking water (CSE, 2020). The 2011 Indian census data showed that 26% of slum dwellers have to search for drinking water outside of their homes. Over half of them are forced to collect drinking water more than 100 meters away from their houses. People are forced to walk through narrow pathways to reach the nearest water sources. These slum pathways are often not even two meters wide making the recommended COVID-19 "social" distancing guidelines impossible to follow (Raju & Ayeb-Karlsson, 2020). Research studies in Mumbai's Kaula Bandar slum show that the lack of access to water has severe implications on people's health, livelihood productivity, and income (Subbaraman et al., 2012).

The compromised living conditions of urban slums contribute to chronic and infectious disease, with slums determined as "unhealthy places" (Ezeh et al., 2017). High population density can result in increased transmission of infectious diseases, such as COVID-19, pneumonia, diarrhea, and tuberculosis (Unger & Riley, 2007). Most slum dwellers reside in one-room homes, often shared with relatives. Residents in urban slums also suffer from chronic illness such as obesity, diabetes, tuberculosis, and respiratory diseases. Furthermore, as non-notified, slum residences were unrecognized by the Public Distribution System leaving many urban poor without food sources during COVID-19 lockdowns (Roy et al., 2020).

Tenuous living situations are coupled with temporary, inadequately regulated, and harsh employment conditions. Many slum dwellers are seasonal or temporary migrant workers, and over 80% of people in India are employed within the informal sector (Bonnet et al., 2019), with no paid leave, insurance, or employment rights (ILO, 2018). These jobs include temporary and seasonal work such as construction work, food- and street vendors, and rickshaw pullers. Millions of people lost their only source of income as the COVID-19 lockdowns closed many industries and street operations across India. Notions of illegality, socio-economic exclusion, informal employment, high population density, weak health services, and inadequate access to water, sanitation, waste management and healthcare services combined to make containing the COVID-19 outbreak a significant challenge (Raju et al., 2021). Collectively they created the social conditions that supported a COVID-19/diabetes mellitus syndemic.

Biomedical Intervention Creates an Opportunity for an Iatrogenic Syndemic

Struggling to contain the surge and working against the biological and social dynamics supporting a syndemic of COVID-19/diabetes mellitus, healthcare professionals began implementing biomedical interventions that played a role in further expanding and exacerbating the syndemic. With oxygen shortages and dwindling supplies of recommended COVID-19 therapies such as remdesivir, doctors began to rely more heavily on steroids to alleviate symptoms. COVID-19 clinical management protocols issued by the Government of India's Ministry of Health and Family Welfare in late May 2021 included the use of inhaled steroids for the management of mild home-based cases. Oral steroids were also recommended, but only if symptoms did not subside over days. For more severe hospitalized cases, parenteral methylprednisolone or dexamethasone were recommended as routine part of therapy. Corticosteroids mitigate the systematic inflammatory response stimulated by COVID-19, which if left untreated can lead to lung injury and multisystem organ dysfunction.

However, even in patients with COVID-19, steroids appeared to have no benefit for those not requiring supplemental oxygen (Group et al., 2021).

Of greater concern, indiscriminate use of corticosteroids, especially in individuals with diabetes, further suppresses the immune systems by raising blood sugars. While increases in blood sugars in response to steroid use were considered temporary, new evidence suggests that steroid use in COVID-19 patients in India stimulated the onset of diabetes, even among people who did not have pre-diabetes (Gandra et al., 2021). Corticosteroids increase insulin resistance, resulting in poorly regulated blood glucose in people with diabetes and the unmasking of diabetes in people with pre-diabetes. In India, patients also resorted to self-medicating with steroids, following the guidance of friends, family, and the media (Ghazi et al., 2021).

Already susceptible to infection due to COVID-19 and diabetes, steroids further suppressed patients' immune responses making them more susceptible to other infections, like mucormycosis. While exposure to mucormycosis is common, prior to the second COVID-19 surge in India, cases of black fungus remained rare. Unregulated blood glucose levels, a combined result of limited access to routine treatment during COVID-19 lockdowns, the effects of COVID-19 on the body, and the additional impact of COVID-19 treatments involving steroids that both worsened existing diabetes and stimulated pre-diabetes, is regarded as the major contributing factor to mucormycosis or black fungus infections. In addition, supplements including zinc, immune system boosters, became part of routine treatment management against COVID-19. Zinc is known to play an important role in fungal growth and development, and positively influences fungal pathogenesis (Staats et al., 2013). The overuse of zinc to respond to a COVID-19 infection could have also contributed to the rise in mucormycosis cases (Gandra et al., 2021).

In addition to the overreliance on steroids as an anti-inflammatory treatment and zinc as an immune system boosting supplement, experts indicate that the humidifiers in COVID-19 wards may have created environments that increased susceptibility to fungal infections (Ghazi et al., 2021). Humidifiers may also have been contaminated with mucormycosis. Similarly, experts speculate that the climate of South Asia, with its high temperatures and humidity, contributes to black fungus infections. The dependence on industrial oxygen created another avenue for black fungus infections as it is not always sterilized (The Times of India, 2021). Prolonged use of the same face masks and breathing tubes, as well as unsterilized medical equipment are also considered causes of black fungus. Beyond the biomedical setting, poverty, low-quality living standards, unhygienic environments, limited access to uncontaminated water, and the cleaning and reuse of cloth facemasks potentially contaminated with mucormycosis, played a role in the COVID-19/diabetes/black fungus iatrogenic syndemic.

In addition, a rising number of cases of *Candida auris*, or "white fungus," have also been reported, with estimates of between 20% and 30% of severely ill, mechanically ventilated COVID-19 patients infected (Biswas, 2021b). *Candida auris* is the most frequently detected germs in critical-care units, has developed drug resistance, and has a mortality rate of 70%. Doctors

Factors contributing to COVID-19 surge
- Lifting of shutdown, social distancing, and face mask mandates
- No limits on Kumbh Mela
- Political rallies held without enforced COVID-19 measures
- Limited urgency placed on vaccine production and national distribution
- Limited social services to address COVID-19-related hardships

COVID-19

Diabetes

Factors contributing to high rates of Diabetes Mellitus
- Urbanization
- Sedentary lifestyles
- Calorie-dense diets
- Limited green space and safe spaces for informal physical activity
- Air pollution

Mucormycosis

Factors contributing to mucormycosis outbreaks
- National policies indicating steroid use of mild and moderate COVID-19 patient management
- Drug and oxygen stock-outs resulting in over-reliance on steroids
- Distribution of steroids in COVID-19 home care kits
- Unregulated blood glucose due to steroid-induced insulin resistance

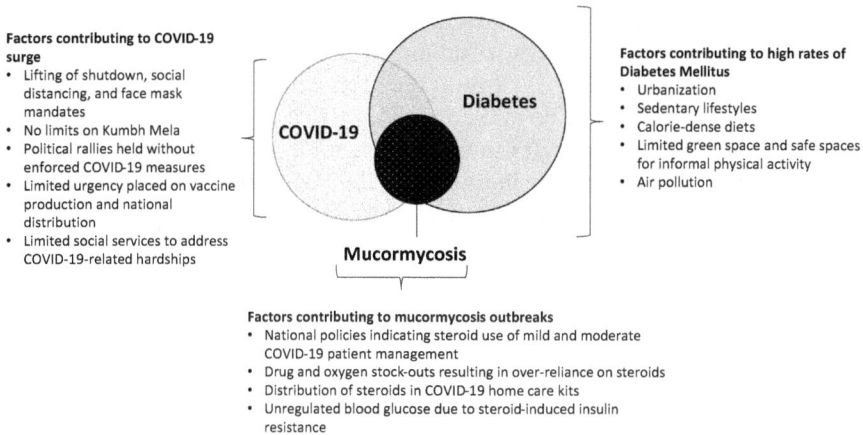

Figure 8.1 An iatrogenic syndemic model of an overburdened health sector and consequent indiscriminate steroid use, COVID-19, diabetes mellitus, and mucormycosis in India.

attribute the rise in *Candida auris* infection to lowered infection control in crowded intensive-care units, a result of fatigue and complacency in overworked healthcare workers during the prolonged pandemic (Biswas, 2021b).

The interaction of these biological and social conditions with the unintended influence of biomedical intervention is considered an iatrogenic syndemic (Singer, 2009; Singer et al., 2017) (see Figure 8.1). Iatrogenesis reflects the adverse effects of medical treatment on health. The schistosomiasis control campaign in Egypt that took place from 1950 to 1980 is one example of iatrogenesis. The use of unsafe intravenously administered therapies during the community-wide schistosomiasis control campaigns led to high numbers of hepatitis C infections (Frank et al., 2000; Strickland, 2006). As a result, Egypt had the highest hepatitis C prevalence in the world, with approximately 5.5 million persons with chronic infections, or 10% of the adult population (Waked et al., 2020). Iatrogenic syndemics are rare, with few fully described. In India, the reliance on steroids and zinc to treat patients with COVID-19, without proper management of blood sugars, as well as the use of unsterilized oxygen, medical equipment, and medical wards, created the conditions that increased the likelihood that patients with pre-diabetes and diabetes succumbed to mucormycosis infections. These interactions are further supported by the social, economic, and political conditions that increased risk for each disease independently and all diseases synergistically.

Recommendations

The COVID-19/diabetes/black fungus iatrogenic syndemic in India serves as a clear warning of the failings of governments globally to develop comprehensive public health programs that extend beyond healthcare delivery to include equity initiatives in economies, infrastructure, environments, and housing. Moving forward, several recommendations, action points, and safeguard measures should be implemented.

First, public health strategies must move away from the neoliberal public health agenda that prioritizes individual behavior change, assumes agency, and consequently places both the responsibility and the burden of health on citizens. Publications in the *Annals of Internal Medicine* (Gandra et al., 2021) and the *American Journal of Hygiene and Tropical Medicine* (Ghazi et al., 2021) examining the black fungus outbreak in India offer solutions that prioritize individual behavior change. Both recommend the wearing of facemasks and physical distancing to prevent COVID-19; vaccination against COVID-19; education on the signs and symptoms of mucormycosis (Gandra et al., 2021); the avoidance of spaces where mucormycosis is common; the wearing of facemasks in places where mucormycosis is likely to be disturbed (e.g., construction sites); wearing protective clothing when handling soil or materials likely infected with mucormycosis; and maintaining personal hygiene (Ghazi et al., 2021). Given the social, economic, and political conditions that place individuals in India at risk for both COVID-19 and mucormycosis, including high density communities preventing physical distancing and limited access to water and sanitation services such recommendations are likely to have limited effect. Governments must ensure healthy environments, increase the availability of improved housing, provide adequate access to quality food and affordable healthcare. Collectively, these efforts to improve underlying social, economic, and political conditions that drive much of the disease will reduce each of the epidemics of COVID-19, diabetes mellitus, and black fungus independently and synergistically.

In addition to the social conditions supporting the epidemics, the indiscriminate use of medications and the overreliance on pharmaceuticals to address social conditions (Ecks, 2020) generated the iatrogenic syndemic. As a first line of intervention, stewardship measures must be implemented to curtail the use of steroids to address COVID-19 both within the formal medical sector and informally as a treatment strategy at home. Policies on the restricted use of steroids should align with recent calls to regulate antibiotic access (Sulis et al., 2021). A time series analysis of antibiotic sales revealed a significant increase in non-child-appropriate formulation antibiotic sales, and particularly azithromycin, during the peak phase of the first COVID-19 epidemic wave in India (Sulis et al., 2021). Strict laws do exist, but they are rarely enforced to regulate the dispensing of drugs by pharmacists and other health establishments that drive patient self-medication (Ghazi et al., 2021). Scholars also call for a system to review, monitor, and regularly audit the treatment and drugs prescribed by physicians as a measure to ensure more judicial future use (Ghazi et al., 2021).

Longer term, governments globally must acknowledge their role in implementing and enforcing measures that ensure public health. At a minimum, this involves investing in basic health and social infrastructures to provide adequate access to healthcare and healthy environments (Yadav et al., 2020), and recognizing that market-driven healthcare systems perpetuate health inequalities and are unable to respond adequately during health crises (Singer & Rylko-Bauer, 2021). To date, while India has successfully achieved a high COVID-19 vaccine coverage rate (New York Times vaccine tracker estimating 69% of the population has been fully vaccinated, https://www.nytimes.com/interactive/2021/world/covid-vaccinations-tracker.html), only 16% of the population has received additional boosters, with no plans presented for the distribution of new variant booster vaccinations. In the medical sector, pandemic preparedness plans need to be developed, ensuring that drug stockouts are minimized and resources can be quickly mobilized.

Cooperation and compliance of citizens during disease outbreaks is necessary, but this requires clear communication and coordinated national strategies, as well as access to resources and structural support beyond the medical sector. Supporting bottom-up approaches by mobilizing grassroots leaders, youth groups, and existing committees proved successful in communicating key health messages and implementing welfare measures through local expertise (Du et al., 2020; Wilkinson et al., 2020). In Kerala, civil society organizations provided services to community members through a "volunteer army" (Dutta & Fischer, 2021). Rapid response of civilian organizations ensured the distribution of food and personal protective equipment to people living in urban slums in Delhi and Mumbai (Shepherd, 2020). Youth in the slums of Nairobi created murals to communicate important prevention measures during the pandemic (UN HABITAT, 2015, 2020). In Mumbai's largest slum, Dharavi, home to approximately 1 million, slum leaders continued their role as problem-solvers to contain the spread of COVID-19 (Auerbach & Thachil, 2021). These strategies ensure people-centered participation (Dutta, 2018; Dutta & Basu, 2011) in both disease containment and management, creating an inclusive rather than hierarchical process (Raju et al., 2021).

Attention also needs to be paid to urban spaces to deliver the aims of the Sustainable Development Goals (SDGS) – including for sustainable cities and communities (SDG11) and for inclusive health and well-being (SDG3). Government development efforts must address urban planning failures and seek solutions to reduce social vulnerabilities, pre-existing as well as future. This includes the provision of adequate and safe housing, improvements in water and sanitation infrastructure, and strategies to address improvements in electricity access. The lack of attention to urban and social vulnerabilities during the COVID-19 outbreak is already proving fatal in India as well as in other countries in the Global South (Raju & Ayeb-Karlsson, 2020; Wilkinson et al., 2020). Collectively, these efforts indicate a need to re-articulate public health principles away from its neoliberal agenda that places the responsibility for health on citizens (Hartmann, 2016; Petersen & Lupton, 1996), and recognize that public and global health transcends beyond the medical sector.

Conclusion

In early 2021, Indian government officials, including Prime Minister Modi, announced that the country had emerged victorious in the fight against COVID-19 (India Today, 2021b, 2021c) prompting complacency. Public health restrictions were relaxed and national vaccine distribution was slow, with a focus on supplying vaccines or vaccine components to other countries (India Today, 2021b). With efforts to prevent infections no longer routinely practiced and vaccine availability limited, Indian citizens became vulnerable to both the new "double-mutant" variant B.1.617 and the variant B.1.1.7 common in the UK and the United States (The New York Times, 2021b). The unanticipated second wave of COVID-19 resulted in an average of 4,000 deaths daily throughout the month of May 2021 (The New York Times, 2021a).

Yet social, economic, and political conditions, not only viral biology, created the context for a new viral surge. No coordinated national public health policies, no enforced COVID-19 prevention measures at well-attended political rallies and religious gatherings including the Kumbh Mela, limited social support structures to alleviate the economic burdens of COVID-19, and a failure to prioritize local access to COVID-19 vaccines created ideal conditions for not only COVID-19 to flourish but epidemic clusters to erupt. Health professionals relied on available treatments which only made the problem worse. The iatrogenic syndemic of COVID-19/diabetes/black fungus in India provides clear indication of what can transpire when a health system is stressed to a point of collapse in a time when public health measures are not prioritized, and governments have not invested in establishing healthy living and working conditions for their constituents.

Note

1 The United Nations defines slums as residential areas where (1) inhabitants have no security of tenure vis-à-vis the land or dwellings they inhabit, with modalities ranging from squatting to informal rental housing, (2) the neighborhoods usually lack, or are cut off from, basic services and city infrastructure and (3) the housing may not comply with current planning and building regulations, and is often situated in geographically and environmentally hazardous areas.

References

Agarwal, S., & Taneja, S. (2005). All slums are not equal: Child health conditions among the urban poor. *Indian Pediatrics*, 42, 233–244.

Anjana, R. M., Pradeepa, R., Deepa, M., Datta, M., Sudha, V., Unnikrishnan, R., Bhansali, A., Joshi, S. R., Joshi, P. P., Yajnik, C. S., Dhandhania, V. K., Nath, L. M., Das, A. K., Rao, P. V., Madhu, S. V., Shukla, D. K., Kaur, T., Priya, M., Nirmal, E., … Icmr-Indiab Collaborative Study Group. (2011). Prevalence of diabetes and prediabetes (impaired fasting glucose and/or impaired glucose tolerance) in urban and rural India: Phase I results of the Indian Council of Medical

Research-INdia DIABetes (ICMR-INDIAB) study. *Diabetologia*, 54(12), 3022–3027. https://doi.org/10.1007/s00125-011-2291-5.

Auerbach, A. M., & Thachil, T. (2021). How does Covid-19 affect urban slums? Evidence from settlement leaders in India. *World Development*, 140, 105304.

Basu, S. (2020). Non-communicable disease management in vulnerable patients during Covid-19. *Indian Journal of Medical Ethics*, 2, 103–105.

Biswas, S. (2021a). Black fungus: India reports nearly 9,000 cases of rare infection. *BBC News*. https://www.bbc.com/news/world-asia-india-57217246.

Biswas, S. (2021b). 'White fungus': Drug-resistant fungal infections pose threat to India patients. *BBC News*. Retrieved June 9, 2021, from https://www.bbc.com/news/world-asia-india-57312832.

Bonnet, F., Vanek, J., & Chen, M. (2019). *Women and men in the informal economy: A statistical brief*. International Labour Office, Geneva, Issue. https://www.ilo.org/wcmsp5/groups/public/---dgreports/---dcomm/documents/publication/wcms_626831.pdf.

CNN. (2021). "Black Fungus" in India: What we know about the disease affecting covid patients. Retrieved May 30, 2021, from https://edition.cnn.com/2021/05/21/india/black-fungus-mucormycosis-covid-explainer-intl-hnk/index.html.

Cornely, O., Alastruey-Izquierdo, A., Arenz, D., Chen, S., Dannaoui, E., Hochhegger, B., Hoenigl, M., Jensen, H.E., Lagrou, K., Lewis, R.E. and Mellinghoff, S.C., M., Mervyn, Pana, Z., Seidel, D., Sheppard, D., Wahba, R., Akova, M., Alanio, A., Al-Hatmi, A., Arikan-Akdagli, S., Chakrabarti, A. (2019). Global guideline for the diagnosis and management of mucormycosis: An initiative of the European Confederation of Medical Mycology in cooperation with the Mycoses Study Group Education and Research Consortium. *The Lancet Infectious Diseases*, 19(12), E405–E421. https://doi.org/10.1016/S1473-3099(10)30312-3.

CSE. (2020). '*Slumming it out*', *down to earth*. https://www.downtoearth.org.in/dte-infographics/slums/index.html?fbclid=IwAR3PiNWh7-84chvlLvUArSevfBPB2k_d-VN5WIUUj_-ILhyRZkg8fY2mDaE.

Diabetes Atlas, 9th Edition. (2019). https://diabetesatlas.org/en/sections/demographic-and-geographic-outline.html.

Du, J., King, R., & Chanchani, R. (2020). *Tackling inequality in cities is essential for fighting COVID-19*. https://thecityfix.com/blog/2020-04-coronavirus-inequality-cities-jillian-du-robin-king-radha-chanchani/.

Dutta, A., & Fischer, H. W. (2021). The local governance of COVID-19: Disease prevention and social security in rural India. *World Development*, 138, 105234.

Dutta, M. J. (2018). Culture-centered approach in addressing health disparities: Communication infrastructures for subaltern voices. *Communication Methods and Measures*, 12(4), 239–259.

Dutta, M. J., & Basu, A. (2011). Culture, communication, and health: A guiding framework. In Teresa L. Thompson, Roxanne Parrott, Jon F. Nussbaum (Eds.) *The Routledge handbook of health communication* (pp. 346–360). Routledge.

Ecks, S. (2020). Multimorbidity, polyiatrogenesis, and COVID-19. *Medical Anthropology Quarterly*, 34(4), 488–503. https://doi.org/10.1111/maq.12626.

Ezeh, A., Oyebode, O., Satterthwaite, D., Chen, Y.-F., Ndugwa, R., Sartori, J., Mberu, B., Melendez-Torres, G. J., Haregu, T., & Watson, S. I. (2017). The history, geography, and sociology of slums and the health problems of people who live in slums. *The Lancet*, 389(10068), 547–558.

Fang, L., Karakiulakis, G., & Roth, M. (2020). Are patients with hypertension and diabetes mellitus at increased risk for COVID-19 infection? *The Lancet Respiratory Medicine, 8*(4), e21.

Frank, C., Mohamed, M. K., Strickland, G. T., Lavanchy, D., Arthur, R. R., Magder, L. S., El Khoby, T., Abdel-Wahab, Y., Anwar, W., & Sallam, I. (2000). The role of parenteral antischistosomal therapy in the spread of hepatitis C virus in Egypt. *The Lancet, 355*(9207), 887–891.

Gamio, L., & Glanz, J. (2021). Just how big could India's true covid toll be? *New York Times.* https://www.nytimes.com/interactive/2021/05/25/world/asia/india-covid-death-estimates.html?smid=em-share.

Gandra, S., Ram, S., & Levitz, S. M. (2021). The "black fungus" in India: The emerging syndemic of COVID-19-associated mucormycosis. *Annals of Internal Medicine.* https://doi.org/10.7326/M21-2354.

Gaur, K., Mohan, I., & Gupta, R. (2017). Syndemic of obesity, hypertension, and hyperglycemia among 15-49 year oldsin Rajasthan: District-level data from national family health survey-4. *RUHS Journal of Health Sciences, 2*(2). http://www.ruhsjhs.in/files/issue/2017/V2N2/original_article_syndemic.pdf.

Geerlings, S. E., & Hoepelman, A. I. (1999). Immune dysfunction in patients with diabetes mellitus (DM). *FEMS Immunology & Medical Microbiology, 26*(3–4), 259–265.

Ghazi, B. K., Rackimuthu, S., Wara, U. U., Mohan, A., Khawaja, U. A., Ahmad, S., Ahmad, S., Hasan, M. M., Dos Santos Costa, A. C., Ahmad, S., & Essar, M. Y. (2021). Rampant increase in cases of mucormycosis in India and Pakistan: A serious cause for concern during the ongoing COVID-19 pandemic. *American Journal of Tropical Medicine and Hygiene, 105*(5), 1144–1147. https://doi.org/10.4269/ajtmh.21-0608.

Group, R. C., Horby, P., Lim, W. S., Emberson, J. R., Mafham, M., Bell, J. L., Linsell, L., Staplin, N., Brightling, C., Ustianowski, A., Elmahi, E., Prudon, B., Green, C., Felton, T., Chadwick, D., Rege, K., Fegan, C., Chappell, L. C., Faust, S. N., … Landray, M. J. (2021). Dexamethasone in hospitalized patients with Covid-19. *The New England Journal of Medicine, 384*(8), 693–704. https://doi.org/10.1056/NEJMoa2021436.

Guan, W.-j., Ni, Z.-y., Hu, Y., Liang, W.-h., Ou, C.-q., He, J.-x., Liu, L., Shan, H., Lei, C.-l., & Hui, D. S. (2020). Clinical characteristics of coronavirus disease 2019 in China. *New England Journal of Medicine, 382*(18), 1708–1720.

Guariguata, L., Whiting, D. R., Hambleton, I., Beagley, J., Linnenkamp, U., & Shaw, J. E. (2014). Global estimates of diabetes prevalence for 2013 and projections for 2035. *Diabetes Research and Clinical Practice, 103*(2), 137–149.

Hartmann, C. (2016). Postneoliberal public health care reforms: Neoliberalism, social medicine, and persistent health inequalities in Latin America. *American Journal of Public Health, 106*(12), 2145–2151. https://doi.org/10.2105/AJPH.2016.303470.

ILO. (2018). *India wage report: Wage policies for decent work and inclusive growth.* https://www.ilo.org/wcmsp5/groups/public/---asia/---ro-bangkok/---sro-new_delhi/documents/publication/wcms_638305.pdf.

India Today. (2021a, May 18, 2021). Karnataka Youth Congress distributing steroids in Covid home isolation kits, says AAP leader. https://www.indiatoday.in/coronavirus-outbreak/video/karnataka-youth-congress-steroids-covid-home-isolation-kits-1803988-2021-05-18.

India Today. (2021b). PM Modi at Davos: Despite doomsday predictions, India defeated Covid and helped 150 other countries. *India Today*. Retrieved June 9, 2021, from https://www.indiatoday.in/india/story/pm-modi-at-davos-despite-doomsday-predictions-india-defeated-covid-and-helped-150-other-countries-1763662-2021-01-28.

India Today. (2021c). Raghuram Rajan explains why Covid 2nd wave took India by surprise. *India Today*. Retrieved June 9, 2021, from https://www.indiatoday.in/business/story/raghuram-rajan-explains-why-covid-2nd-wave-took-india-by-surprise-1798699-2021-05-04.

India Today. (2021d). Shortage of antifungal drug as mucormycosis cases rise in India, states press panic button. Retrieved May 30, 2021, from https://www.indiatoday.in/coronavirus-outbreak/story/mucormycosis-amphotericin-b-drug-shortage-symptoms-treatment-1803854-2021-05-18.

Jeong, W., Keighley, C., Wolfe, R., Lee, W. L., Slavin, M. A., Kong, D. C. M., & Chen, S. C. (2019). The epidemiology and clinical manifestations of mucormycosis: A systematic review and meta-analysis of case reports. *Clinical Microbiology and Infection*, 25(1), 26–34. https://doi.org/10.1016/j.cmi.2018.07.011.

Kluge, H. H. P., Wickramasinghe, K., Rippin, H. L., Mendes, R., Peters, D. H., Kontsevaya, A., & Breda, J. (2020). Prevention and control of non-communicable diseases in the COVID-19 response. *The Lancet*, 395(10238), 1678–1680.

Kontoyiannis, D., & Lewis, R. (2015). Agents of mucormycosis and entomophthoramycosis. In J. Bennett, R. Dolin, & M. Blaser (Eds.), *Principles and practices of infectious diseases* (8th ed., pp. 2909–2919). Elsevier.

Nanditha, A., Ma, R., Ramachandran, A., Snehalatha, C., Chan, J., Chia, K., Shaw, J., & Zimmet, P. (2016). Diabetes in Asia and the Pacific: Implications for the global epidemic. *Diabetes Care*, 39(3), 472–485. https://doi.org/10.2337/dc15-1536.

National Geographic. (2021). A rare black fungus is infecting many of India's COVID-19 patients—Why? Retrieved May 30, 2021, from https://www.nationalgeographic.com/science/article/a-rare-black-fungus-is-infecting-many-of-indias-covid-19-patientswhy.

Nolan, L., Bloom, D. E., & Subbaraman, R. (2017). Legal status and deprivation in India's urban slums: An analysis of two decades of national sample survey data. https://cdn1.sph.harvard.edu/wp-content/uploads/sites/1288/2012/11/Legal-Status-andDeprivation-in-Indias-Urban-Slums.pdf.

Osrin, D., Das, S., Bapat, U., Alcock, G. A., Joshi, W., & More, N. S. (2011). A rapid assessment scorecard to identify informal settlements at higher maternal and child health risk in Mumbai. *Journal of Urban Health*, 88(5), 919–932.

Pal, R., & Bhadada, S. K. (2020). COVID-19 and non-communicable diseases. *Postgraduate Medical Journal*, 96(1137), 429–430.

Palejwala, S. K., Zangeneh, T. T., Goldstein, S. A., & Lemole, G. M. (2016). An aggressive multidisciplinary approach reduces mortality in rhinocerebral mucormycosis. *Surgical Neurology International*, 7, 61–61. https://doi.org/10.4103/2152-7806.182964.

Petersen, A., & Lupton, D. (1996). *The new public health: Health and self in the age of risk*. Sage Publications, Inc.

Prakash, H., & Chakrabarti, A. (2019). Global epidemiology of mucormycosis. *Journal of Fungi*, 5(1), 26.

Raju, E., & Ayeb-Karlsson, S. (2020). COVID-19: How do you self-isolate in a refugee camp? *International Journal of Public Health*, 65(5), 515–517.

Raju, E., Dutta, A., & Ayeb-Karlsson, S. (2021). COVID-19 in India: Who are we leaving behind? *Progress in Disaster Science, 10*, 100163. https://doi.org/https://doi.org/10.1016/j.pdisas.2021.100163.

Raut, A., & Huy, N. T. (2021). Rising incidence of mucormycosis in patients with COVID-19: Another challenge for India amidst the second wave? *The Lancet Respiratory Medicine, 9*(8), e77.

Rocha, I. C. N., Hasan, M. M., Goyal, S., Patel, T., Jain, S., Ghosh, A., & Cedeño, T. D. D. (2021). COVID-19 and mucormycosis syndemic: Double health threat to a collapsing healthcare system in India. *Tropical Medicine & International Health, 26*(9), 1016–1018. https://doi.org/10.1111/tmi.13641.

Roden, M. M., Zaoutis, T. E., Buchanan, W. L., Knudsen, T. A., Sarkisova, T. A., Schaufele, R. L., Sein, M., Sein, T., Chiou, C. C., Chu, J. H., Kontoyiannis, D. P., & Walsh, T. J. (2005). Epidemiology and outcome of zygomycosis: A review of 929 reported cases. *Clinical Infectious Diseases, 41*(5), 634–653. https://doi.org/10.1086/432579.

Roy, D., Boss, R., & Pradhan, M. (2020). *How India's food-based safety net is responding to the COVID-19 lockdown.* https://www.ifpri.org/blog/how-indias-food-based-safety-net-responding-covid-19-lockdown.

Shepherd, A. (2020). Delhi prepares to hit 500,000 covid-19 cases. *BMJ, 370*, m2817. https://doi.org/10.1136/bmj.m2817.

Singer, M. (2009). *Introduction to syndemics: A critical systems approach to public and community health.* John Wiley & Sons.

Singer, M., Bulled, N., Ostrach, B., & Mendenhall, E. (2017). Syndemics and the biosocial conception of health. *The Lancet, 389*(10072), 941–950. https://doi.org/10.1016/S0140-6736(17)30003-X.

Singer, M., & Rylko-Bauer, B. (2021). The syndemics and structural violence of the COVID pandemic: Anthropological insights on a crisis. *Open Anthropological Research, 1*(1), 7–32. https://doi.org/doi:10.1515/opan-2020-0100.

Singh, A. K., Singh, R., Joshi, S. R., & Misra, A. (2021). Mucormycosis in COVID-19: A systematic review of cases reported worldwide and in India. *Diabetes & Metabolic Syndrome: Clinical Research & Reviews, 15*(4), 102146.

Skiada, A., Pavleas, I., & Drogari-Apiranthitou, M. (2020). Epidemiology and diagnosis of mucormycosis: An update. *Journal of Fungi, 6*(4), 265.

Staats, C. C., Kmetzsch, L., Schrank, A., & Vainstein, M. H. (2013). Fungal zinc metabolism and its connections to virulence. *Frontiers in Cellular and Infection Microbiology, 3*, 65.

Strickland, G. T. (2006). Liver disease in Egypt: Hepatitis C superseded schistosomiasis as a result of iatrogenic and biological factors. *Hepatology, 43*(5), 915–922. https://doi.org/10.1002/hep.21173.

Subbaraman, R., O'brien, J., Shitole, T., Shitole, S., Sawant, K., Bloom, D. E., & Patil-Deshmukh, A. (2012). Off the map: the health and social implications of being a non-notified slum in India. *Environment and Urbanization, 24*(2), 643–663.

Sulis, G., Batomen, B., Kotwani, A., Pai, M., & Gandra, S. (2021). Sales of antibiotics and hydroxychloroquine in India during the COVID-19 epidemic: An interrupted time series analysis. *PLoS Medicine, 18*(7), e1003682. https://doi.org/10.1371/journal.pmed.1003682.

Thakur, J. (2020). Novel coronavirus pandemic may worsen existing global noncommunicable disease crisis. *International Journal of Noncommunicable Diseases, 5*(1), 1.

The Lancet. (2021). India's COVID-19 emergency. *The Lancet, 397*(10286), 1683. https://doi.org/10.1016/S0140-6736(21)01052-7.

The New York Times. (2021a). Tracking coronavirus in India: Latest map and case count. *New York Times.* Retrieved June 9, 2021, from https://www.nytimes.com/interactive/2021/world/india-covid-cases.html.

The New York Times. (2021b). What to know about India's coronavirus crisis. *New York Times.* Retrieved June 9, 2021, from https://www.nytimes.com/article/india-coronavirus-cases-deaths.html.

The Times of India. (2021). Sharing oxygen cylinders cause for black fungus, say experts. Retrieved May 30, 2021, from https://timesofindia.indiatimes.com/city/bengaluru/karnataka-sharing-oxygen-cylinders-cause-for-mucormycosis-say-experts/articleshow/82927895.cms.

UN HABITAT. (2015). *Issue paper on informal settlements.* https://unhabitat.org/sites/default/files/download-manager-files/Habitat-III-Issue-Paper-22_Informal-Settlements-2.0%20%282%29.pdf.

UN HABITAT. (2020). *Youth in Nairobi slum use murals to educate the community about COVID-19.* https://unhabitat.org/youth-in-nairobi-slum-use-murals-to-educate-the-community-about-covid-19.

Unger, A., & Riley, L. W. (2007). Slum health: From understanding to action. *PLoS Medicine, 4*(10), e295.

Waked, I., Esmat, G., Elsharkawy, A., El-Serafy, M., Abdel-Razek, W., Ghalab, R., Elshishiney, G., Salah, A., Abdel Megid, S., Kabil, K., El-Sayed, M. H., Dabbous, H., El Shazly, Y., Abo Sliman, M., Abou Hashem, K., Abdel Gawad, S., El Nahas, N., El Sobky, A., El Sonbaty, S., ... Zaid, H. (2020). Screening and treatment Program to eliminate hepatitis C in Egypt. *New England Journal of Medicine, 382*(12), 1166–1174. https://doi.org/10.1056/NEJMsr1912628.

Wang, D., Hu, B., Hu, C., Zhu, F., Liu, X., Zhang, J., Wang, B., Xiang, H., Cheng, Z., & Xiong, Y. (2020). Clinical characteristics of 138 hospitalized patients with 2019 novel coronavirus–infected pneumonia in Wuhan, China. *Jama, 323*(11), 1061–1069.

Wilkinson, A., Ali, H., Bedford, J., Boonyabancha, S., Connolly, C., Conteh, A., Dean, L., Decorte, F., Dercon, B., & Dias, S. (2020). Local response in health emergencies: Key considerations for addressing the COVID-19 pandemic in informal urban settlements. *Environment and Urbanization, 32* (2): 503–522.

World Health Organization. (2020). *COVID-19 significantly impacts health services for noncommunicable diseases.* https://www.who.int/news-room/detail/01-06-2020-covid-19-significantly-impacts-health-services-for-noncommunicable-diseases.

World Heart Federation. (2020). *COVID 19 and CVD: World Heart Federation.* https://www.world-heart-federation.org/covid-19-and-cvd/.

Wrapp, D., Wang, N., Corbett, K. S., Goldsmith, J. A., Hsieh, C.-L., Abiona, O., Graham, B. S., & McLellan, J. S. (2020). Cryo-EM structure of the 2019-nCoV spike in the prefusion conformation. *Science, 367*(6483), 1260–1263.

Yadav, U. N., Rayamajhee, B., Mistry, S. K., Parsekar, S. S., & Mishra, S. K. (2020). A syndemic perspective on the management of non-communicable diseases amid the COVID-19 pandemic in low- and middle-income countries. *Frontiers in Public Health, 8,* 508–508. https://doi.org/10.3389/fpubh.2020.00508.

Yang, J., Zheng, Y., Gou, X., Pu, K., Chen, Z., Guo, Q., Ji, R., Wang, H., Wang, Y., & Zhou, Y. (2020a). Prevalence of comorbidities in the novel Wuhan coronavirus

(COVID-19) infection: A systematic review and meta-analysis. *International Journal of Infectious Diseases*, 94(1), 91–95.

Yang, X., Yu, Y., Xu, J., Shu, H., Liu, H., Wu, Y., Zhang, L., Yu, Z., Fang, M., & Yu, T. (2020b). Clinical course and outcomes of critically ill patients with SARS-CoV-2 pneumonia in Wuhan, China: A single-centered, retrospective, observational study. *The Lancet Respiratory Medicine*, 8(5), 475–481.

9 COVID-19 Lockdown and "Shadow Pandemic" of Gender-Based Violence in Nigeria

Chiemezie S. Atama and Obinna J. Eze

Gender-Based Violence as a Global Pandemic

Gender-based violence (GBV) is a global pandemic that affects one in three women in their lifetime (The World Bank, 2019). It is both a social and public health problem (Wada et al., 2022). GBV transcends continental, national, ethnic, racial, religious, educational, socioeconomic class, and age boundaries. Although women can be abusive in their relationships, the evidence indicates that women are mostly at the receiving end of GBV (Ifemeje, 2012; Tenkorang et al., 2013). In the United States, both women and men report having been perpetrators and victims of partner aggression (Carney et al., 2006; Straus, 2007; Straus & Ramirez, 2007). In Zimbabwe, about 35% of women reported having experienced physical violence from the age of 15, and 14% had experienced sexual violence at least once in their lifetime (Mukamana et al., 2020). In Ghana, one in three women experienced some form of GBV (Alangea et al., 2018). In India, 56% of the women in a survey approved of wife beating in situations when a wife cooks bad food, shows disrespect to in-laws, leaves home without her husband's permission, or if a wife produces more daughters than sons (Aihie, 2009). These sentiments are shared across many African communities.

GBV depicts a pattern of abusive behaviors by one or both partners in an intimate relationship such as marriage, dating, family, friends, or cohabitation (United Nations, 2010). It has many forms including physical aggression (hitting, kicking, biting, shoving, restraining, throwing objects) or threats thereof (Iliyasu et al., 2011). Other types of GBV include sexual abuse, emotional abuse, controlling or domineering behavior, intimidation, stalking, passive/covert abuse, and economic deprivation (United Nations, 2010). GBV is manifested through a multitude of actions, including the forced marriage of young girls, human trafficking, female genital mutilation, rape and attempted rape, purdah or the screening of women from men, violence directed at individuals with different sexual orientations, sexual violence, verbal abuse, and laws and regulations that limit the rights of women and their access to health and social services due to gender.

DOI: 10.4324/9781003365358-10

Traditional gender roles create platforms for violence against women in sub-Saharan Africa. African culture demands that women should not only be submissive to their husbands but also respectful, dutiful, and serviceable to the extent that challenges to abuse may be interpreted as attempting to subvert the authority of men. Such cultural norms have projected African societies as inherently patriarchal, ones that condone male superiority, the basis for which all forms of GBV may sometimes be legitimized (Tenkorang et al., 2013).

The threat of interpersonal violence violates human rights, constrains choice, and negatively impacts a person's ability to participate in, contribute to, and benefit from personal, community, and national development. It has a profound impact on physical and psychological health (The World Bank, 2019). In addition to causing injury, violence increases the long-term risk of depression (Heise et al., 2002). High rates of violence against women have serious consequences for family stability, the mental health of mothers and children, post-traumatic stress, self-harm, and eating and sleep disorders (WHO, 2012). Increasingly, research has highlighted the health burdens, intergenerational effects, and demographic consequences of such violence. Children who witness violence are more likely to tolerate violence and commit violent acts as adults (Hashemi et al., 2022; Woollett & Thomson, 2016). The intergenerational effects of violence on children include risky sexual behaviors, emotional instability, poor mental health, poor academic performance, and substance abuse (Fork et al., 2019). Children who experience violence are twice as likely to become violent as adults (Chanda, 2019). Despite these clear concerns, efforts to address GBV globally and at national levels have been largely ineffective to date.

GBV as an Ongoing Public Health Problem in Nigeria

A high prevalence of GBV has been reported throughout Nigeria (National Population Commission & ICF International, 2019). GBV in Nigeria is rooted in culture and religious norms and beliefs, ritualism, poverty, and unemployment (Nigerian Women Trust Fund, 2020). GBV is linked to the polygamous marriage system (Anderson et al., 2007). It is experienced more by women who are young, have low income, and are divorced or separated (Oladepo et al., 2011). GBV has also been linked to the lifestyle of husbands such as smoking and alcohol consumption (Saidi et al., 2008). Thus, drivers of GBV in Nigeria are diverse and complex.

Although the struggle for equivalent sociocultural, political, and economic rights by gender has been a shared long-term global battle, it is particularly problematic in Nigeria (Mshelia, 2021). For example, in the Cross Rivers State of Nigeria, women are denied funds for essentials and self-care, denied access to own cash crops, and are only allowed to own farms with cassava and vegetables, even when they have limited economic value (Nigerian Women Trust Fund, 2020). In parts of southeast Nigeria, women may be allowed to inherit moveable properties but are strictly restricted from inheriting land.

Patriarchal cultural permissiveness justifies men's physical aggression toward women in the country (Oladepo et al., 2011).

There is a shared understanding that issues concerning families and intimate relationships should not be made public (Okolo & Okolo, 2018; Oladepo et al., 2011). As such, many cases of GBV remain unreported, and the true national burden of GBV is unrecognized. Nigerian law enforcement does not possess the tools to adequately respond to GBV cases. Many police officers lack the knowledge and training to deal with GBV cases effectively and others presume that such cases are domestic matters, outside their jurisdiction. Some women suffer intimidation and assault from dubious police officers upon filing rape reports.

Nigeria's legal system possesses insufficient mechanisms to protect citizens against GBV. Nigeria's age of consent portrays a similar degree of inconsistency. Popular opinion generally places Nigeria's age of consent at 11 years old, the lowest in the world. This stems from Section 7(2) of the 2015 Sexual Offences Bill, which states that "A person who commits an offense of defilement with a child aged eleven years or less shall upon conviction be sentenced to imprisonment for life." Nevertheless, a complete reading of sub-sections (3) and (4) of Section 7 within the same Bill reveals that it penalizes sexual activity with a child "between the age of twelve and fifteen years" and "between the age of sixteen and eighteen years," respectively.

In northern Nigeria, the concurrent application of Western and Islamic Jurisprudence (Sharia Law) can also limit judicial convictions for GBV since perpetrators often find safe havens within Sharia Law. In Bauchi State, for instance, convicted rapists can file counterclaims on grounds of "character defamation" and ultimately avoid punishment while shifting blame to victims. The combination of ambiguous laws, weak enforcement as well as many states' failure to pass progressive legislation poses a significant obstacle in Nigeria's attempts to combat GBV in the country.

COVID-19 Pandemic and "Shadow Pandemic" of GBV in Nigeria

The first COVID-19 case was recorded in Lagos, Nigeria, on February 27, 2020 (Federal Ministry of Health, 2020). Initial curtailment strategies applied by the Nigerian government, as given by Nigerian Center for Disease Control (NCDC), included maintaining physical distance, hand washing and use of hand sanitizers, and avoiding groups of more than 50 individuals (NCDC, 2020). These, by implication, required the closing of churches, mosques, and marketplaces, and significantly limiting the size of marriage and burial functions and other public gatherings. Growing case numbers ultimately resulted in a national lockdown enforced on March 30, 2020 (Ibrahim et al., 2020).

The national COVID-19 lockdown aimed to abate the spread of the pandemic. However, it caused significant hardship, particularly among already marginalized communities. This lockdown restricted movement outside the household, closed schools, and shut down many means of earning. Women working as day laborers or in the informal market were particularly affected. In addition, as unpaid childcare typically falls on women, this reality, coupled with school closures, added additional weight to an already heavy burden. Economic difficulty and loss of livelihood during the lockdown increased women's dependency on partners, increased the likelihood of women engaging in transactional sex, which heightened exposure to sexually transmitted diseases, sexual exploitation, unwanted pregnancies, and GBV. Furthermore, COVID-19 lockdowns severely limited access to essential health services, including reproductive care. GBV facilities were also difficult to access during the lockdown period. Mirabel Centre, a sexual assault referral center in Lagos, Nigeria, indicated that many GBV survivors in Lagos were unable to access the shelter during lockdown.

The lockdown in Nigeria resulted in a significant upswing in criminal activity and victimization. The spike in GBV cases reported during the COVID-19 pandemic in the country has been unprecedented. A United Nations (2020) report on GBV in Nigeria indicated a 56% increase nationally. Between April and May 2020, the Women's Aid Collective Enugu (WACOL) reported approximately 156 cases of GBV in Enugu state. As evidenced in the statement of the Inspector General of Police in June 2020, the Nigerian Police recorded 717 rape cases between January and May 2020 (Ngbokai, 2020).

In the three Nigerian locations that pioneered the lockdown, namely Lagos, Abuja, and Ogun, the number of domestic violence cases rose three-fold in a single month, from 60 in March to 238 in April 2020. By contrast, states that observed less stringent lockdowns such as Benue, Ebonyi, and Cross River saw only a 53% increase in reported GBV cases between March and April 2020. This alarming rise in GBV cases during lockdown strongly points to a positive correlation between lockdown and rising GBV incidence. The incidence of physical abuse toward minors and teens also increased during the COVID-19 pandemic. The Lagos State Domestic and Sexual Violence response team in Nigeria recorded a 10% rise in the physical abuse of children in March 2020, with hotline reports averaging 13 calls per day. The team suggested that many people, particularly women, commit violence toward children to transfer aggression from previous trauma. If we consider that most crimes go unreported in Nigeria, it is likely that the figures of GBV during the lockdown period were significantly more than is officially documented.

GBV has been termed a "shadow pandemic" by the WHO and United Nations (2020), who recognize that COVID-19 lockdowns resulted in a significant increase in GBV globally. Given institutional closures, many cases remained unreported, with few services available to those suffering.

Syndemic of COVID-19 Lockdown and GBV

The unexpected emergence of the COVID-19 pandemic and the subsequent public health policy for disease containment in the form of a national lockdown created triggers, such as income deficits, ruined businesses, or being stuck at home for unusually long hours. While providing protection from COVID-19 infection, victims were trapped with their abusers. The stressors triggered by the lockdown coupled with existing social norms of gender inequality influenced rates of GBV in Nigeria. In so doing, the lockdown exposed millions of women and girls to greater levels of violence than even the high level before the pandemic (Young & Aref-Adib, 2020). As evidenced in reviews of the literature and published reports, similar situations have been reported globally (Chanda, 2019; Mittal & Singh, 2020).

The impact became more devastating in Nigeria due to high degrees of poverty and economic instability, inadequate access to resources, and legal mechanisms that allowed for the proliferation of GBV cases as offenders evaded punishment (UK AID, 2020). The social impacts of the COVID-19 lockdown and GBV interacted syndemically, with the former increasing rates of the latter. As noted by Stark and colleagues (2020, p. 1), describing a syndemic of COVID-19, Ebola, and GBV in the Democratic Republic of the Congo, "it is not the infection of COVID-19 that increases the risk of GBV but rather the gender-insensitive systems and policies that magnify the risk." At the same time, GBV increased the risk of exposure to COVID-19 as biological-biological interaction (see Singer et al., 2017). For this interaction, we draw on Singer (2011) and Douglas-Vail (2015) to show the biosocial interaction of COVID-19 and GBV in Nigeria.

The syndemics of the COVID-19 lockdown and GBV is multifaceted, existing face-to-face and online, with girls and young women reporting harassment and abuse on the internet (Jatmiko et al., 2020). The decision to stop the use of social media or to self-censor to avoid abuse was considered by many girls. This puts the onus on girls and women to change their behavior, rather than the perpetrators. However, violence is the sole responsibility of the perpetrator, who must be held accountable according to national and international legislation. Fear or threat of violence must not restrict girls from living free and full lives or realizing their full potential. Certain groups are more vulnerable to violence, including girls and young women from poor, rural, or indigenous communities, those who are or are perceived to be lesbian, gay, bisexual, and transgender (LGBTQ+), those living with disabilities, and girls and women who speak out about political, social, and cultural issues regarding gender inequality.

Conclusion and Recommendations

GBV has been on the front burner as a major health issue affecting women, especially in low-income countries. Yet, more needs to be done to ameliorate this threat, especially in light of the added abuse ushered in by the COVID-19 lockdown. GBV affects mostly women and girls, as such, the term has been used interchangeably with "violence against women." The root cause of GBV lies in unequal power relations between women and men.

As a result, a variety of factors on the individual level, and at levels of community and society, can combine to raise the likelihood of GBV. GBV knows no social, economic, or national boundaries as it occurs in both the public and private spheres, including homes, workplaces, schools, religious environments, or on the streets. GBV affects all categories of women and young girls: rich and poor, old and young, Christian and Muslim, and people from diverse ethnic backgrounds. Still, economically poor, and socially marginalized women and girls have the fewest resources to escape abuse and suffer the greatest consequences and perhaps the greatest incidence of GBV.

In most cases, the perpetrators of GBV are people known to the victims, people they love and trust. The effects of GBV are far-reaching and extend beyond the individual survivor to communities and society in general. Thus, potential social responses to GBV are most effective when there is a common understanding of the nature and causes of GBV and it is addressed from all angles, through the participation of multiple sectors and entire communities.

Women cannot be excluded from national or global development. They constitute more than half of the world's population with vital roles as leaders, workers, homemakers, caregivers, healers, and custodians of fundamental, social, and cultural values of society. Full community development is impossible without their insights, cooperation, and participation. Considering the importance of women as mothers, primary earners, teachers, and guardians, they deserve respect, recognition, and better treatment. GBV happens on daily basis in Nigeria; yet, it is one of the most hidden categories of crimes as it is often unreported and even when reported is not acted on by authorities. The consequent adverse effects on society are not properly documented or responded to at the policy level. We recommend the following policy changes to address the rising threat of a COVID-19-GBV syndemic:

Skill acquisition for women: Most incidents of GBV are tied to poor economic status. Reproductive and productive roles of women often place them at the bottom of the socioeconomic ladder. Women mostly perform low-paying jobs, which rob them of power to participate in decision-making within the socio-economic, political, and cultural spheres. In some parts of Nigeria, the input of a girl child's earnings into the family income is so high that it becomes economically unwise to allow such a child to go to school. Girls contribute to the family income by hawking food items, helping with household chores, working as maids for wealthier families, and looking after their younger siblings. These activities can expose them to further victimization. However, if girls acquire employable skills, they can work outside the home, become more independent, or contribute significantly to the family income. As such, the Ministry of Women's Affairs and other stakeholders should embark on strategies that facilitate girls' and women's educational, economic, social, and political empowerment.

Evidence-based culturally centered interventions to address gender power dynamics: Revisit the patriarchal nature of Nigerian society by implementing interventions that are developed by women to address issues they experience. By so doing, women will be able to stand their ground on issues directly affecting them rather than remaining docile or accepting male-focused harmful cultural practices. This is no small task, and it will face resistance, but it is vital to curbing GBV and the harm it does not only to women but to the whole of society.

Coalition of government and civil society organizations: Partnerships between the government and civil society organizations are needed to handle issues of GBV. The police, who usually are the first point of call for women experiencing GBV, has been marred with mistrust in Nigeria. Consequently, civil society organizations now serve as the first contact point, and they take up cases of GBV for indigent individuals. Thus, there is a need for collaboration between the government and civil society organizations in changing the pattern of GBV.

Criminal justice reforms and commitment to the existing legal framework on GBV: Reforms of the criminal justice system are necessary to clear gray areas that still impede the speedy management of GBV cases in law courts. While notable reforms have been recorded toward tackling GBV in Nigeria, there needs to be a greater effort toward the application of these legal frameworks.

Engagement of faith-based organizations: Most Nigerians are adherent to faith-based organizations. Taking advantage of these organizations to alter social norms involves incorporating faith-based leaders in advocacy efforts.

The COVID-19 lockdown exposed millions of at-risk women and girls to even greater levels of violence than the high-level incidents before the pandemic, creating a syndemic. Incidents of GBV globally are largely attributed to general economic struggles emanating from access to education and employment. However, gender inequities, orchestrated by patriarchy, place countries including Nigeria, at particularly high risk for GBV. Remedying GBV will require urgency in policy implementation (Roy et al., 2022). Cultural beliefs that support gender power imbalances must be addressed, and law enforcement and legislation on GBV must be clearer and supportive of GBV case reporting.

References

Aihie, O.N. (2009). Prevalence of domestic violence in Nigeria: implication for counseling. *Edo Journal of Counseling*, 2(1), 1–8.

Alangea, D.O., Addo-Lartey, A.A., Sikweyiya, Y., Chirwa, E.D., Coker-Appiah, D., Jewkes, R., & Adanu, R.M.K. (2018). Prevalence and risk factors of intimate partner violence among women in four districts of the central region of Ghana: baseline findings from a cluster randomized controlled trial. *PLoS ONE*, 13(7), e0200874. https://doi.org/10.1371/journal.pone.0200874.

Anderson, N., Ho-foster, A., Mitchell, S., Scheepers, E., & Goldstien, S. (2007). Risk factors for domestic physical violence: national cross-sectional household surveys in eight southern African countries. *British Medical Journal on Women's Health*, 7, 11.

Carney, M., Buttell, F., & Dutton, D. (2006). Women who perpetrate intimate partner violence: a review of the literature with recommendations for treatment. *Aggression and Violent Behavior*, 12, 108–115.

Chanda, F. (2019). The impact of gender based violence on child development in Livingstone district of Zambia. *Texila International Journal of Academic Research*, 6(1), 1–6. https://doi.org/10.21522/TIJAR.2014.06.01.Art002.

Douglas-Vail, M. (2015). Syndemic theory and its applications to HIV/AIDS public health interventions. *International Journal of Medical Sociology and Anthropology*, 6(1), 1–10.

Federal Ministry of Health. (2020). Health minister: first case of COVID-19 confirmed in Nigeria. https://www.health.gov.ng/index.php?option=com_k2&view=item&id=613:health-minister-first-case-of-covid-19-confirmed-in-nigeria.

Fork, C.M., Catallozi, M., Localio, A.R., Grisso, J.A., Wiebe, D.J., & Fein, J.A. (2019). Intergenerational effects of witnessing domestic violence: health of the witnesses and their children. *Preventive Medicine Reports*, 15, 100942. https://doi.org/10.1016/j.pmedr.2019.100942.

Hashemi, L., Fanslow, J., Gulliver, P., & McIntosh, T. (2022). Intergenerational impact of violence exposure: emotional-behavioural and school difficulties in children aged 5–17. *Frontiers Psychiatry*, 12, 771834. https://doi.org/10.3389/fpsyt.2021.771834.

Heise, L., Ellsberg, M., & Gottmoeller, M. (2002). A global overview of gender-based violence. *International Journal of Gynecology & Obstetrics*, 78, S5–S14. https://doi.org/10.1016/S0020-7292(02)00038-3.

Ibrahim, R.L., Ajide, K.B., & Olatunde, J.O. (2020). Easing of lockdown measures in Nigeria: implications for the healthcare system. *Health Policy Technology*, 9(4), 399–404. https://doi.org10.1016/j.hlpt.2020.09.004.

Ifemeje, S.C. (2012). Gender-based domestic violence in Nigeria: a socio-legal perspective. *Indian Journal of Gender Studies*, 19(1), 137–148.

Iliyasu, Z., Abubakar, I.S., Babashani, M., & Galadanc, H.S. (2011). Domestic violence among women living with HIV/AIDS in Kano, Northern Nigeria. *African Journal of Reproductive Health*, 15(3), 41–50.

Jatmiko, M.I., Syukron, M., & Mekarsari, Y. (2020). Covid-19, harassment and social media: a study of gender-based violence facilitated by technology during the pandemic. *The Journal of Society and Media*, 4(2), 319–347. https://doi.org/10.26740/jsm.v4n2.p319-347.

Mittal, S., & Singh, T. (2020). Gender-based violence during COVID-19 pandemic: a mini-review. *Frontiers in Global Women's Health*, 1. https://doi.org/10.3389/fgwh.2020.00004.

Mshelia, I.H. (2021). Gender based violence and violence against women in Nigeria: a sociological analysis. *International Journal of Research and Innovation in Social Sciences*, 5(8), 2454–6186.

Mukamana, J.I., Machakanja, P., & Adjei, N.K. (2020). Trends in prevalence and correlates of intimate partner violence against women in Zimbabwe, 2005–2015. *BMC International Health and Human Rights*, 20(2), 1–11. https://doi.org/10.1186/s12914-019-0220-8.

National Population Commission (NPC) [Nigeria] & ICF International. (2019). *Nigeria Demographic and Health Survey 2018*. Abuja and Rockville, MD: NPC and ICF International.

NCDC. (2020). Coronavirus (COVID-19) highlights. National Centre for Disease Control. https://covid19.ncdc.gov.ng.

Nigerian Women Trust Fund. (2020). Analysis of the root causes of violence against women and girls in Nigeria: a leadership strategy. https://nigerianwomentrustfund. org/wp-content/uploads/NWTF-Violence.pdf.

Ngbokai. R. (2020). Nigeria records 717 rape incidents in 5Months—IGP Nigeria records 717 rape incidents in 5 months—IGP. *Daily Trust*, Monday, 15 January.

Okolo, N.C., & Okolo, C.P.W. (2018). Gender based violence in Nigeria: a study of Makurdi metropolis in Benue state. *Nigeria Injury Prevention*, 24, A99. https://doi. org/10.1136/injuryprevention-2018-safety.273.

Oladepo, O., Yusuf, O.B., & Arulogun, O.S. (2011). Factors influencing gender based violence among men and women in selected states in Nigeria. *African Journal of Reproductive Health*, 15(4), 78–86.

Roy, C.M., Bukuluki, P., Casey, S.E., Jagun, M.O., John, N.A., Mabhena, N., Mwangi, M., & McGovern, T. (2022). Impact of COVID-19 on gender-based violence prevention and response services in Kenya, Uganda, Nigeria, and South Africa: a cross-sectional survey. *Frontiers of Global Women's Health*, 2, 780771. https://doi.org/10.3389/fgwh.2021.780771.

Saidi, H, Awori, K.O, & Odula P. (2008). Gender associated violence at a woman's hospital in Nairobi. *East African Medical Journal*, 85(7), 347–354.

Singer, M. (2011). Toward a critical biosocial model of ecohealth in Southern Africa: the HIV/AIDS and nutrition insecurity syndemic. *Annals of Anthropological Practice*. https://doi.org/10.1111/j.2153-9588.2011.01064.x/ful.

Singer, M., Bulled, N., Ostrach, B., & Mendenhall, E. (2017). Syndemics and the biosocial conception of health. *Lancet*, 389(10072), 941–950. https://doi.org/10.1016/S0140-6736(17)30003-X.

Stark, L., Meinhart, M., Vahedi, L., Carter, S.E., Roesch, E., Scott Moncrieff, I. Palaku, P.M., Rossi, F., & Poulton, C. (2020). The syndemic of COVID-19 and gender-based violence in humanitarian settings: leveraging lessons from Ebola in the Democratic Republic of Congo. *BMJ Global Health*, 5(11), e004194. https://doi.org/10.1136/bmjgh-2020-004194.

Straus, M.A. (2007). Dominance and symmetry in partner violence by male and female university students in 32 nations. *Children and Youth Services Review*, 30, 252–275.

Straus, M.A., & Ramirez, I.L. (2007). Gender symmetry in prevalence, severity, and chronicity of physical aggression against dating partners by university students in Mexico and USA. *Aggressive Behavior*, 33, 281–290.

Tenkorang, E.Y., Owusu, A.Y., Yeboah, E.H., & Bannerman, R. (2013). Factors influencing domestic and marital violence against women in Ghana. *Journal of Family Violence*, 28, 771–781. https://doi.org/10.1007/s10896-013-9543-8.

The World Bank. (2019). Gender-based violence (violence against women and girls). 25 September. https://www.worldbank.org/en/topic/socialsustainability/brief/violence-against-womenandgirls#:~:text=Gender%2Dbased%20violence%20(GBV),3%20women%20in%20their%20lifetime.

UK AID. (2020). Effect of COVID-19 on gender-based violence. *Advisory Note*, September2020.

United Nations. (2010). Convention on the elimination of all forms of discrimination against women, CEDAW. http://www.un.org/womenwatch/daw/cedaw/text/econvention.html.

United Nations. (2020). Gender-based violence in Nigeria during the COVID-19 crisis: the shadow pandemic. Brief prepared by UN Women with UNFPA, UNODC and UNICEF on behalf of the UN System in Nigeria.

Wada, O.Z., Olawade, D.B., Amusa, A.O., Moses, J.O., & Eteng, G.J. (2022). Gender-based violence during COVID-19 lockdown: case study of a community in Lagos, Nigeria. *African Health Sciences*, 22(2), 79–87. https://doi.org/10.4314/ahs.v22i2.10.

WHO. (2012). Intimate partner violence. http://www.who.int/about/licensing/copyright_form/en/index.html.

Woollett, N., & Thomson, K. (2016). Understanding the intergenerational transmission of violence. *South African Medical Journal*, 106(11), 1068–1070. https://doi.org/10.7196/SAMJ.2016.v106i11.12065.

Young, J.C., & Aref-Adib, C. (2020). The shadow pandemic: gender-based violence and COVID-19. https://www.theigc.org/blog/the-shadow-pandemic-gender-based-violence-and-covid-19/.

10 Ecosyndemics, COVID-19, and Child Health in the Anthropocene

Merrill Singer

The World Health Organization (WHO) and other global monitors of child health, including UNICEF and the World Bank, have celebrated findings indicating that the global under-five mortality rate declined significantly between 1990 and 2018 while acknowledging that improvements have not been evenly distributed across richer and poorer populations. In 2022, however, the WHO and several collaborating organizations published a report entitled "Protect the Promise: 2022 Progress Report on the Every Woman, Every Child Global Strategy for Women's, Children's and Adolescents' Health (2016–2030)" (WHO et al., 2022). The report shows that children's health has suffered globally in recent years. Of the 137 million children born every year, 3.8% still die before they reach the age of five, or about 15,000 child deaths every day (Suzuki & Kashiwaste, 2019). In 2020, 5 million children died before reaching the age of five. Africa has the highest under-five mortality rate, about nine times higher than that in Europe. Similarly, while childhood morbidity from conditions like diarrheal diseases was reduced from 4.6 million to 0.8 million in recent decades, most of this reduction was in high-income countries, suggesting that significant inequities between countries persist. Children born in low-income countries now have an average life expectancy at birth of about 63 years, compared to 80 years in high-income countries, a 17-year disparity in longevity. In 2020, it is estimated that over 40 million children suffered from life-threatening acute malnutrition. Almost 75% of these children lived in lower or middle-income countries in the Global South. Six countries in the Global South – Afghanistan, the Democratic Republic of the Congo, Ethiopia, Sudan, Syria, and Yemen are among the top ten food-insecure countries. Asserts H.E. Ms. Kersti Kaljulaid, the former president of Estonia, "There is a crisis of inequity that is piling on already increasing and compounding threats. In a world where too many children, adolescents and women are dying, equity, empowerment and access are what needs urgent focus" (WHO et al., 2022).

Notably, the WHO reports that harmful environmental conditions are a major contributor to current childhood morbidity, mortality, and disability, particularly in the Global South. Children are especially vulnerable to various environmental risks, including climate change, air pollution, inadequate

DOI: 10.4324/9781003365358-11

potable water, lack of sanitation and hygiene, toxic chemical exposures, and e-waste. Climate change and other anthropogenic modifications of the environment threaten "to reverse the gains in global child health and the reductions in global child morbidity and mortality made over the past 25 years" (Philipsborn & Chan, 2018). Notably, these environmental adversities do not exist in isolation but co-occur and interact, often with a significant increase in harm to human health (Singer, 2021).

One understudied aspect of the rising environmental health risks of children is ecosyndemics. Ecosyndemics refers to biosocial threats to public health that involve adverse interactions among two or more diseases or other health conditions that are promoted by ecocrises. Ecocrises and ecocrises interactions, ever more common events in the Anthropocene, promote adverse synergies among two or more diseases or other health conditions that threaten public health. While there has been a growing policy interest in the interactions between global environmental change and the quality of human health, comparatively little attention has been paid to the interactions between environmental change and infectious disease emergence, despite growing evidence that causally links these two health-related phenomena (Allen et al., 2017; Singer, 2014). Of note, it is estimated that about 70% of emergent infectious disease, including almost all recent pandemics including COVID-19, originate in animals (mostly wildlife), and their emergence occurs often because of human penetrations of and disturbances to environments, such as deforestation and expansion of agricultural land, and intensification of livestock production (McFarlane et al., 2013; Weiss & Mc-Michael, 2004). Indeed, the COVID-19 pandemic "reminds us that many emerging diseases arise from complex interactions between humans, wildlife, and domestic animals, resulting from changes in land use or food systems" (Haines et al., 2020).

Ecocrises disproportionately affect children, especially poor children, magnifying existing disparities in social determinants of health. In a time of COVID-19 and climate change, two environmentally linked threats to health, the purpose of this chapter is to call attention to the value of assessing and responding to the ecosyndemics of childhood in overcoming barriers to improving child health in the Global South.

Child Health and Climate Change

Despite political and corporate denial or equivocation, climate change is adversely affecting every region on Earth, and in multiple and often synergistic ways. According to the 2022 Intergovernmental Panel on Climate Change (IPCC) – the United Nations organization charged with monitoring and assessing the emerging science related to climate change:

> Withering droughts, extreme heat and record floods already threaten food security and livelihoods for millions of people. Since 2008,

devastating floods and storms have forced more than 20 million people from their homes each year. Since 1961, crop productivity growth in Africa shrunk by a third due to climate change.

(Levin et al., 2022)

To really fathom the complexity of the impact of climate change on child health, we need to consider a wide array of factors, including (but not limited to) changing temperatures on land and precipitation patterns, increases in ocean temperatures and acidity, melting of glaciers and sea ice and resulting sea level rise and coastal flooding, changes in the frequency, intensity, and duration of extreme weather events like hurricanes and droughts, shifts in ecosystem characteristics, like the length of the growing season, timing of plant blooms, and migration and extinction of species (including disease vectors and food animals), the buildup of greenhouse gases in our atmosphere and its effects on pollution, and climate feedback loops: e.g., raising temperatures → melting tundra → release of greenhouse gases stored in tundra → further rising temperatures.

Scientists, across many disciplines and countries, agree that climate change is real, and they also concur about its causes and impacts. At this point, the evidence is overwhelming, solid, and clear. Humans and their diverse interactions with the environment are the primary current driver of climate change but these actions are not evenly distributed across human populations and groups. For example, three billion people in poorer nations use less energy on an annual per capita basis than a standard American refrigerator does in a year. At a broader level, it is evident that global unequal consumption and global unequal environmental destruction reflect the dominant economy in the world system. As Chomsky argues, under the global neoliberal economic regime which has reigned supreme for the last half century, capital "is 'free' to exploit and destroy with abandon, as it has been doing, including – we should not forget – destroying the prospects for organized human life" (Polychroniou, 2022). When neoliberalism became the dominant economic force globally in the 1980s, global temperatures began increasing at an alarming rate. Neoliberalism, which views markets as the primary mechanism to allocate scarce resources, commodified the planet's resources leading corporations and the wealthy to overexploit Earth's assets and cause multifaceted environmental destruction ostensively in the name of efficiency, but in reality, in the service of profit. The richest 20 corporations, for example, are among the biggest producers of carbon emissions and constitute a polluting elite (Di Duca, 2021).

While the ideology of neoliberalism called for the withdrawal of the state from social welfare programs (e.g., policies to keep basic food costs down), many corporate sectors continued to demand and to receive significant government subsidies. In the U.S., for example, the federal government continued to provide billions of tax dollars for research into fossil fuel extraction that benefited polluting oil companies. According to Oil Change International (2021), a research, communication, and advocacy organization, internationally, governments provide at least $775 billion to $1 trillion annually in subsidies to the fossil fuel industry.

The basic message taught to us by climate and environmental scientists is that when we damage the planet, we harm ourselves and our children (Singer & Mendenhall, 2022). The health implications of this message are echoed by public health leaders. In 2021, 600 organizations representing 47 million global health professionals issued a letter declaring that climate change is "the single biggest health threat facing humanity" (GCHA Newsletter, 2021). The WHO estimates that between the years 2030 and 2050, at least 250,000 people will die each year (beyond those that would have died of various factors) because of climate change. Moreover, as stressed by Bhutta, Aimone, and Akhtar (2019), "Children pay a disproportionate price for climate change, with some estimates suggesting up to 88 percent of the burden of disease related to it." This excess morbidity is related to a combination of physiological vulnerability, especially among young children, as well as their level of risk of exposure.

Environmental threats to children's health come from the multiple disruptions wrought by climate change, including rising global temperatures. Global temperatures rose about 1.8°F (1°C) from 1901 to 2020 (Lindsey & Dahlman, 2022). As a result, India saw a 55% rise in deaths due to extreme heat between 2000–2004 and 2017–2021 (Romanello et al., 2022). The study by Romanello and co-workers notes that vulnerable populations including children are most at risk from extreme heat. Because of climate change, around the globe, children under one year old collectively experienced 600 million more days of heatwaves (4.4 more days per child) in 2012–2021, compared to 1986–2005.

Drought is another expression of the heat-effects of climate change. The Horn of Africa, for example, is currently enduring the worst drought in recorded history, with no end in sight (Button, 2022). Many aid agencies believe that a declaration of famine is imminent. Famine declarations are only made under extreme conditions: when a full third of a region's children are severely malnourished, a fifth of the population has no access at all to food, and there are two hunger-related deaths per 10,000 people each day. Children are hit particularly hard during famines because of the nutrient demands of their developing body systems. Children in hunger crises experience a condition called "wasting" in which their bodies are too thin, and their immune systems are weak. Children suffering wasting are vulnerable to developmental delays, disease, and death. A child experiencing wasting is over ten times more likely to die than a healthy child, often from diarrhea or infection. As noted by United Nations Children's Fund (UNICEF, 2020), "The number of children who suffer from wasting can increase dramatically as a result of conflict, epidemics and food insecurity, including that caused by climate change-induced droughts and flooding."

Children also are especially vulnerable to severe heat because of suffering compromised thermoregulatory function at extreme temperatures (Perera &

Nadeau, 2022). Moreover, children depend on adults to protect them from extreme weather, something that can be difficult, especially for poorer parents and those forced to flee disasters and conflict. Extreme heat can quickly sicken children in several ways. It can cause dehydration, heat exhaustion, heat cramps, and heat stroke. High heat can also encumber the helping capacity of children's caregivers (Davies, 2022). Heat-related child mortality in Africa increased to 11,000 deaths annually in the years between 1995 and 2004, of which 5,000 were linked to the negative impacts of climate change. In the 2011–2020 decade, heat-related deaths jumped from 8,000 to 19,000 per year on the continent (Chapman et al., 2022).

Sea-level rise has accelerated from 1.7 mm/year throughout most of the 20th century to 3.2 mm/year since 1993 (Climate.gov, 2022). This increase is driven by the melting of land-based ice-like glaciers. Glaciers are shrinking. The average thickness of 30 well-studied glaciers has decreased more than 60 feet since 1980 (Climate.gov, 2020). The Children's Climate Risk Index (CCRI) reveals 240 million children are now highly exposed to coastal flooding due to sea-level rise. According to Henrietta Fore, UNICEF's executive director,

> For the first time, we have a complete picture of where and how children are vulnerable to climate change, and that picture is almost unimaginably dire. Climate and environmental shocks are undermining the complete spectrum of children's rights, from access to clean air, food and safe water; to education, housing, freedom from exploitation, and even their right to survive. Virtually no child's life will be unaffected.
>
> (UNICEF, 2021)

Climate change-intensified monsoon rain is another cause of flooding. Flooding, due to very heavy rain in Pakistan and melting glaciers in Pakistan's northern mountain regions in 2022, caused flood waters to inundate nearly the entire country and resulted in at least 1,500 deaths (including hundreds of children). In the aftermath, in Pakistan's Sindh Province – a center of the worst flooding – more than ten children are now dying every day at the Mother and Child Healthcare Hospital alone. According to Aadarsh Leghari, UNICEF's Communication Officer in Pakistan, "Many children are not even reaching hospitals because the medical facilities they could access are either underwater or just not accessible" (Saifi et al., 2022). UN Population Fund estimates that there are more than 127,000 pregnant women in Pakistan, about 2,000 of whom are giving birth every day, many under unhygienic conditions on the side of the road because of the flooding (Wallen & Yusufzai, 2022). Numerous child deaths are the consequence of water-related ailments. Standing water is an ideal breeding ground for mosquitoes, which are currently spreading malaria and dengue fever in Pakistan. Dengue causes flu-like symptoms, including piercing headaches, muscle and joint pains, fever, and rashes. Extreme cases can cause bleeding, shock, organ failure, and potentially death. Additionally, respiratory illnesses are now rampant in Pakistan's children because of the flooding. At the same time, flooded agricultural land and loss of food storage are causing widespread malnutrition in children. In Nigeria, climate-linked flooding in 2022 caused the worst floods in a decade impacting over 3 million people across the country, of which an estimated 60% were children, and left 1.4 million Nigerians displaced while claiming 500 lives. The devastating floods injured over 1,500 people and destroyed over 70,000 hectares of farmland (UNICEF, 2022a).

COVID-19 and Children

While children have not been the face of the COVID-19 pandemic, they are at risk of becoming one of its biggest victims. Among the 4.1 million COVID-19 deaths reported through 2021, only 0.4% (or about 16,100) occurred in children and adolescents under 20 years of age (UNICEF, 2022b). Of these child deaths, 53% occurred among adolescents ages ten to nineteen, and 47% among children ages 0 to nine. In the Global South, particularly, however, the pandemic has changed children's lives in profound ways, including through the implementation of mitigation policy measures that may inadvertently have done more harm than good. These negative impacts are proving to be most damaging for children in the poorest countries, and in the poorest neighborhoods in poorer countries, and for those who are already in disadvantaged or vulnerable situations.

Compounding the toll on children is school loss due to the pandemic. Analysis by Save the Children has identified the extent of this threat to children's health. According to Inger Ashing, chief executive officer of Save the Children:

> As with every crisis, the biggest victims of the COVID-19 pandemic are children, and our analysis shows that when it comes to school closures, the poorer the country, the bigger the impact... Especially in lower-income countries, where children have far fewer days of schooling in their lifetime to begin with and where there's less access to remote learning, it's vital that children can get back to school as soon as it's safe to do so... Sadly, girls are more likely than boys to have disproportionately missed out on their schooling, as all too often girls leave school early due to child marriage, pregnancy, or having to work.
>
> (Save the Children, 2021)

Being out of school, children lose the protections and support that schools offer in addition to the education they receive. Save the Children found that children in poorer countries have lost 66% more of their lifetime number of schooldays during the COVID-19 outbreak compared to children in wealthier countries. On average, girls in poorer countries missed 22% more days in school than boys. During the pandemic, children in some of the poorest countries in the world have lost up to 20% of their lifetime days in school. For example, in Guinea, children have missed 22% of their total lifetime number of school days on average. Boys lost an average of around 15% of their lifetime schooldays; girls lost a notable 39%. In Burkina Faso, children suffered the loss of over 20% of their total lifetime of schooldays, with boys missing out of 14% of their schooldays, and girls 29%. In Afghanistan, the figure is almost 13% on average, with around 9% for boys and 21% for girls. Finally, in South Sudan, up to 27% of children did not return to school even once they were allowed to do so.

In other words, although children are not the age group hardest hit by SARS-CoV-2 that causes COVID-19, the indirect effects stemming from the pandemic, like school loss, have significantly disadvantaged children in the Global South. In addition, direct stress on health systems and disruptions to life-saving health services like immunization and antenatal care, as well as drops in food security, have produced devastating increases in child morbidity and mortality. During the pandemic, disadvantaged children in poorer countries are at increased risk of missing essential routine childhood vaccinations. Analysis by Causey and colleague (2020) found that worldwide from January to December 2020, about 30 million children missed their DTP3 (diphtheria, tetanus, and pertussis) doses and over 27 million children missed MCV1 (measles-containing-vaccine) doses for measles (Roberts, 2020). Missed treatment and preventive healthcare is expected to contribute to increasing mortality and morbidity due to childhood infectious diseases like measles, malaria, and pneumonia (Chandir et al., 2020; Fore et al., 2020; Nghochuzie et al., 2020; Spencer, 2021).

Significantly contributing to the impact of the pandemic on children is the illness and (often sudden) death of parents and other caregivers/breadwinners. Two years into the pandemic, Oxfam International (2022) reports that "Every minute, four children around the world have lost a parent or caregiver to COVID." Using mortality and fertility data to model minimum estimates and rates of COVID-19-associated deaths, for the period from March 1, 2020, to April 30, 2021, Hillis and colleagues (2021) estimate that over a million children suffered the death of primary caregivers, including at least one parent or custodial grandparent. The 21 countries in their study with the highest primary caregiver death rates (involving the death of at least one per 1,000 children) were mostly in the Global South. These included Peru (10.2 per 1,000 children), South Africa (5.1), Mexico (3.5), Brazil (2.4), Colombia (2.3), Iran (1.7), and Argentina (1.1). Between two and five times more children lost fathers to COVID-19 than mothers. More broadly, it is estimated that the number of children who have experienced the loss of a parent or caregiver due to COVID-19-related deaths is over 10 million globally as of May 1, 2022 (CDC, 2022). Hillis and colleagues (2021) label orphanhood and caregiver deaths as the "hidden pandemic resulting from COVID-19." This less visible component of the pandemic nonetheless has a tragic emotional and economic impact on children's health. Generally, it is known that losing primary caregivers is associated with higher risks of experiencing mental health problems; physical, emotional, and sexual violence; and family poverty (Kidman & Palermo, 2016). Kidman and Palermo (2016) report that paternally orphaned children are more at risk than non-orphans to experience sexual violence, potentially linked to household economic vulnerability.

As Hillis emphasizes, "You have this constellation of abuses or adversities piling up on the individual child" (McKeever, 2022). That compounding of adversities can result in a condition known as toxic stress. Under normal conditions, the body copes with stressors by increasing the heart rate and flooding the body with stress hormones. If stress conditions are prolonged or severe, the body may experience a cascade of harmful biological responses—including impaired neuronal synapses of the brain. Toxic stress can put a child at risk for long-term complications from diseases like diabetes and Parkinson's. Also, it can damage the body's immune system and its ability to fight off disease while increasing the risk of dying from heart disease or an infection. Orphaned children also are at higher risk of suicide.

Exemplary is the case of 14-year-old Ivo who lives in the small town of Pasaman in the Indonesian province of West Sumatra. Ivo passes the cemetery where her father is buried every day on her way to school (McKeever, 2022). She visits his grave site so often that the flowers she picks from the bougainvillea in her front yard and leaves at his grave are still fragrant when she returns with a fresh bunch the next day. Her father died of kidney failure while suffering from COVID-19. The younger of his two children, Ivo remembers how they were inseparable. She wants to be a policewoman when she grows up because her father was a security guard. "I really miss him getting mad at me," Ivo says as tears stream down her cheeks. Without him, Ivo's family has fallen on difficult economic times. Her mother, the only breadwinner for the family of three, struggles to stretch the small amount of money she earns working at a local grocery store. Under these circumstances, Ivo's diet has suffered.

Similar is the case of Nitish Kumar and his two sisters who live in the small village of Madhulata in the poor Indian state of Bihar. When their mother died of COVID-19, the children buried her in the backyard; she was only 32 years old. Their father had died of COVID-19 just a few months earlier. With COVID stigma rife in the local community, no neighbors or relatives came forward to help with the burial or to care for the children. Instead, Kumar and his sisters found themselves grieving orphans alone and scared. At the age of 14, Kumar is now the only possible breadwinner in the family and worries that he will have to drop out of school to make money to feed his sisters. He explained,

I wanted to become a doctor. But my first priority now is to arrange food for my sisters rather than continuing with my studies. Right now, we are surviving on relief materials being donated by social workers, but they will not be available all the time. I will have to work. With their death, my dream too was buried.

His sister, Soni, shared her fears for the future without their parents: "We have no sources of income," she said. "We will have to do something to keep us alive" (Ellis-Petersen & Chaurasia, 2021).

As families lose their sources of income due to COVID-19 and the resulting recession in the global economy, households already on the edge are falling further into poverty. A joint analysis by Save the Children and UNICEF found that the number of children living in poor households in the Global South could increase by 11–15% or 63–86 million children due to the pandemic (Fiala & Delamonica, 2020). Vulnerable children are becoming malnourished because of the deteriorating quality of their diets and the multiple shocks created by the pandemic and its containment measures. Efforts to mitigate the transmission of COVID-19 have complicated the crisis by disrupting food systems, upending health and nutrition services, and threatening food security. In short, the biggest impact of COVID-19 on children's health has not been directly caused by the virus but rather by the pandemic as a highly disruptive – literally world-shaking – socioeconomic crises for which the global community and poor countries in particular were not prepared.

The COVID-19 Ecosyndemic among Children: The Case of Lagos

As this discussion suggests, the pandemic has had both direct and indirect effects and shorter- and longer-term impacts on children in the Global South including on their health and well-being. The most damaging effects probably have been those with enduring consequences, including malnutrition, toxic stress, physical and emotional trauma, loss of a sense of security, grief, and missing prophylactic inoculations. All these factors make children highly vulnerable. No doubt, during the pandemic many children have suffered multiple adversities as well as the consequences of their interaction. For example, malnutrition and infection are mutually reinforcing and their co-occurrence puts children at heightened risk for particularly adverse outcomes. Malnutrition is the primary cause of immunodeficiency worldwide, and infants, children, and adolescents (as well as the elderly) are the most at risk. There is a two-way relationship between malnutrition and infection because poor nutrition leaves children underweight, weakened, and vulnerable while infection contributes to malnutrition, creating a vicious cycle (Katona & Katona-Apte, 2008). As summarized by Nelson and colleagues (2020),

> Growing evidence indicates that in the first three years of life [especially], a host of biological (e.g., malnutrition, infectious disease) and psychosocial (e.g., maltreatment, witnessing violence, extreme poverty)

hazards can affect a child's developmental trajectory and lead to increased risk of adverse physical and psychological health conditions.

The health effects of enduring multiple biopsychosocial challenges occur across various body systems damaging cardiovascular, immune, metabolic, and brain health, and may, if a child survives, persist into adulthood and influence an individual's life course and longevity.

As a result of climate change and other environmental crises, the challenges facing children in the Global South are further compounded in that disruptions of the environment can produce many of the same threats to children's health as the pandemic. In effect, some children, especially those in the poorest families and communities, are experiencing a complex storm of dangers from the polluted air they breathe to the ravages of extreme summer heat episodes or the flooding of the family's farm plot, and from the emotional burden of losing a parent to COVID-19 to inadequate nutrient intake and loss of emotional security because of being orphaned by parental death. How children respond to such a landslide of threats varies by individual and social capacities and resiliency. Manderson and Warren (2016) introduced the term "recursive cascades" to refer to the ways poverty and social exclusion can create the preconditions for multiple, often entwined and interacting chronic health problems, and how, in turn, these chronic health problems can increase disadvantage for individuals and their households. The result of a recursive cascade of experiencing one problem after another is an inevitable trajectory of increasing ill health and growing impoverishment. As Pennea and colleagues (2021) argue, "The intersection between climate change and COVID-19 exacerbates … existing disparities by impacting children's physical and mental health that are a direct product of poverty and structural racism." Similarly, Kurtz and colleagues (2022) point out that:

> Environmental factors, including climate and geographical conditions, and social-economic factors are determinants of production, availability, and access to food. Because a person is a social being in constant interaction with the environment, air pollution is not merely a factor that could add to malnutrition aggravating the baseline condition but is a causal factor of malnutrition.

As these comments indicate, various threats to health are intimately linked and mutually causal, especially so for children because of their vulnerability and dependency.

Syndemics can emerge within recursive cascades as co-occurring or sequential diseases (as noted for malnutrition and infection) and their effects interact adversely and further complicate the health burden of a population and its children. Because resulting child morbidity and mortality are not a direct consequence of suffering SARS-CoV-2 infection, they may never be counted in COVID-19 statistics in countries with significant child health problems like Nigeria, India, Pakistan, the Democratic Republic of the Congo, and Ethiopia. Rather deaths may be attributed to single causes like pneumonia, diarrhea, or malaria. Analyses, however, show that children in poor countries often suffer multiple interacting health problems (Pappachan & Choonara, 2017).

An example of a child health ecocrisis/COVID-19 syndemic forming as part of a recursive cascade can be seen among the poor of Lagos, Nigeria (see Chapter 1 in this volume). The nation's capital and commercial and economic hub, Lagos has a population of 23.3 million and is growing by 3.2% a year. Rapid urbanization and industrialization have exposed the majority of the city's population to dangerous levels of air pollution. Moreover, as many as 70% of city residents live below the poverty line on about US$1 a day. Millions live in crowded informal settlements constructed with whatever materials can be scavenged from the city. As the World Bank (2022) reports, "climate and conflict shocks – which disproportionately affect Nigeria's poor – are multiplying, and their effects have been compounded by COVID-19."

At the center of the city's ecocrisis is air pollution. Cars, trucks, and other road vehicles comprise the primary sources of ambient air pollution in Lagos. Each day it is estimated that over 225 vehicles clog every kilometer of road in the city. Most vehicles in Lagos are over 15 years old and are powered by old emission technologies and fuel with high sulfur levels (200 times higher than current U.S. standards for diesel) (World Bank, 2020). A second source of pollution is industrial emissions. There are several commercial industrial zones in Lagos, like Apapa, Idumota, Ikeja, and Odogunyan, where various production activities are concentrated, including cement, chemicals, furniture, refinery, and steel manufacturing. These crowded centers of production have especially high levels of pollution. In Odogunyan, for example, a PM2.5 concentration of 1,770 $\mu g/m^3$ was recorded in 2020 (World Bank, 2020). Long-term exposure to fine particulate matter with an aerodynamic diameter of less than 2.5 micrometers is especially harmful to health, as these small particles can pass the barriers of the lung and enter into the bloodstream, causing premature deaths as well as respiratory and cardiovascular diseases (Brook et al., 2010). Generators, which supply half of Lagos' total energy demand, are a third major source of air pollution. The poor combustion of the gasoline and oil used to operate the generators contributes to the heavily polluted air breathed by Lagos residents. Air pollution in Lagos is between six and ten times the maximum level recommended by the WHO.

These already difficult conditions are exacerbated by climate change. It has been well established that in the presence of heat and sunlight, chemical emissions from vehicles and factories react to form ground ozone, which is a highly reactive, oxidative gas, and a harmful pollutant. As average temperatures rise due to climate change, ground ozone levels go up. The primary ingredients for ground ozone are nitrogen oxides and volatile organic compounds. These are produced when fossil fuels are burned. Sunlight and heat, however, are key. Epidemiological studies have shown that an increase of

10 µg/m³ in ground ozone over a two-day period triggered an increased risk of death by 0.18%. This translated to 6,262 additional deaths in cities that have been studied (Vicedo-Cabrera et al., 2020).

Ozone is particularly dangerous to children because their lungs are still developing, and they often spend more time outdoors than adults. As noted by Lee et al. (2021), ozone can inflame the cells that line a child's upper airways and lungs. Long-term exposure has also been linked to the development of asthma in children, but even short-term exposure can be quite harmful, making it more difficult to breathe due to asthma, chronic bronchitis, and acute lower respiratory infections in children (Hunt et al., 2016). Of note, under five mortalities due to lower respiratory infections (from all causes combined) in Nigeria is the second highest in the world after India (Croitoru et al., 2020). A World Bank (2014) study in Nigeria, which did not consider the added adverse effect of climate change, estimated that pollution in Lagos is responsible for 30,000 premature deaths, half of them among children under one-year-old, as well as causing up to 350,000 lower acute respiratory diseases.

The risk to children's health in Lagos has been further compromised by the pandemic, which has had a devastating impact on livelihoods and access to food. Early in the pandemic, the Nigerian government imposed a five-week lockdown, resulting in loss of work and income, an economic downturn, and rising food prices. This left many households struggling to feed their families. The five-week lockdown, which restricted movement and required all except essential services to close, had a significant economic impact. The crisis for many Lagosians is illustrated by the case of Okuomo. Before the pandemic, she had worked over a decade cleaning dormitories at the University of Lagos, earning about US$44 a month. But the university shut down in March 2020 to prevent the spread of the virus. Deemed a nonessential worker, Okuomo lost her income. Within a few months, she had used up her limited savings and was unable to adequately feed her children. She explained, "We don't eat like we used to. People who used to eat three meals are now eating one … We [have] our fill in the morning, and sometimes at night we just soak two handfuls of *garri* [a staple made from cassava] and sleep" (Adelaja, 2021). Although most people were able to resume economic activity once the lockdown ended, many saw their overall incomes fall while food prices remained high. According to Mohammed Yunus, a volunteer with the Nigerian Slum/Informal Settlements Federation, in October 2020: "People have started working again, but not fully. Then there's inflation, the increasing price of food and commodities. People tell us that they only have enough income to make food once a day." Falling incomes, rising food prices, and the absence of government economic or food support combined to leave many people hungry. As noted above, under such conditions it is children who suffer most. In sum, the child health ecocrisis/COVID-19 syndemic in Lagos consisted of the interaction between COVID-19, air pollution, malnutrition, and intense poverty (Choji et al., 2021). These combined to disrupt families and shorten the lives and well-being of children.

Conclusion

The issue of ecosyndemics remains understudied despite the growing day-by-day advance during the Anthropocene of the degradation of the environment on which we depend for life. Ecosyndemic research calls attention to the ways human activities not only damage ecosystems but lead to the damaging interaction of ecocrises (e.g., such as the interaction of climate change and resulting heating and acidification of the oceans in combination with over-fishing is destroying coral reefs on which families in many parts of the world depend on for their livelihoods). Children are particularly at risk in ecocrisis syndemics, especially economically poor and socially marginalized children. These complex events rob them of nutrients, healthy air, and clean water, while exposing them to toxins and infectious diseases. The consequences can be seen in the failure to achieve desired improvements in child health in the Global South despite considerable international and national efforts in recent years. With climate change and the pandemic even gains that had been made are starting to slip away. To quote Greta Thunberg (2022),

> We are approaching a precipice. And I would strongly suggest that those of us who have not yet been greenwashed out of our senses stand our ground. Do not let them drag us another inch closer to the edge. Not one inch. Right here, right now, is where we draw the line.

References

Adelaja, T. (2021). "Between Hunger and the Virus" The Impact of the Covid-19 Pandemic on People Living in Poverty in Lagos, Nigeria. *Human Rights Watch*. https://www.hrw.org/report/2021/07/28/between-hunger-and-virus/impact-covid-19-pandemic-people-living-poverty-lago.

Allen, T., Murray, K.A., Zambrana-Torrelio, C., Morse, S.S., Rondinini, C., Di Marco, M., Breit, N., Olival, K.J., & Daszak, P. (2017). Global Hotspots and Correlates of Emerging Zoonotic Diseases. *Nature Communication*, 8(1), 1124. https://doi.org/10.1038/s41467-017-00923-8.

Bhutta, Z.A., Aimone, A., & Akhtar, S. (2019). Climate Change and Global Child Health: What Can Paediatricians Do? *Archives of Disease in Childhood*, 104(5), 417–418. https://doi.org/10.1136/archdischild-2018-316694.

Brook, R., Rajagopalan, S., Pope III, A., Brook, J.R., Bhatnagar, A., Diez-Roux, A.V., Holguin, F., Hong, Y., Luepker, R., Mittleman, M., Peters, A., Siscovick, D., Smith, S., Whitsel, L, Kaufman, J. (2010). Particulate Matter Air Pollution and Cardiovascular Disease. *Circulation*, 121(21), 2331–2378. https://doi.org/10.1161/CIR.0b013e3181dbece1.

Button, H. (2022). Famine Projected in Somalia as Widespread Areas of Eastern Horn Face Extreme Need. *Agrilinks*. https://agrilinks.org/post/famine-projected-somalia-widespread-areas-eastern-horn-face-extreme-need.

Causey, K., Fullman, N., Sorensen, R., Galles, N., Zheng P., Aravkin, A., Danovaro-Holliday, M.., Martinez-Piedra, R., Sodha, S., Velandia-González, M., Gacic-Dobo, M., Castro, E., He, J., Schipp, M., Deen, A., Hay, S.I., Lim, S.S., Mosser, J.F.

(2020). Estimating Global and Regional Disruptions to Routine Childhood Vaccine Coverage during the COVID-19 Pandemic in 2020: A Modelling Study. *Lancet*, 398(10299), 522–534.

CDC. (2022). Global Orphanhood Associated with COVID-19. https://www.cdc.gov/globalhealth/covid-19/orphanhood/index.html.

Chapman, S., Birch, C.E., Marsham, J.H., Part, C., Hajat, S., Chersich, M.F., Ebi, K.L., Luchters, S., Nakstad, B., & Kovat, S. (2022). Past and Projected Climate Change Impacts on Heat-Related Child Mortality in Africa. *Environmental Research Letters*, 17(7). https://doi.org/10.1088/1748-9326/ac7ac5.

Chandir, S., Siddiqui, D., Mehmood, M., Setayesh, H., Siddique, M., Mirza, A., Soundardjee, R., Dharma, V., Shah, M., Abdullah, S., Akhter, M., Ali Khan, A., Khan, A. (2020). Impact of COVID-19 Response on Uptake of Routine Immunization in Sindh, Pakistan: An Analysis of Provincial Immunization Registry Data. *Vaccine*, 38, 7146–7155.

Choji, I., Etukudoh, N., Adeyem, O., & Ophelia, J. (2021). Covid-19 and the and the Nigerian Environment: The Way Forward. *Journal of Innovative Science and Research Technology*, 6(6), 2456–2156.

Climate.gov. (2020). Climate Change: Mountain Glaciers. https://www.climate.gov/news-features/understanding-climate/climate-change-mountain-glaciers.

Climate.gov. (2022). Climate Change: Global Sea Level. https://www.climate.gov/news-features/understanding-climate/climate-change-global-sea-level.

Croitoru, L., Chang, J.C., & Kelly, A. (2020). *The Cost of Air Pollution in Lagos*. Washington, DC: The World Bank Group.

Davies, D. (2022). Extreme Heat: Keeping Kids Safe When Temperatures Soar. *HealthyChildren.Org*. https://www.healthychildren.org/English/safety-prevention/at-home/Pages/Protecting-Children-from-Extreme-Heat-Information-for-Parents.aspx.

Di Duca, M. (2021). How Neoliberalism Destroyed the Planet and Why Capitalism Won't Save Us. *Global Social Challenges*. https://sites.manchester.ac.uk/global-social-challenges/2021/05/04/how-neoliberalism-destroyed-the-planet-and-why-capitalism-wont-save-us/.

Ellis-Petersen, H., & Chaurasia, M. (2021). 'My Dream Was Buried': The Children of India Orphaned by Covid. *The Guardian*. https://www.theguardian.com/world/2021/jun/11/my-dream-was-buried-the-children-of-india-orphaned-by-covid.

Fiala, O., & Delamonica, E. (2020). Children in Monetary-Poor Households: COVID-19's Invisible Victims. *UNICEF*. https://data.unicef.org/data-for-action/children-in-monetary-poor-households-covid-19s-invisible-victims/.

Fore, H., Ghebreyesus, T., Watkins, K., Greenslade, L., Berkley, S., Bassat, Q., Duneton, P., Klugman, K., & Golden, A. (2020). Leveraging COVID 19 Response to End Preventable Deaths from Child Pneumonia. *Lancet*, 396, 1709–1711.

GCHA Newsletter (Global Climate and Health Alliance). (2021). Letter from 46 Million Health Workers Calling for Global Climate Action Delivered to COP26 & COP27 Presidencies. https://climateandhealthalliance.org/press-releases/letter-delivered-to-world-leaders-from-46-million-health-workers-calling-for-global-climate-action/.

Haines, A., Scheelbeek, P., & Abba, K. (2020). The Health Case for Urgent Action on Climate Change. *British Medical Journal*, 368. https://doi.org/10.1136/bmj.m1103.

Hillis, S., Unwin, H.J.T., Chen, Y., Cluver, L., Sherr, L., Goldman, P.S., Ratmann, O., Donnelly, C., Bhatt, S., Villaveces, A., Butchart, A., Bachman, G., Rawlings, L.,

Green, P., Nelson, C., Flaxman, S. (2021). Global Minimum Estimates of Children Affected by COVID-19-Associated Orphanhood and Deaths of Caregivers: A Modelling Study. *Lancet.* https://doi.org/10.1016/S0140-6736(21)01253-8.

Hunt, A., Ferguson, J., Hurley, F., & Searl, A. (2016). *OECD Environment Working Papers Social Costs of Morbidity Impacts of Air Pollution.* Paris: OECD Publishing. https://www.oecd-ilibrary.org/content/paper/5jm55j7cq0lv-en.

Kidman, R., & Palermo, T. (2016). The Relationship between Parental Presence and Child Sexual Violence: Evidence from Thirteen Countries in Sub-Saharan Africa. *Child Abuse and Neglect*, 51, 172–180.

Lindsey, R., & Dahlman, L. (2022). Climate Change: Global Temperature. *climate. gov.* https://www.climate.gov/news-features/understanding-climate/climate-change-global-temperature.

Katona, P., Katona-Apte, J. (2008). The interaction between nutrition and infection. *Clinical Infectious Diseases* 46(10), 1582–1588. https://doi.org/10.1086/587658.

Kurtz, M., Lezon, C., Boyer, P., & Tasat, D. (2022). Malnutrition and Air Pollution in Latin America: Impact of Two Stressors on Children's Health. *Intechopen.* https://doi.org/10.5772/intechopen.104656.

Lee, Y., Lee, P, Choi, S., An, M., Jang, A. Effects of Air Pollutants on Airway Diseases. *International Journal of Environmental Research and Public Health.* 2021 Sep 20;18(18), 9905. https://doi.org/10.3390/ijerph18189905.

Levin, K., Boehm, S., & Carter, R. (2022). 6 Big Findings from the IPCC 2022 Report on Climate Impacts, Adaptation and Vulnerability. World Resources Institute. https://www.wri.org/insights/ipcc-report-2022-climate-impacts-adaptation-vulnerability.

Manderson, L., & Warren, N. (2016). "Just One Thing after Another": Recursive Cascades and Chronic Conditions. *Medical Anthropology Quarterly*, 30(4), 479–497.

McFarlane, R., Sleigh, A., & McMichael, A. (2013). Land-Use Change and Emerging Infectious Disease on an Island Continent. *International Journal of Environmental Research & Public Health*, 10, 2699–2719.

McKeever, A. (2022). COVID-19's Hidden, Heartbreaking Toll: Millions of Orphaned Children. *National Geographic.* https://www.nationalgeographic.com/science/article/covid-19-hidden-heartbreaking-toll-millions-of-orphaned-children.

Nelson, C.A., Scott, R.D., Bhutta, Z.A., Harris, N.B., Danese, A., & Samara, M. (2020). Adversity in Childhood Is Linked to Mental and Physical Health throughout Life. *British Medical Journal*, 371, m3048. https://doi.org/10.1136/bmj.m3048.

Nghochuzie, N., Olwal, C., Udoakang, A., Amenga-Etego, L., & Amambua-Ngwa, A. (2020). Pausing the Fight against Malaria to Combat COVID 19 Pandemic in Africa: Is the Future of Malaria Bleak? *Frontiers in Microbiology*, 11, 1476. https://doi.org/10.3389/fmicb.2020.01476.

Oil Change International. (2021). Fossil Fuel Subsidy Overview. https://priceofoil.org/fossil-fuel-subsidies/.

Oxfam International. (2022). COVID-19 Death Toll Four Times Higher in Lower-Income Countries Than Rich Ones. https://www.oxfam.org/en/press-releases/covid-19-death-toll-four-times-higher-lower-income-countries-rich-ones.

Pappachan, B., & Choonara, I. (2017). Inequalities in Child Health in India. *BMJ Paediatrics Open*, e000054. https://doi.org/10.1136/bmjpo-2017-000054.

Pennea, E., Anderson, L., Moore, C., & McDermott, L. (2021). The Nexus of Climate Change, COVID-19, and Environmental Justice on Children's Health. *Journal of Applied Research on Children*, 12(1).

Perera, F., & Nadeau, K. (2022). Climate Change, Fossil-Fuel Pollution, and Children's Health. *New England Journal of Medicine*, 386, 2303–2314.

Philipsborn, R., & Chan, K. (2018). Climate Change and Global Child Health. *Pediatrics*, 141(6), e20173774.

Polychroniou, C. (2022). Noam Chomsky: "We're on the Road to a Form of Neofascism." *TruthOut*. https://truthout.org/articles/noam-chomsky-were-on-the-road-to-a-form-of-neofascism/?eType=EmailBlastContent&eId=a1e885af-5d26-47eb-a0c1-.

Roberts, L. (2020). Pandemic Brings Mass Vaccinations to a Halt. *Science*, 368(3487), 116–117.

Romanello, M., Di Napoli, C., Drummond, P., Green, C., Kennard, H., Lampard, P., Scamman, D., Arnell, N., Ayeb-Karlsson, S., Ford, L.B., Belesova, K., Bowen, K., Cai, W., Callaghan, M., Campbell-Lendrum, D., Chambers, J., van Daalen, K.R., Dalin, C., Dasandi, N., Dasgupta, S., Davies, M., Dominguez-Salas, P., Dubrow, R., Ebi, K.L., Eckelman, M., Ekins, P., Escobar, L.E., Georgeson, L., Graham, H., Gunther, S.H., Hamilton, I., Hang, Y., Hänninen, R., Hartinger, S., He, K., Hess, J.J., Hsu, S.C., Jankin, S., Jamart, L., Jay, O., Kelman, I., Kiesewetter, G., Kinney, P., Kjellstrom, T., Kniveton, D., Lee, J.K.W., Lemke, B., Liu, Y., Liu, Z., Lott, M., Batista, M.L., Lowe, R., MacGuire, F., Sewe, M.O., Martinez-Urtaza, J., Maslin, M., McAllister, L., McGushin, A., McMichael, C., Mi, Z., Milner, J., Minor, K., Minx, J.C., Mohajeri, N., Moradi-Lakeh, M., Morrissey, K., Munzert, S., Murray, K.A., Neville, T., Nilsson, M., Obradovich, N., O'Hare, M.B., Oreszczyn, T., Otto, M., Owfi, F., Pearman, O., Rabbaniha, M., Robinson, E.J.Z., Rocklöv, J., Salas, R.N., Semenza, J.C., Sherman, J.D., Shi, L., Shumake-Guillemot, J., Silbert, G., Sofiev, M., Springmann, M., Stowell, J., Tabatabaei, M., Taylor, J., Triñanes, J., Wagner, F., Wilkinson, P., Winning, M., Yglesias-González, M., Zhang, S., Gong, P., Montgomery, H., & Costello, A. (2022). The 2022 Report of The Lancet Countdown on Health and Climate Change: Health at the Mercy of Fossil Fuels. https://www.preventionweb.net/publication/2022-report-lancet-countdown-health-and-climate-change-health-mercy-fossil-fuels.

Save the Children. (2021). COVID-19: Kids in World's Poorest Countries Lost 66% More of Lifetime at School Than Richer Peers. *Save the Children*. https://www.savethechildren.net/news/covid-19-kids-world's-poorest-countries-lost-66-more-lifetime-school-richer-peers-save-children.

Singer, M. (2014). *The Anthropology of Infectious Disease*. Walnut Creek, CA: Left Coast Press.

Singer, M. (2021). *Ecocrises Interactions: Human Health and the Changing Environment*. New York: Wiley.

Singer, M., & Mendenhall, E. (2022). Syndemics in Global Health. In *A Companion to Medical Anthropology*, Singer, M., Erickson, P., & Abadia-Barrero, C., eds. Hoboken, NY: Wiley Blackwell.

Saifi, S., Mogul, R., Coren, A., Sidhu, S., Iqbal, J., & Mandhro, S. (2022). First Came the Floods. Now, Pakistan's Children Face a New Disaster. *CNN*. https://www.cnn.com/2022/09/25/asia/pakistan-floods-children-water-borne-disease-intl-hnk-dst/index.html.

Spencer, N. (2021). Children of the Syndemic. *Çocuk Dergisi - Journal of Child*, 21(3), 270–274.

Suzuki, E., & Kashiwaste, H. (2019). Despite Remarkable Progress, 15,000 Children and 800 Women Still Die Every Day Mostly of Preventable Or

Treatable Causes. *World Bank Blogs.* https://blogs.worldbank.org/opendata/despite-remarkable-progress-15000-children-and-800-women-still-die-every-day-mostly.

Thunberg, G. (2022). *The Climate Book.* London: Allen Lane.

UNICEF. (2020). Nutrition and Care for Children with Wasting. https://www.unicef.org/nutrition/child-wasting.

UNICEF. (2021). One Billion Children at 'Extremely High Risk' of the Impacts of the Climate Crisis - UNICEF. https://www.unicef.org/press-releases/one-billion-children-extremely-high-risk-impacts-climate-crisis-unicef.

UNICEF. (2022a). Nigeria: Emergence Flood Response. https://www.unicef.org/media/130026/file/Nigeria%20Flash%20Update%20(Flood)%20for%20September%20–%20November%202022..pdf.

UNICEF. (2022b). COVID-19 Confirmed Cases and Deaths. https://data.unicef.org/resources/covid-19-confirmed-cases-and-deaths-dashboard/.

Vicedo-Cabrera, A., Sera, F., Liu, C., Armstrong, B., Milojevic, A., & Guo, Y. (2020). Short Term Association between Ozone and Mortality: Global Two Stage Time Series Study in 406 Locations in 20 Countries. *British Medical Journal,* 368. https://doi.org/10.1136/bmj.m108.

Wallen, J., & Yusufzai, A. (2022). Women Forced to 'Give Birth by the Side of the Road' after Floods Devastate Pakistan. *The Telegraph.* https://www.telegraph.co.uk/authors/a/ap-at/ashfaq-yusufzai/.

Weiss, R., & McMichael, A. (2004). Social and Environmental Risk Factors in the Emergence of Infectious Diseases. *Nature Medicine,* 10, S70–S76. https://doi.org/10.1038/nm1150.

World Bank. (2014). Diesel Power Generation: Inventories and Black Carbon Emissions in Nigeria. https://openknowledge.worldbank.org/handle/10986/28419.

World Bank. (2020). The Cost of Air Pollution in Lagos. https://www.worldbank.org/en/topic/environment/publication/the-cost-of-air-pollution-in-lagos.

World Bank. (2022). Deep Structural Reforms Guided by Evidence Are Urgently Needed to Lift Millions of Nigerians Out of Poverty, Says New World Bank Report. https://www.worldbank.org/en/news/press-release/2022/03/21/afw-deep-structural-reforms-guided-by-evidence-are-urgently-needed-to-lift-millions-of-nigerians-out-of-poverty.

WHO, UN Children's Fund UNICEF, the UN Sexual and Reproductive Health Agency, UNFPA, Partnership for Maternal, Newborn & Child Health, and Countdown to 2030. (2022). *Protect the Promise.* Berlin: WHO and UNICEF.

Conclusion
COVID Syndemics in the Global South

Merrill Singer, Nicola Bulled, and Inayat Ali

Pestilence is in fact very common, but we find it hard to believe in a pestilence when it descends upon us. There have been as many plagues as wars in history; yet always plagues and wars take people equally by surprise.

Albert Camus, The Plague

Although starting in December 2019 in Wuhan, China, the World Health Organization (WHO) officially declared the SARS-CoV-2 outbreak a Public Health Emergency of International Concern on January 30, 2020, and a global pandemic on March 11, 2020. Countries were urged to quickly implement strict physical distancing, quarantine, isolation, and lockdown measures to protect the public from the contagious virus. Despite all efforts, the disease engulfed the nations of the world within a few months, and partly because of the unintended consequences of lockdown initiatives, left scarring impacts on the health and mental health of global populations and on the functioning of prevention, treatment, and other care and social systems. As a result, in addition to causing the death of millions and causing untold suffering, COVID-19 altered the fabric of social lives and meanings.

Despite warnings of imminent pandemic disease and multiple simulation events to guide pandemic disease preparations, the world was caught off guard in one way or another and ill-prepared for COVID-19. The prior series of emergent infectious diseases from the first SARS outbreak in 2003 to Zika in 2016 did not trigger recognition of the need for a new era in global infectious disease preparation and cooperation. Even in the Global North, with its comparatively abundant resources, warnings went unheeded. In January 2017, Anthony Fauci, director of the U.S. National Institute of Allergy and Infectious Diseases, for example, cautioned members of the incoming Trump administration about the inevitability of a "surprise outbreak" of a new disease and urged preparations be initiated immediately. During a speech at Georgetown University in Washington, D.C., Fauci stated, "There is no question that there will be a challenge to the coming administration in the arena of infectious diseases," adding, "the thing we're extraordinarily confident about is that we're going to see this in the next few years." Fauci pointed

DOI: 10.4324/9781003365358-12

to the risks presented by unknown diseases, in addition to those from re-emergent ones (Soonamaker, 2020). Multiple pandemic simulation exercises, including Clade X, run with Trump White House and US Congress leaders in May 2018, highlighted systemic deficiencies in public health systems and the need for robust and coordinated efforts across multiple government and private sector actors.

Why was COVID-19 so devastating? There are several reasons, but the primary concern in this volume is interaction with other diseases and health conditions, and institutionalized disparities resulting in magnified negative health outcomes. The latter was of equal concern to the contributors to this collection is the unequal distribution of resources and power across the so-called Brandt Line dividing the wealthier countries of the Northern Hemisphere from the poorer countries of the Southern Hemisphere. While this rough categorization is recognized as faulty (e.g., countries like Australia, New Zealand, and Argentina), the designation caught on because it captures broad outlines in the divide in investment in healthcare systems, substantial evidence that inequality between the world's richest and poorest countries is widening, and inequality within countries is growing.

The preceding chapters detail the serious synergistic health and social impacts of COVID-19 and efforts to control this highly infectious and potentially lethal disease across countries of the Global South including within diaspora or oppressed populations from the Global South found living under difficult conditions in the Global North. The adoption of a syndemic framework offers an opportunity for systems-level thinking and public health planning that considers the full complexity of human-disease interactions, which is useful in informing future pandemic preparations and responses. This approach allows for better informed and positioned programming and reality-based policy that can address the unique contextual factors that create the supporting conditions for adverse COVID-19 disease interactions.

One model for beginning to implement global syndemics planning and preparation is suggested by the Washington State Department of Health's (2023) Syndemic Planning Group. The mission of this body is to study disease outbreaks and recommend statewide strategies, funding priorities, communications needs, research, and evaluation activities to enhance prevention, diagnosis, treatment, care, and response to emergent or re-emergent diseases while reducing health inequities and disparities related to these conditions and proactively addressing and dismantling oppressive systems and practices, utilizing a syndemic approach to statewide coordination of prevention and care.

Chapters in this volume examine the lived experience of COVID-19 locally but often present only a limited critical gaze on the global geopolitical dynamics that enhanced local crises. For example, vaccine distribution remained highly unequal, with 80% of citizens in the Global South still waiting for the vaccine in September 2022 when 80% of citizens in the Global North were vaccinated. Such inequities increased health burdens, reduced economic productivity, and contributed to the development of new variants that threatened everyone (Steinert et al., 2022).

Solutions, however, must look at how unique local conditions are influenced by the global. Now is the time for implementing pandemic preparation efforts on a global scale, enhancing monitoring of disease outbreaks, assessing local capacities to respond, coordinating communications, sharing resources, and addressing infrastructure needs. The WHO's technology transfer hub, for example, supported the reproduction of Moderna's mRNA COVID-19 vaccine, without the involvement of Afrigen Biologics and Vaccines in Cape Town, South Africa. Increasing the capacity to develop vaccines in the Global South will contribute to enhanced regional distribution.

The WHO should also reconsider established initiatives such as the benefits-sharing provisions applied to commercial entities under the Pandemic Influenza Preparedness Framework, in which pharmaceutical companies are required to provide 10% of their supply of real-time vaccine manufacturing capacity to the WHO to distribute to low-resource countries. Of note, 75% of the world's population lives in the Global South. Furthermore, wealthy countries in the Global North can establish Advance Purchase Agreements, sleeping contracts with vaccine manufacturers that lay dormant until triggered by a predetermined event, such as a WHO announcement of a pandemic disease emergency. While encouraged, Advance Purchase Agreements are cost prohibitive for most countries in the Global South, further limiting their ability to compete in the global market and acquire the vaccines needed during a crisis.

Also, of need is expanded research on the nature of syndemics, the pathways of interaction among diseases, patterns of disease clustering, bio-social interaction in disease formation, and the identification of effective syndemic prevention and intervention strategies. The economic burden for this transition to foundational recognition of the keen threat posed by runaway syndemics must be borne by the countries of the Global North. They have the wealth, no small part of which was and is extracted from the Global South.

References

Soonamaker, T. (2020). Fauci Warned the Trump Administration of a Potential Epidemic Way Back in 2017. *Science Alert*. https://www.sciencealert.com/niaid-director-warned-us-government-of-a-surprise-outbreak-in-2017.

Steinert, J.I., Sternberg, H., Veltri, G.A., & Büthe, T. (2022). How Should COVID-19 Vaccines Be Distributed between the Global North and South: A Discrete Choice Experiment in Six European Countries. *eLife*, 11, e79819. https://doi.org/10.7554/eLife.79819.

Washington State Department of Health. (2023). Syndemic Planning Group. https://doh.wa.gov/you-and-your-family/illness-and-disease-z/hiv/syndemic-planning-group.

Index

For Product Safety Concerns and Information please contact our EU
representative GPSR@taylorandfrancis.com
Taylor & Francis Verlag GmbH, Kaufingerstraße 24, 80331 München, Germany

www.ingramcontent.com/pod-product-compliance
Lightning Source LLC
Chambersburg PA
CBHW060258220326
41598CB00027B/4147